Critical Problems in Vascular Surgery

Critical Problems in Vascular Surgery

Edited by

Frank J. Veith, M.D.
Chief, Division of Vascular Surgery
Professor of Surgery
Montefiore Hospital and Medical Center—
Albert Einstein College of Medicine
New York, N.Y.

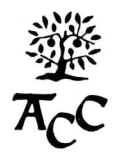

APPLETON-CENTURY-CROFTS/New York

Copyright © 1982 by APPLETON-CENTURY-CROFTS
A Publishing Division of Prentice-Hall, Inc.

All rights reserved. This book, or any parts thereof, may not be used or reproduced in any manner without written permission. For information, address Appleton-Century-Crofts, 292 Madison Avenue, New York, N.Y. 10017.

82 83 84 85 86 / 10 9 8 7 6 5 4 3 2 1

Prentice-Hall International, Inc., London
Prentice-Hall of Australia, Pty. Ltd., Sydney
Prentice-Hall of India Private Limited, New Delhi
Prentice-Hall of Japan, Inc., Tokyo
Prentice-Hall of Southeast Asia (Pte.) Ltd., Singapore
Whitehall Books Ltd., Wellington, New Zealand

Library of Congress Cataloging in Publication Data
Main entry under title:

Critical problems in vascular surgery.

　Papers from the Seventh Annual Symposium on Current Critical Problems in Vascular Surgery, held Nov. 13–15, 1980 at the Grand Hyatt Hotel, New York, N.Y., and sponsored by the Dept. of Surgery, Montefiore Hospital and Medical Center and the Albert Einstein College of Medicine, Bronx, New York.
　Includes bibliographies and index.
　1. Cardiovascular system—Surgery—Congresses.
2. Cardiovascular system—Surgery—Complications and sequelae—Congresses.　I. Veith, Frank J.　II. Symposium on Current Critical Problems in Vascular Surgery (7th: 1980: New York, N.Y.)　III. Montefiore Hospital and Medical Center. Dept. of Surgery.　IV. Albert Einstein College of Medicine.　[DNLM: 1. Vascular surgery.　WG 170 C934]
RD597.C74　　　617'.413　　　81–8010
ISBN 0-8385-1245-3　　　　　　　AACR2

Cover and text design: Jean M. Sabato

PRINTED IN THE UNITED STATES OF AMERICA

Contributors

F. Gregory Baumann, Ph.D.
Research Assistant Professor of Surgery,
New York University Medical Center,
New York, New York

John J. Bergan, M.D.
Magerstadt Professor of Surgery,
Chief, Division of Vascular Surgery,
Northwestern University Medical School,
Chicago, Illinois

Victor M. Bernhard, M.D.
Professor of Surgery,
Director, Vascular Surgery,
Medical College of Wisconsin,
Milwaukee, Wisconsin

Eugene F. Bernstein, M.D.
Professor of Surgery,
Head, Vascular Surgery,
University of California, San Diego,
San Diego, California

Michael A. Bettman, M.D.
Assistant Professor of Radiology,
Harvard Medical School,
Peter Bent Brigham Hospital,
Boston, Massachusetts

Scott J. Boley, M.D.
Director, Pediatric Surgery,
Professor of Surgery,
Montefiore Hospital and Medical Center—
Albert Einstein College of Medicine,
New York, New York

Laurence J. Brandt, M.D.
Co-Director, Division of Gastroenterology,
Montefiore Hospital and Medical Center,
Associate Professor of Medicine,
Albert Einstein College of Medicine,
New York, New York

James Chang, M.D.
Assistant Professor of Clinical Radiology,
New York University School of Medicine,
Chief of Cardiovascular Radiology,
St. Vincent's Hospital and Medical Center of New York,
New York, New York

W. Andrew Dale, M.D.
Professor of Clinical Surgery,
Vanderbilt Medical School,
Nashville, Tennessee

Dominic A. DeLaurentis, M.D.
Director, Department of Surgery,
The Pennsylvania Hospital,
Professor of Surgery,
University of Pennsylvania School of Medicine,
Philadelphia, Pennsylvania

Ralph DePalma, M.D.
Chairman and Professor,
Department of Surgery,
University of Nevada,
School of Medicine,
Reno, Nevada

James A. DeWeese, M.D.
Chairman and Professor,
Division of Cardiothoracic Surgery,
Strong Memorial Hospital of
The University of Rochester,
Rochester, New York

William R. Flinn, M.D.
Assistant Professor of Surgery,
Northwestern University Medical School,
Chicago, Illinois

Wilson V. Garrett, M.D.
Associate Attending Surgeon,
Baylor University Medical Center,
Clinical Instructor in Surgery,
University of Texas Southwestern Medical School,
Dallas, Texas

Sushil K. Gupta, M.D.
Assistant Attending, Department of Surgery,
Montefiore Hospital and Medical Center,
Assistant Professor of Surgery,
Albert Einstein College of Medicine,
New York, New York

Henry Haimovici, M.D.
Chief Emeritus, Division of Vascular Surgery,
Montefiore Hospital and Medical Center, Bronx, New York;
Clinical Professor of Surgery,
Albert Einstein College of Medicine,
New York, New York

John P. Harris, M.D.
Jobst Fellow in Peripheral Vascular Surgery,
Northwestern University Medical School,
Chicago, Illinois

Ronald D. Harris, M.D.
Associate Clinical Professor of Radiology,
University of California at San Diego,
La Jolla, California;
Chief, Division of Ultrasound and Body Computerized Tomography,
Scripps Clinic Medical Institutions,
La Jolla, California

Robert W. Hobson, II, M.D.
Director, Division of Vascular Surgery,
Professor and Vice-Chairman, Department of Surgery,
College of Medicine and Dentistry of New Jersey,
New Jersey Medical School,
Newark, New Jersey

Anthony M. Imparato, M.D.
Professor of Surgery,
Director of the Division of Vascular Surgery,
New York University Medical Center;
Visiting Surgeon,
Bellevue Hospital,
New York, New York

Zafar Jamil, M.D.
Assistant Professor of Surgery,
College of Medicine and Dentistry of New Jersey,
New Jersey Medical School,
Newark, New Jersey

Barry T. Katzen, M.D.
Attending Radiologist,
Alexandria Hospital, Alexandria, Virginia;
Associate Clinical Professor of Radiology,
George Washington University School of Medicine,
Washington, District of Columbia

George R. Leopold, M.D.
Professor of Radiology,
Head, Division of Ultrasound,
University of California at San Diego,
La Jolla, California

Thomas G. Lynch, M.D.
Assistant Professor of Surgery,
Division of Vascular Surgery,
College of Medicine and Dentistry of New Jersey,
New Jersey Medical School,
Newark, New Jersey

Wesley S. Moore, M.D.
Professor of Surgery,
Chief, Section of Vascular Surgery,
University of California, Los Angeles,
Los Angeles, California

R. Don Patman, M.D.
Attending Surgeon,
Baylor University Medical Center,
Clinical Assistant Professor of Surgery,
University of Texas Southwestern Medical School,
Dallas, Texas

Malcolm O. Perry, M.D.
Professor of Surgery,
Chief, Vascular Surgery,
Cornell University Medical College,
New York, New York

John M. Porter, M.D.
Professor of Surgery,
Head, Division of Vascular Surgery,
University of Oregon Health Sciences Center,
Portland, Oregon

Neil D. Rudo, M.D., Ph.D.
Fellow in Peripheral Vascular Surgery,
Northwestern University Medical School,
Chicago, Illinois

Edwin W. Salzman, M.D.
Professor of Surgery,
Harvard Medical School;
Associate Director of Surgery,
Beth Israel Hospital,
Boston, Massachusetts

Seymour Sprayregen, M.D.
Head, Division of Vascular Radiology,
Montefiore Hospital and Medical Center, Bronx, New York;
Professor of Radiology,
Albert Einstein College of Medicine,
New York, New York

Horace C. Stansel, Jr., M.D.
Professor of Surgery and Pediatrics,
Cardiothoracic Surgery,
Vascular Surgery,
Yale University,
New Haven, Connecticut

Ronald J. Stoney, M.D.
Professor of Surgery,
University of California Medical Center, San Francisco,
San Francisco, California

David S. Sumner, M.D.
Professor of Surgery and
Chief, Section of Peripheral Vascular Surgery,
Southern Illinois University School of Medicine,
Springfield, Illinois

C. M. Talkington, M.D.
Associate Attending Surgeon,
Baylor University Medical Center;
Clinical Assistant Professor of Surgery,
University of Texas Southwestern Medical Center,
Dallas, Texas

Jesse E. Thompson, M.D.
Attending Surgeon and Director,
Graduate Education in Vascular Surgery,
Baylor University Medical Center at Dallas;
Clinical Professor of Surgery,
University of Texas Southwestern Medical School,
Dallas, Texas

Frank J. Veith, M.D.
Chief, Division of Vascular Surgery,
Professor of Surgery,
Montefiore Hospital and Medical Center—
Albert Einstein College of Medicine,
New York, New York

James S. T. Yao, M.D., Ph.D.
Associate Professor of Surgery,
Director, Blood Flow Laboratory,
Northwestern University Medical School,
Chicago, Illinois

Contents

Contributors v

Preface. xv

1. Landmarks in Vascular Surgery: Past Triumphs and Present Challenges/*Henry Haimovici* 1

I/NEW TECHNIQUES IN DIAGNOSIS AND MANAGEMENT

2. Echography and Computed Tomography in the Diagnosis and Evaluation of Abdominal Aortic Aneurysms/*Eugene F. Bernstein, Ronald D. Harris, and George R. Leopold* 31

3. Diagnosis of Deep Vein Thrombosis of the Lower Extremities/*Michael A. Bettman and Edwin W. Salzman* . . . 45

4. Transcatheter Therapeutic Embolization/*James Chang and Barry T. Katzen* 59

5. The Current Status of Percutaneous Transluminal Angioplasty/*Seymour Sprayregen* 83

6. Update on Polytetrafluoroethylene Vascular Grafts I/*John J. Bergan, John P. Harris, Neil D. Rudo and James S. T. Yao*. 105

7. Update on Polytetrafluoroethylene Vascular Grafts II/*Horace C. Stansel, Jr.* **123**

II/GRAFT FAILURES

8. Pathogenesis and Prevention of Intimal Hyperplasia/*Anthony M. Imparato and F. Gregory Baumann*. **133**

9. Anastomotic Neointimal Fibrous Hyperplasia: Pathogenesis and Prevention/*James A. DeWeese* **151**

10. Thrombosis of Infrainguinal Grafts/*Frank J. Veith, and Sushil K. Gupta* **159**

11. Indications for Use of Alternative Vascular Prostheses in Infrainguinal Arterial Reconstruction/ *Robert W. Hobson II, Zafar Jamil and Thomas G. Lynch* **175**

III/RECONSTRUCTIVE VENOUS SURGERY

12. Reconstructive Venous Surgery: Diagnosis and Techniques/*John J. Bergan, Neil D. Rudo, John P. Harris, and James S. T. Yao* **185**

13. Reconstructive Venous Surgery/*W. Andrew Dale* **199**

IV/DIFFICULT PROBLEMS WITH EXTREMITY ISCHEMIA

14. Amputations Below the Knee for Gangrene with Occlusive Disease Below the Inguinal Ligament/*Ronald J. Stoney* **217**

15. Management of Gangrene in Patients without a Suitable Outflow Tract Below the Inguinal Ligament: Definition of True Unreconstructibility/*Wesley S. Moore*. **229**

16. Fate of Patients with a Blind Popliteal Artery Segment: Limb Loss with a Patent Femoropopliteal Graft/*Sushil K. Gupta and Frank J. Veith* **241**

17. Limitations of Profunda Femoris Vascularization/ *Victor M. Bernhard*. **251**

18. Present Role of Lumbar Sympathectomy in the Treatment of Lower Limb Ischemia/*James S. T. Yao and William R. Flinn* **263**

19. Upper Extremity Ischemia: Role of the Vascular Surgeon in Raynaud's Syndrome and Finger Gangrene/ *John M. Porter* **277**

V/MISCELLANEOUS TOPICS

20. New Developments in Surgery of the Visceral Circulation/*Scott J. Boley and Lawrence J. Brandt* **299**

21. Management of Posttraumatic Pain Syndromes: Causalgia and Reflex Sympathetic Dystrophy/*Jesse E. Thompson and R. Don Patman* **321**

22. Arterial Injuries Caused by Blunt Trauma/*Malcolm O. Perry*. **329**

VI/PROBLEMS IN CAROTID SURGERY

23. Role of Noninvasive Testing and Imaging in Carotid Disease/*David S. Sumner* **341**

24. Re-stenosis Following Carotid Endarterectomy/*Jesse E. Thompson, R. Don Patman, C. M. Talkington, and Wilson V. Garrett*. **361**

VII/PROBLEMS IN AORTIC SURGERY

25. Management of Infected Aortic Grafts/*Frank J. Veith and Sushil K. Gupta* **371**

26. The Use of Autogenous Tissues in the Management of Infected Aortic Prosthetic Grafts/*Ronald J. Stoney* **387**

27. Aortoduodenal and Other Aortoenteric Fistulas/*Victor M. Bernhard* **399**

28. The Hypoplastic Aortoiliac Syndrome/*Dominic A. DeLaurentis*. **411**

29. Etiology and Management of Sexual Problems Related to Aortoiliac Disease and Surgery/*Ralph G. DePalma*. **429**

30. Thrombosis of Aortofemoral, Axillofemoral, or Femorofemoral Grafts/*Wesley S. Moore*. **445**

Index. **463**

Preface

This book is an attempt to analyze in some depth the critical problems currently facing vascular surgeons. It is designed to appeal to the serious vascular surgeon who deals with vascular surgery on a daily basis. For this reason it takes a hard look at new items, difficult problem areas, and controversies, rather than the simpler, better known material covered in other volumes. In several instances chapters are included from two authorities with differing points of view on controversial topics so that the present state of the art can be appraised in the most complete fashion. In essence, this book should provide the greatest possible amount of important information that is not otherwise available to those whose practices are largely or significantly devoted to vascular surgery.

To arrive at this cutting edge of vascular surgery, authors have been selected on the basis of their large and recent experience with their topics as well as the clarity of their thinking and presentation. Because these authors have usually had long-standing interest in their subjects and are recognized authorities, their current thinking is presented in the best possible perspective with regard to prior advances. Important key references are included so that this book can serve as a starting point for those who wish to probe a subject in greater depth. The historical perspective of each chapter is further enhanced by Henry Haimovici's chapter on "Landmarks in Vascular Surgery." This informative and engrossing chapter provides many new insights into the way key developments in vascular surgery occurred or evolved and is, in many instances, based on the author's personal contact with the pathfinders or innovators.

The book represents a summation of the 1980 Montefiore-Einstein Vascular Symposium. As such, its purpose is not to examine all important problem areas in vascular surgery—only those deemed to be of critical importance and utmost interest at the present time. An attempt has been made to avoid the presentation of another multiauthored, loosely edited symposium proceedings with chapters of varying quality and value and limited organization and theme. All contributions have been carefully edited and integrated so that this volume should provide not only high quality background information for those who attended the symposium, but also and more importantly, the greatest numbers of answers to the most difficult questions most often asked by serious vascular surgeons today. My appreciation extends to Steven Abramson for his expert advice and editing on this volume.

Critical Problems in Vascular Surgery

ONE
Landmarks in Vascular Surgery: Past Triumphs and Present Challenges

Henry Haimovici

> *If the science of medicine is not to be lowered to the rank of a mere technical profession, it must preoccupy itself with its history.*
>
> Emile Littré (1801–1881)

At the turn of this century most of the basic principles and techniques in vascular surgery had already been conceived in the experimental laboratory. In spite of these early contributions, a wide gap elapsed before their clinical applications. It was not until the late 1940s that clinical vascular surgery could expand and fulfill its great potential, due in large part to concurrent major developments in angiography, antibiotics, anticoagulants, blood transfusions, and other areas, as well.[32]

To gain a proper perspective of the seeds that led to the present-day progress in vascular surgery, an insight into some of its major landmarks may be illuminating. The early achievements in this field, consisting, among others, primarily of preventing thrombosis or hemorrhage in the reconstruction of diseased vessels, represented real triumphs. They are still viewed as such today.

The legacy of the original pathfinders enabled their successors to pave the way for new and more brilliant accomplishments. The historical link between our present knowledge and the efforts of the pioneers of yesteryear is best expressed by an old aphorism attributed to Issac Newton: "If I have seen farther," he said, "it is by standing on the shoulders of giants."[46]

The objectives of this chapter will be limited to a brief survey of the early pioneering milestones, and will deal mostly with some of the basic principles rather than with technologic details of vascular surgery.

VASCULAR SUTURES, ANASTOMOSES, AND GRAFTING OF VESSELS

One of the earliest reported anastomosis between two vessels was carried out in 1877 by Nikolai Eck between the portal vein and the inferior vena cava. He worked out this shunt by means "of more than 60 vivisections." Eck "conducted these experiments with the purpose of clarifying some physiological problems as well as to determine whether it would be possible to treat some cases of mechanical ascites by means of forming such a fistula." This contribution remained buried for a long time and was rediscovered with the advent of the treatment of decompression for portal hypertension.[13]

Towards the end of the nineteenth century, there was a gradually increasing interest in the methods of blood vessel suturing.[36,37,39] Without going into all of their technical aspects, suffice it to say that *one* of the problems dealing with repair and anastomosis of blood vessels revolved around the proper method of dealing with the intima. The early investigators avoided penetrating it for fear of injuring its endothelium and causing thrombosis (Fig. 1). It was not until 1899 that Dörfler adopted the technique of penetrating all layers of the vessel.[18] From his experience, he concluded that aseptic silk thread in the lumen of the blood vessel does not necessarily lead to thrombosis, and therefore, the penetration of the intima was not contraindicated. This was the first important step in the technique of vascular sutures.

A more comprehensive investigation of vascular sutures and anastomoses had to await the beginning of this century. In 1902 Carrel published a paper (Fig. 2) entitled "Surgical Technique of Vessel Anastomosis and Transplantation of Organs," which proved to be a most notable contribution to this field.[5] This brief article, written by Carrel only two years after he received his medical degree, marks the beginning of his wide-ranging scientific achievements.

In this article, among other aspects, he described the anastomosis of vessels as follows:

> The method herein described is very simple. It is applicable to arteries and veins, to large and small vessels. It respects the integrity of the endothelium. The anastomosis is absolutely watertight and does not cause any narrowing in the calibre of the vessel. It permits to achieve with equal ease an end-to-side as well as an end-to-end anastomosis. Its performance is simple.

Ueber Arteriennaht.

Von

Dr. Julius Dörfler,
approb. Arzt aus Weissenburg a/S.

Der gewaltige Aufschwung, den die Chirurgie in den letzten Jahrzehnten dank einer vervollkommneten Asepsis, einer fortgeschrittenen Technik und nicht zuletzt der Kühnheit der Chirurgen auf allen Gebieten genommen hat, hat auch die Chirurgie des Gefässsystems ganz ausserordentlich gefördert.

Der Schrecken, den uns sonst Verletzungen des Herzens und der grossen Blutgefässe einflössten, hat bedeutend an Nachdruck verloren, seitdem uns gezeigt worden, dass wir in der e i n f a c h e n N a h t ein Hilfsmittel besitzen, diesen schwersten Verletzungen auf das Erfolgreichste zu begegnen. So sehen wir Verletzungen des Herzens des öfteren durch die Naht geheilt, sehen die Venennaht als bewährte Methode wohl allgemein geübt und finden endlich in den letzten Jahren auch eine kleine Zahl erfolgreicher Arteriennähte verzeichnet. Während nun die Naht unter den Behandlungsarten von

FIGURE 1. First page of original article by Dorfler (published in 1899).[18]

In his original work, as mentioned above, Carrel attempted to avoid including the intima in the suture, but changed later to the technique used by Dörfler. Except for this point, Carrel brought several operative improvements, one of which was the use of the three-stay suture technique, or as it is otherwise known, the "triangulation method."

Carrel started his experimental work in Lyon, France, either alone, or with Morel and others. Among these was a junior member, René Leriche, with whom he unsuccessfully attempted replacement of an occluded femoral artery with a vein graft.

After coming to the United States, Carrel continued his laboratory work with Guthrie for two years (1905–1906) during which period they coauthored 21 publications.[6,7,12] Either alone or with Guthrie,[28] he performed and devised every conceivable vascular transplant using autogenous, homo-, and heterologous grafts.[8] One of their joint contributions (Fig. 3) was a significant publication entitled "Anastomosis of Blood Vessels by the Patching Method and Transplantation of the Kidney."[12] This experimental work demonstrated the feasibility of a surgical technique, the usefulness of which found its clinical application only in the 1950s.

The importance of Carrel's laboratory findings during these two short years became rapidly known. Impressed by them, Halsted invited him

LA TECHNIQUE OPÉRATOIRE DES ANASTOMOSES VASCULAIRES ET LA TRANSPLANTATION DES VISCÈRES.

Par le Dr CARREL, prosecteur à la Faculté.

Pendant les derniers mois de l'année 1901, j'ai commencé des recherches sur le manuel opératoire des anastomoses vasculaires, dans le but de réaliser la transplantation de certains organes.

Cette transplantation consiste à prendre une glande, corps thyroïde ou rein, par exemple, à l'enlever avec son artère et sa veine, puis à greffer ces vaisseaux sur un autre point de l'appareil circulatoire. Simple curiosité opératoire aujourd'hui, la transplantation d'une glande pourra peut-être un jour avoir un certain intérêt pratique.

Nous n'étudierons ici que la technique employée pour obtenir une bonne réunion de vaisseaux souvent très petits.

La méthode, que je vais décrire, est très simple. Elle convient également aux artères et aux veines, aux vaisseaux de gros ou de petit calibre. Elle respecte l'intégrité de la tunique endothéliale. L'anastomose présente une étanchéité absolue, et ne provoque aucune diminution du calibre du vaisseau. Elle permet de réaliser aussi facilement une réunion termino-latérale, qu'une réunion termino-terminale. Son exécution est facile.

FIGURE 2. First page of Carrel's original article, which appeared in 1902.[5]

to deliver a lecture at Johns Hopkins on his experiments. His presentation had a great impact and was enthusiastically received.

Later that year, Carrel accepted an appointment at the Rockefeller Institute where he worked from 1906 to the end of 1939. During his association with the Rockefeller Institute his research encompassed cellular aging, intrathoracic surgery,[10] and cellular and organ cultures. Also together with Charles Lindbergh they devised a blood perfusion pump capable of supporting organs in vitro culminating in a model of an artificial heart.

Of the investigations during this period, Carrel was the first to study the functional and histological results of the use of preserved homografts

RÉSULTATS DU PATCHING DES ARTÈRES,

par ALEXIS CARREL et C.-C. GUTHRIE.

Le *patching* consiste à oblitérer une perte de substance de la paroi d'une artère ou d'une veine à l'aide d'un lambeau emprunté à une artère, à une veine ou au péritoine. La présente note traite seulement du patching des artères.

Cette opération est employée dans les réparations de la paroi artérielle, à la suite d'une résection partielle, et dans certaines transplantations artérielles uniterminales.

Il existe trois sortes de patching des artères, suivant que le lambeau est artériel, veineux ou péritonéal.

1° *Patching par un lambeau artériel.* — On régularise les bords de l'ouverture artérielle qu'il s'agit de fermer et on lui donne une forme à

FIGURE 3. First page of original article by Carrel and Guthrie on patching method of blood vessels which appeared in French in 1906 (Compt. Rend. So. Biol., 60, 1009, 1906).

(Fig. 4).[9] In 1910 he reported his extensive efforts to preserve arterial grafts in a so-called viable state. To achieve this goal he used various electrolyte solutions, serum, defibrinated blood, and refrigeration at minus 4 C. Although Carrel reached the conclusion that blood vessels could be preserved in a condition of "latent life," later evidence showed that these grafts underwent morphologic changes, and that they ultimately acted only as scaffolding for the ingrowth of fibrous tissue along with the so-called spread of a neointima from the living host vessel. The same process of graft integration into the host is well known today in biologic and synthetic grafts.[29]

Illustrating this point is Carrel's description of the biologic changes of the venous graft in the arterial system, which he ascribed to "arterialization" of the vein.[11] Although the current, more sophisticated findings relating to the morphologic alterations of transplanted venous tissue have disputed some of Carrel's interpretations, his basic observations remain valid.

The present widespread use of venous autogenous grafts as arterial substitutes deserves a few comments about the development of this aspect of vascular surgery. Following Carrel's experimental demonstration in 1902, Goyanes performed in 1906 the first clinical interposition of a venous autograft after excision of a popliteal aneurysm.[23] Subsequently Murphy,[48] Stitch,[53] Lexer,[42] and others reported the use of venous autogenous grafts, either for occlusive or aneurysmal disease. In this coun-

RÉSULTATS ELOIGNES
DE LA TRANSPLANTATION DES VEINES
SUR LES ARTÈRES

Par Alexis CARREL.

J'ai proposé il y a cinq ans la transplantation de segments veineux dans le traitement des anévrismes et de certaines lésions traumatiques des artères (1). Je m'appuyais alors sur les résultats d'expériences que j'avais faites à Lyon avec Morel (2) et à Chicago avec Guthrie (3). Ces expériences avaient démontré que, dans certaines conditions, les anastomoses artérioveineuses restent perméables,

FIGURE 4. First page of original article by Carrel on long term results of transplantation of veins in the arteries which appeared in 1910.[11]

try, Bernheim,[2] stimulated by Halsted, was the first to replace successfully a popliteal aneurysm with a segment of saphenous vein. He later achieved recognition through his monograph "Surgery of the Vascular System,"[1] published in 1913. But in spite of these early but sporadic successes, veins were rarely used as an arterial substitute except for some attempts during World War I.

The significance of the basic principles established by Carrel emerged only much later, and fully justified his laboratory efforts in more than one way. It can be truly said that the principles and techniques of all modern vascular grafting, including organ transplants, stem from the exhaustive investigations of this pioneering work. Sterling Edwards,[21] in the preface of his biography on Carrel, mentions advice given over the past 30 years to young investigators, that illustrates the vastness of his contributions: "If you think you've invented a new technique in heart or blood vessel surgery, you'd better check to see if Dr. Alexis Carrel didn't try the same thing 50 years ago."

Carrel's contributions had a tremendous impact on the medical world of his time because of their innovations and their clinical implications. In 1912 he was awarded the Nobel Prize in Medicine "in recognition of his work on vascular suture and the transplantation of blood vessels and organs."

RECENT SURGICAL CONTRIBUTIONS

The modern revival of vascular surgery was ushered in in 1938 by the successful ligation of a patent ductus by Robert Gross.[24] That was followed by another milestone in this field: Blalock's first operation for tetralogy of Fallot in 1944, in which he anastomosed the left subclavian to the left pulmonary artery by an end-to-side technique.[4] Shortly thereafter Crafoord[14] of Stockholm and Gross[26] independently performed the first corrections of the coarctation of the aorta with and without graft replacements.

Although these procedures are designed for congenital cardiovascular abnormalities, they are mentioned here only as a background to the historical development of vascular surgery. After extensive laboratory investigations of methods for preservation and transplantation of grafts (all inspired from Carrel's earlier research), Gross published in 1948 and 1949 his observations on the use of human arterial homografts in the treatment of coarctation of the aorta and of tetralogy of Fallot (Fig. 5).

Thus began truly the modern phase of vascular grafting. The impetus provided by revival of Carrel's principles led to similar applications in other parts of the vascular system.

It was shortly thereafter that Jacques Oudot of Paris performed the first successful resection of the aortic bifurcation and its replacement with a homograft (Fig. 6).[49] The idea for such a procedure had already been conceived by Leriche in 1923: "The ideal treatment of the thrombosis of the terminal abdominal aorta should consist of a resection of the occluded segment, and reestablishment of arterial continuity by a graft."[41] What seemed unobtainable in 1923 was achievable in 1950 by Oudot. It is of some interest to note that the right limb of the graft thrombosed and required, subsequently, a crossover shunt from the left external iliac to the right. This type of vascular graft provided the principle for extraanatomic procedures 10 years later.

Jacques Oudot was exceptional in more than one way. The same year he pioneered the first successful replacement of an aortic bifurcation with a homograft, he was a member of the French mountain climbing team which ascended the Annapurna in Nepal.[34] Maurice Herzog, in his book entitled *Annapurna,* recounts the heroic conquest of the highest mountain ever climbed by man up to that time. As the surgeon of the expedition, Oudot treated frostbite lesions of several of the members with intraarterial priscoline and procaine, along with digital amputations under the most trying conditions. Unfortunately Oudot's career came to a sudden tragic end[50] in a car accident in 1953, a few weeks before the Second International Cardiovascular Meeting in Lisbon, where he

8 Critical Problems in Vascular Surgery

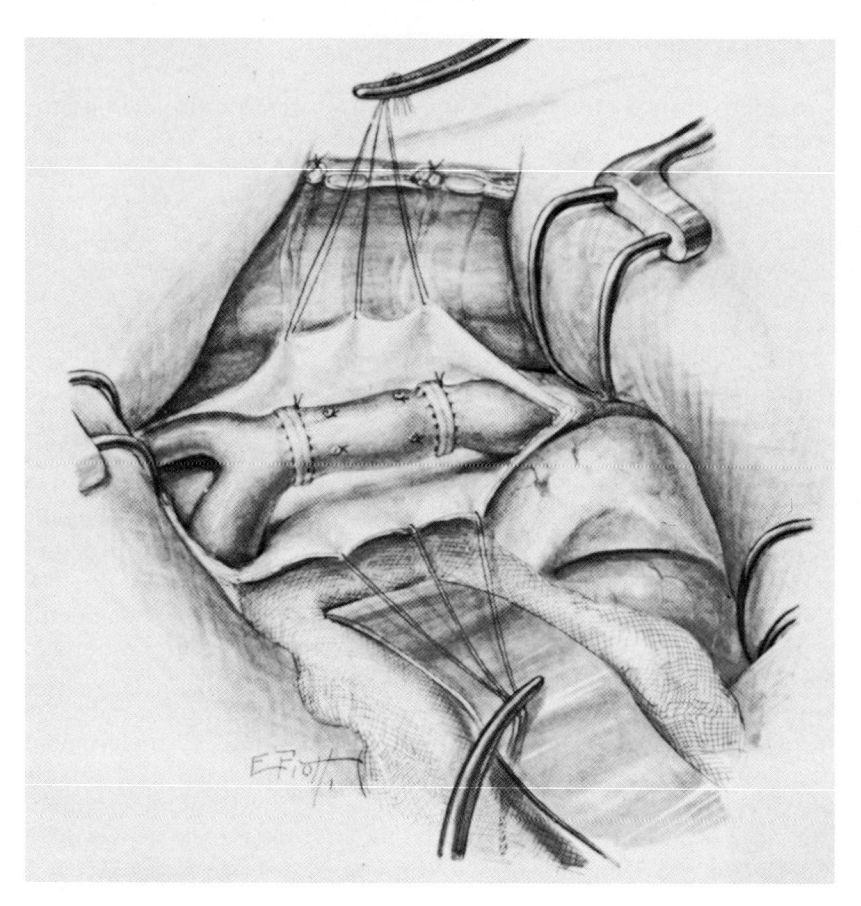

FIGURE 5. Illustration from the original article by Gross et al. depicting insertion of a human aortic graft following removal of a narrowed segment of the aorta for the treatment of coarctation of the aorta.[26]

was to present a movie about his surgical experience with occlusive and aneurysmal disease of the terminal abdominal aorta.

Leriche and the French school, under his influence, devised many of the pioneering operations for repair of occlusive and aneurysmal lesions. I would be remiss for not indicating even briefly his leading role in the early period of this modern era of vascular surgery. He became best known for advocating the use of sympathectomy for a wide range of vascular diseases, later incorporated in his classic book on *Surgery of Pain*. His trips to the United States before World War I, and after World War II, resulted in his association with the leading American surgeons of the day, Halsted, Matas, Cushing, and Carrel among others (Fig.

| 234 | LA PRESSE MEDICALE, 21 Février 1951 | 1951 — 59 — N° 12 |

LA GREFFE VASCULAIRE DANS LES THROMBOSES DU CARREFOUR AORTIQUE

Par Jacques OUDOT
(Paris)

FIGURE 6. Title of the first page of the article by Oudot describing the first vascular graft for the bifurcation of the aorta which appeared in 1951.[49]

7). The latter, who was his early mentor in France, introduced him to the American audience. Although currently Leriche's name remains attached mostly to the syndrome of occlusion of the aortic bifurcation, his many other achievements have assured him of a select place in the history of vascular surgery.

THROMBOENDARTERECTOMY

This procedure, originally designed for simple removal of thrombi under heparin cover, turned out to be more than a simple thrombectomy. Because of its new conceptual impact on the development of vascular surgery, a brief historical background may provide an insight into how an accidental finding may open a new avenue in scientific thinking.

Disobstruction of occluded arteries by simple thrombectomy was not new. Severeanu in 1880, Jianu[39] in 1909, and Delbet[16] in 1906 and again in 1911, are credited with attempting thrombectomy for arterial disobliteration. The latter stated rather optimistically that "the easiest operation that can be done to cure arterial obstructions is incision of the artery, extraction of the thrombus, and closure of the vessel." The results obviously rarely supported such views.

Indeed, these early attempts were relegated to oblivion until 1946 when J. Cid Dos Santos decided to do this operation under heparin cover, which obviously was unavailable in earlier attempts.[19,20] To test this concept he first did arterial embolectomies in a few delayed cases. Their successful outcome led him to conclude that "at this moment, embolectomy, and generally speaking the whole of vascular surgery, is on the verge of a new period which found its origin in the practice of anticoagulant therapy with heparin." Then, as a further step he "considered for the first time the possibility of removing the old central organized thrombus of an endarteritis obliterans. "Exactly what I had in mind was to find the plane of cleavage between the old thrombus and the intima, leaving a devastated intimal wall to be coated by a newly built endothelium while anticoagulation was active" (Fig. 8). Being con-

10 Critical Problems in Vascular Surgery

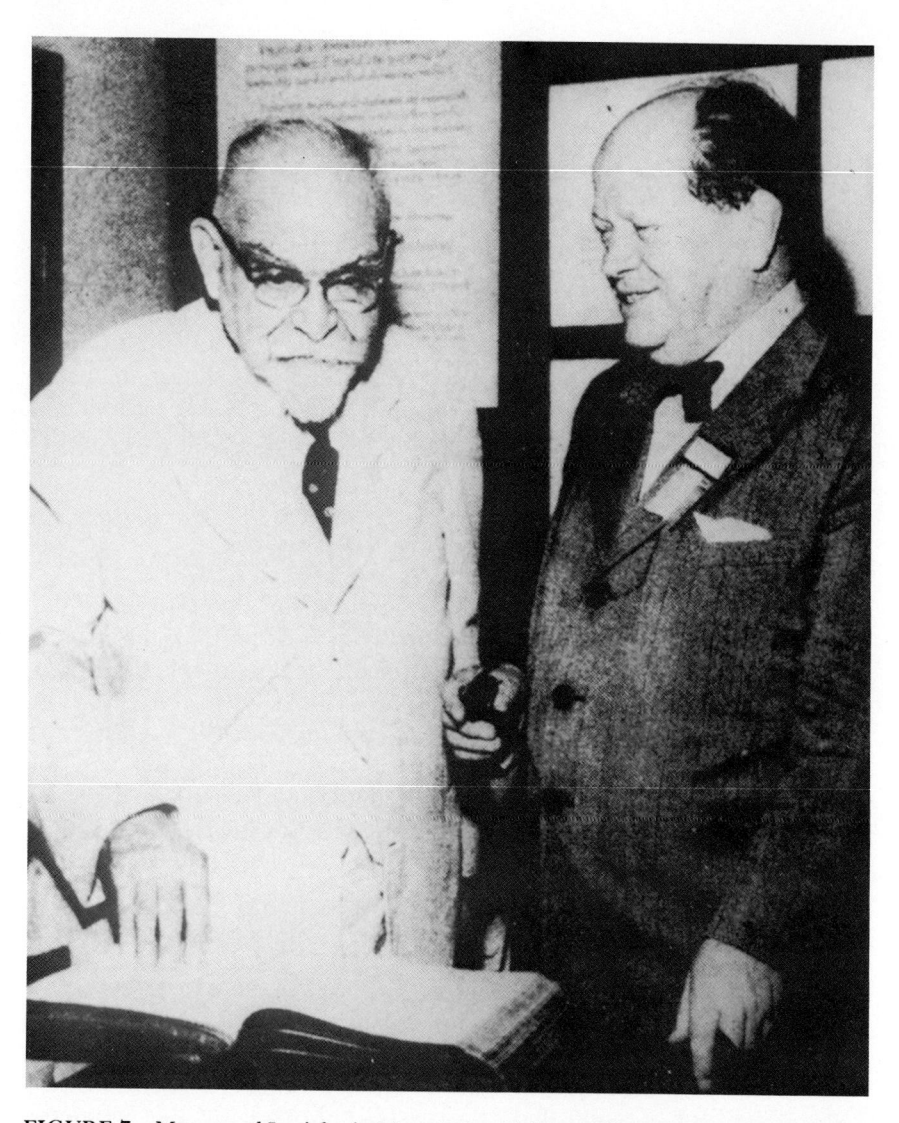

FIGURE 7. Matas and Leriche in Matas' New Orleans office (1949). (Illustration from *Rudolph Matas* by Isidore Cohn, M.D. Copyright © 1960 by Isidore Cohn and Hermann B. Deutsch. Reprinted by permission of Doubleday & Co., Inc.)

cerned "of the consequences," Dos Santos settled for a lost case to start with. So the first patient was a 66 year-old man, with a left ischemic limb, due to an iliofemoral occlusion. The procedure resulted in patency of the vessels, lasting three days, when the patient died of advanced uremia. The arteriogram taken before and after the procedure, both in vivo and postmortem, confirmed the patency of the iliofemoral vessels.

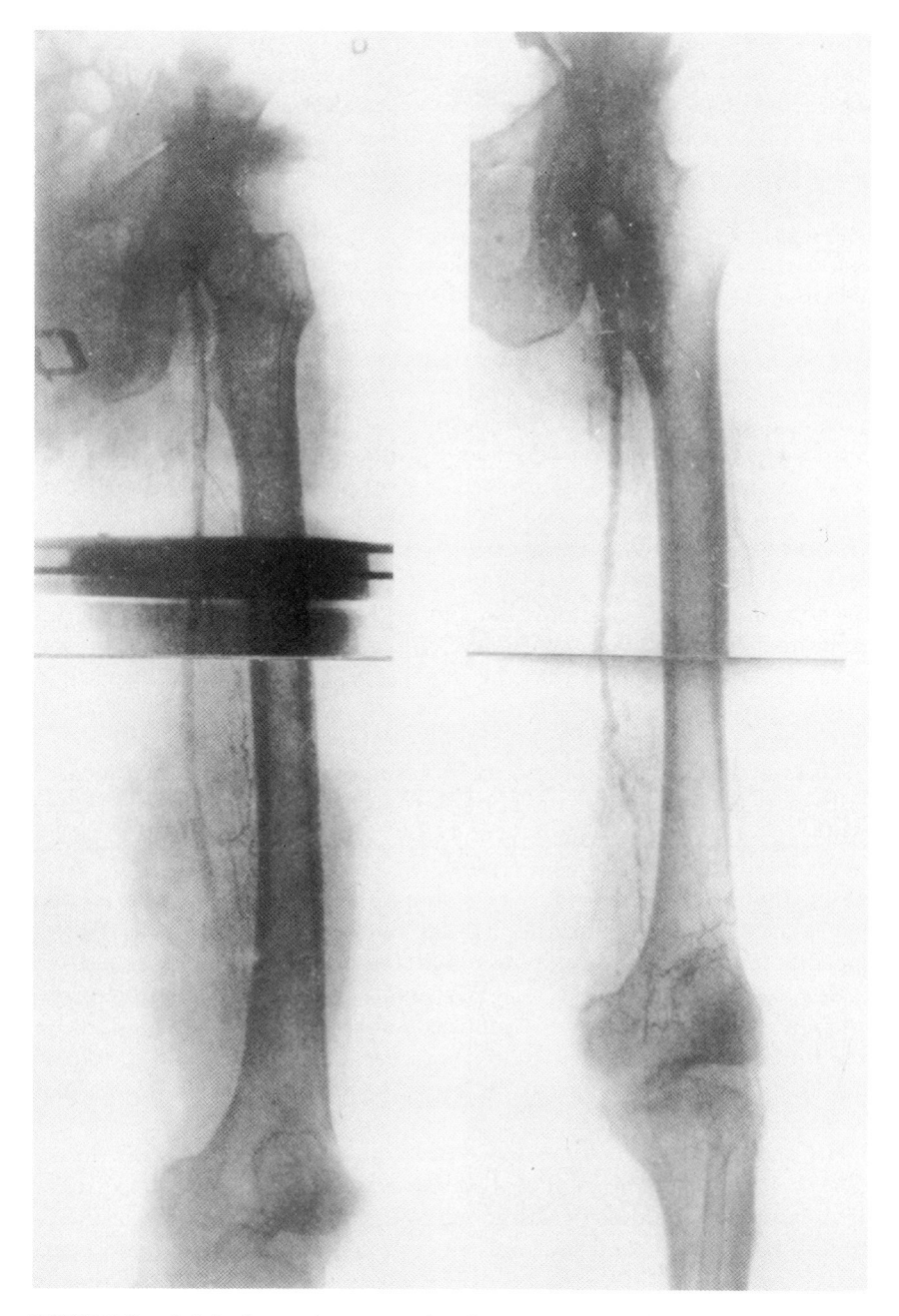

FIGURE 8. Original arteriograms taken by Dos Santos[20] immediately after thromboendarterectomy *(left)* and at post mortem *(right)*. Patency of the arterial tree which was disobstructed by the endarterectomy technique is demonstrated.

Histopathologic examination, however, to his great astonishment, showed not only the thrombus but also the whole intima and part of the media. And in spite of this there was no rethrombosis. This at the time, as stated by Dos Santos, "was unbelievable."

These findings encouraged him to try next a more appropriate patient, a 35-year-old woman with a subclavian-axillary arterial thrombosis, associated with a cervical rib. Again, the histopathologic findings were similar to those in the first case. The clinical recovery with patency of subclavian-axillary persisted for 29 years, as of the date of his publication.

The data provided by these two cases were quite revealing. While Dos Santos originally planned and thought that he had done a thrombectomy, the histology disclosed otherwise, as already mentioned. So Dos Santos stated: "I really had performed a different operation from the one I originally intended to do; and I could conclude that, under heparin action, blood could flow against muscle without giving place to a thrombosis. It seemed unbelievable." Thus, Dos Santos felt that the integrity of the intima as a requirement for a successful surgical procedure is no longer tenable. This new procedure, which later was called "thromboendarterectomy," showed that blood could flow in the absence of an intima, even without heparin and above all, without inducing thrombosis. He further stated that the general and indisputable conclusion is that "direct arterial surgery in itself has no need of the presence of the intima, in order to achieve vascular patency."

This new technique appeared as a revolutionary idea because it seemed to negate the prevailing concept according to which an injured intima leads inevitably to vascular thrombosis. Indeed, unlike embolectomy in which only the thrombus is removed, in thromboendarterectomy both the thrombus and the endartery (intima and part of the inner media) are excised. In the history of vascular surgery, this procedure holds a special place because of its physiologic implications.

Dos Santos in his presidential address to the 12th International Congress of the ICVS, given a few months before his death, in summarizing the impact of this operation stated with great conviction, and justifiably so, "that endarterectomy is at the origin of modern peripheral vascular surgery."[20]

Historically, there is little doubt of its impact on the impetus it provided by originating new concepts in intravascular clotting in the absence of an endothelial lining.[30,32] Although thromboendarterectomy as an operation is still indicated, but only in certain specific arterial lesions, its initial usefulness was displaced by the bypass grafts introduced shortly after the publication of Dos Santos's first cases.

The accidental finding that arterial thrombosis does not necessarily occur after removal of the intimal lining and a portion of the media is a typical example of serendipity. An accidental finding, as stated by Pasteur, favors an investigator only if his mind is well prepared to receive it. Dos Santos was obviously well qualified to interpret the significance of his findings, and thus opened a new chapter in this field.

THE BYPASS PRINCIPLE

Although known only since 1948, the bypass principle was not entirely new. It was first advocated by Ernest Jeger of Germany in 1913, for managing peripheral aneurysms.[38] This principle remained undoubtedly buried in his book "Die Chirurgie der Blutgefasse und des Herzens" (Fig. 9). It was not until 1948 that Jean Kunlin of Paris, an associate of R. Leriche, independently reported this procedure in the management of femoropopliteal occlusive arterial disease.[40]

Up to 1948, the conventional technique for managing arterial lesions consisted theoretically of excision of the lesions with interposition of a graft. The bypass approach was entirely novel, and had significant advantages. Its rationale was based on a twofold improvement over the previous technique: 1) avoidance of operative trauma or damage to adjacent veins or nerves, and 2) preservation of collaterals. Today, it is widely applied in managing all sorts of arterial lesions, but especially those below the groin and in the coronary arteries.

How did Kunlin conceive this approach? The inside story as related to me by Kunlin many years ago is based on the operative findings in his first case (Fig. 10). This patient was a 54-year-old man who had already had previously an arteriectomy of the superficial femoral artery. This latter procedure was based on Leriche's concept that removal of an occluded arterial segment would result in peripheral vasodilatation. The ischemia was not relieved, however, and Kunlin decided then to implant a venous graft. Exposure of the previous operative area in the thigh disclosed a tremendous fibrotic reaction around the resected arterial ends, precluding an end-to-end approach. This left Kunlin with no other alternative but an end-to-side implantation of the venous graft. And so was born the bypass procedure. This was perhaps a fortuitous decision, and illustrates another example of serendipity.

ANEURYSMS

Until 1951 the surgical management of aneurysms was occasionally palliative, and most often ineffective in preventing either thrombosis with loss of limb or rupture. Few surgeons have achieved prominence

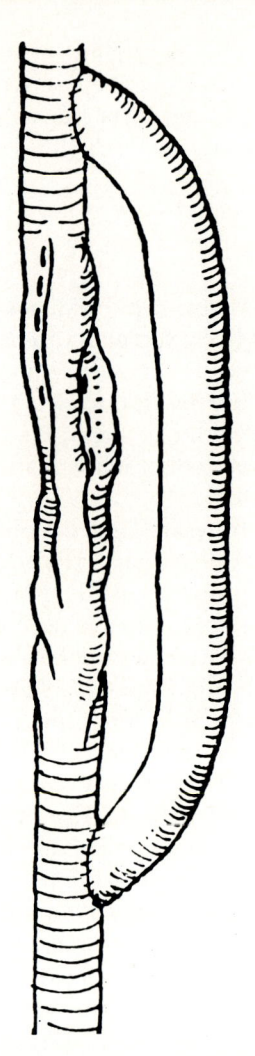

FIGURE 9. Diagram of bypass principle described by E. Jeger in 1913.[38]

in their own time for their heroic operative attempts in dealing with peripheral, thoracic, or abdominal aneurysms. Antyllus, the most remarkable surgeon of the second century, introduced ligation of the artery above and below the aneurysmal sac, opening the latter, evacuating the clot, and allowing the wound to heal by granulation. Much later, in 1710, Annell applied a ligature immediately above the aneurysm without disturbing the sac. In 1785, John Hunter, realizing that the walls of the arteries were diseased close to the sac, advocated their ligature

Le traitement de l'artérite oblitérante par la greffe veineuse (*)

J. KUNLIN Paris

La transplantation d'un segment de veine dans le but de remplacer une partie lésée du canal artériel a été pratiquée dès le début de ce siècle. Ce sont surtout les remarquables travaux expérimentaux de Carrel qui ont, à cette époque, donné un essor considérable à la chirurgie vasculaire. Carrel a mis au point la technique de la suture vasculaire et a fixé les règles de sa réussite.

La première greffe vasculaire chez l'homme a été faite par Goyanes (de Madrid), en 1906, en vue de rétablir la circulation après la résection d'un anévrysme poplité. Cette technique ne s'est pas imposée, à cause de ses difficultés, sauf en Allemagne où elle compte de chauds partisans (Lexer, E. Rehn) et elle a, en général, cédé le pas à la méthode de Matas (endoanévrysmorraphie).

C'est mon Maître, le Professeur R. Leriche qui le premier a tenté de remplacer un segment d'artère thrombosée par une veine. En 1909, étant chef de clinique d'Antonin Poncet, il explora, avec Carrel, une thrombose fémoro-poplitée, mais devant l'étendue de l'oblitération renonça à son projet.

Cette tentative ne fut, semble-t-il, pas renouvelée à cause des résultats heureux de la sympathectomie et de l'artérectomie, et aussi en raison des risques de thrombose dans des greffons de grande étendue. On pensait que seules des greffes de quelques centimètres pouvaient être faites avec succès. Le mauvais état de la paroi artérielle de l'artérite, d'autre part, était une raison de plus de renoncer.

Depuis plus d'un an un nouvel essor a été donné par Juan Cid Dos Santos aux méthodes de revascularisation des membres. La thrombend-artérectomie, qu'avec M. Leriche nous avons pratiquée sur 23 malades et au développement de laquelle MM. Bazy, Huguier, Reboul et Pierre Laubry ont beaucoup contribué, donne des résultats immédiats très intéressants et représente un net progrès dans le traitement des artérites.

Il nous a semblé qu'avec l'aide des anticoagulants comme l'héparine et la coumarine on pouvait de nouveau tenter de rétablir une circulation défectueuse due à une oblitération artérielle en amenant, par un canal veineux de dérivation, le sang de la partie de l'artère située en amont de la thrombose dans la partie distale libre de l'artère.

Nous avons tenté notre première greffe chez un artéritique grave, âgé de 54 ans, ne pouvant plus travailler depuis un an, ayant déjà subi la sympathectomie lombaire et l'artérectomie fémorale, l'amputation du gros orteil. Ce malade souffrait de plus en plus surtout depuis l'apparition d'œdème et d'ulcérations gangréneuses du dos du pied gauche.

Le 3 juin 1948, nous avons uni l'artère fémorale commune à l'artère poplitée par l'intermédiaire d'un segment veineux saphénien long de 26 cm 1/2. La transformation du malade a été immédiate. Les ulcérations ont guéri en deux semaines. Les douleurs ont disparu dès l'opération. Le pied qui était froid

* Soc. Fr. de Cardiologie, 19 déc. 1948.

FIGURE 10. First page of the original article on bypass graft by Kunlin published in 1949.

at a distance well above the aneurysmal dilatation. The operation he performed was for a popliteal aneurysm of a patient who had been symptomatic for three years. The extremity had progressed to severe distal ischemia. The arterial ligatures were placed within the fascial tunnel, formed in the anterior thigh, between the femoral triangle and the opening in the adductor magnus muscle, this compartment being since then commonly called "Hunter's canal." When the patient died 15 months later, the aneurysmal sac was thoroughly thrombosed.

John Hunter achieved great prominence for many and varied contributions. The famous "Hunterian Collection" includes thousands upon thousands of specimens—animals as well as plants—monsters and mummies—skulls of five grade divisions of the human race, and the famous skeleton of the Irish giant. This collection, in addition to all his scientific accomplishments, placed Hunter among the giants of the eighteenth century. This was recognized many years after his death when his body was transferred to Westminster Abbey. The brass plaque over his grave is inscribed with the words, "the founder of scientific surgery."

In 1888, Matas introduced a new procedure of epoch-making significance,[43] which later in 1909 he designated as "endoaneurysmorrhaphy." His principles still find application today. His first case was that of a traumatic aneurysm of the left brachial artery (Fig. 11). As stated by Matas in his report, the ligature immediately above and below the sac completely failed to check the circulation in the aneurysm. He then opened the sac and closed the orifices of the collaterals leaving or entering the sac itself. He felt that "it is in accomplishing this last result that we have an opportunity to observe the advantage gained by the improvement of the present day." Matas subsequently devised three types of operations: restorative endoaneurysmography, for saccular aneurysms; reconstructive endoaneurysmorraphy, in which a new vessel is made out of the old one; and obliterative endoaneurysmorraphy, for fusiform aneurysms (Fig. 12).[44,45] In his report to the American Surgical Association in 1940, of a total of 620 operations for aneurysms 101 had been treated by the various methods of endoaneurysmorraphy. Today, some of Matas' principles are still applicable in the technique of aneurysmectomy. Closure of ostia of lumbar or intercostal branches within the sac remains an important step.

William Stewart Halsted, originally from New York, was the first full-time chief of the department of surgery at Johns Hopkins University School of Medicine. Halsted, one of the giants of American surgery, famous for many innovations, has left his imprint also on vascular surgery. Among his many contributions, he was particularly interested in the thoracic outlet syndrome associated with cervical ribs.[33] In 1916 he was able to collect from the literature 716 cases of cervical ribs (Fig.

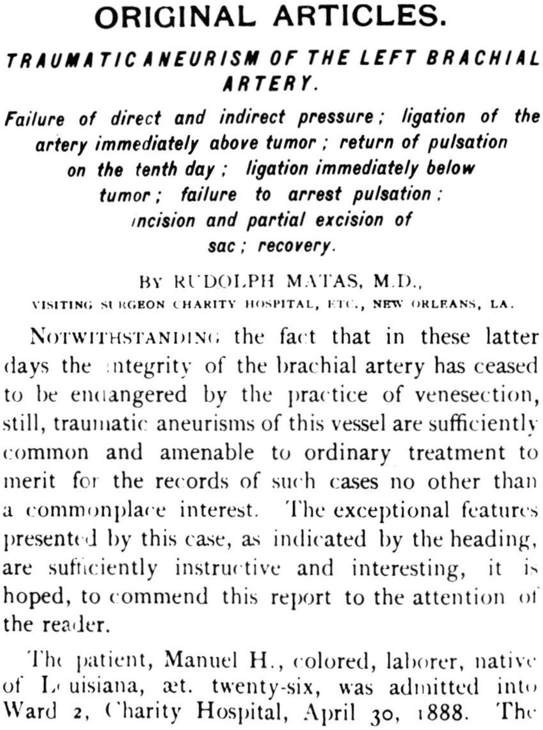

ORIGINAL ARTICLES.

TRAUMATIC ANEURISM OF THE LEFT BRACHIAL ARTERY.

Failure of direct and indirect pressure; ligation of the artery immediately above tumor; return of pulsation on the tenth day; ligation immediately below tumor; failure to arrest pulsation: incision and partial excision of sac; recovery.

BY RUDOLPH MATAS, M.D.,
VISITING SURGEON CHARITY HOSPITAL, ETC., NEW ORLEANS, LA.

NOTWITHSTANDING the fact that in these latter days the integrity of the brachial artery has ceased to be endangered by the practice of venesection, still, traumatic aneurisms of this vessel are sufficiently common and amenable to ordinary treatment to merit for the records of such cases no other than a commonplace interest. The exceptional features presented by this case, as indicated by the heading, are sufficiently instructive and interesting, it is hoped, to commend this report to the attention of the reader.

The patient, Manuel H., colored, laborer, native of Louisiana, æt. twenty-six, was admitted into Ward 2, Charity Hospital, April 30, 1888. The

FIGURE 11. First page of the article by Matas on the treatment of traumatic aneurysm of the left brachial artery by means of his technique of endoaneurysmorrhaphy performed in 1888.[43]

13). Of these, 525 were clinical cases, the rest being autopsy and museum specimens. Three hundred sixty presented symptoms of compression, of which 125 cases of cervical ribs presented with vascular symptoms. In 27 of the latter, or 21.6 percent, there were subclavian aneurysms. This review led Halsted to investigate the cause of the subclavian aneurysm formation and the mechanism of the poststenotic dilatation. Based on his experiments, he attributed the latter to two main factors: 1) a "whirlpool-like play of the blood below the site of the constriction and 2) to the lowered blood pressure." Later Emile Holman, one of his former residents, confirmed essentially the mechanism of the poststenotic dilatation by attributing it to mural structural fatigue, secondary to the turbulent flow that induces vibrations leading to the histologic changes of the artery.

While most of the preceding attempts in dealing with peripheral and central aneurysms are today only of historic interest, nevertheless they

18 Critical Problems in Vascular Surgery

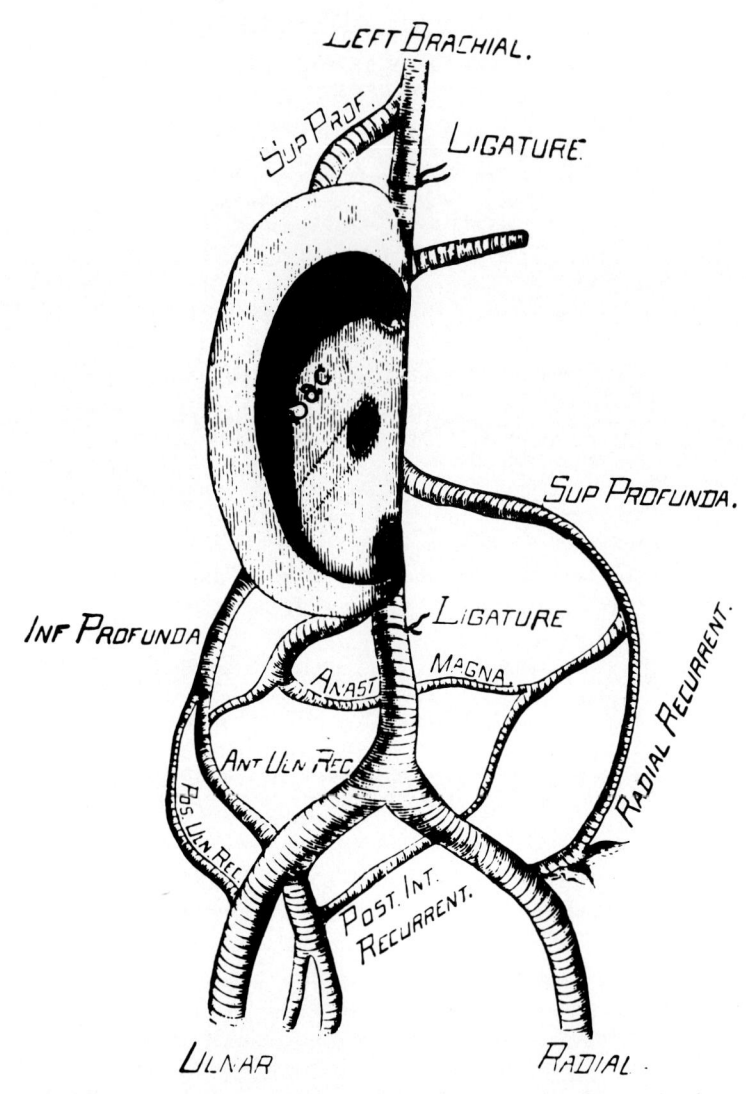

Schematic representation of the collateral circulation in the case of M. H.

FIGURE 12. Drawing of the first endoaneurysmorrhaphy performed by Matas in 1888 for a large traumatic aneurysm of the brachial artery. Note the large collateral circulation.[43]

AN EXPERIMENTAL STUDY OF CIRCUMSCRIBED DILATION OF AN ARTERY IMMEDIATELY DISTAL TO A PARTIALLY OCCLUDING BAND, AND ITS BEARING ON THE DILATION OF THE SUBCLAVIAN ARTERY OBSERVED IN CERTAIN CASES OF CERVICAL RIB.*

By W. S. HALSTED, M.D.

(From the Department of Surgery of the Johns Hopkins University, Baltimore.)

PLATES 16 TO 19.

(Received for publication, June 27, 1916.)

No one, since Deitmar,[1] has attempted to collate the cases of dilation of the subclavian artery associated with cervical rib. Deitmar cites five cases (Adams, Coote, Poland, Baum, and von Heinecke), including one (von Heinecke's) which I have tabulated as doubtful. Streissler's review[2] is perhaps the fullest in the literature on the subject of cervical rib. Although it appeared less than 3 years ago no addition is made by this author to Deitmar's list.

FIGURE 13. First page of the original article by Halsted on cervical ribs including experimental and clinical data on the topic.[33]

provided the impetus and the inspiration to the subsequent generations for managing these dreadful conditions. Ultimately in 1951 the excisional therapy of abdominal aneurysm, by Dubost and his associates, ushered in the current era of curative surgery of aneurysms (Fig. 14). The excisional technique described by Dubost was subsequently modified by incorporating some of the Matas principles in dealing with the lumbar vessels and leaving part of the sac to be wrapped around the graft. The development of the surgery for all sorts of aneurysms is now history.

DISSECTING ANEURYSMS

The first surgical attempt to correct this condition was made in 1935 by Gurin,[27] and later in 1955 by Shaw.[52] The discovery of the physiopathology is another example of serendipity. Gurin's case presented with a picture of acute arterial insufficiency of the right external iliac artery. The operation disclosed an infiltration of dark blood in its lateral third, extending as far as could be seen in both directions. Upon entering the true lumen of the artery, it was found narrowed by the dissecting hematoma (aneurysm), and completely occluded by an atheromatous mass. The intima and media opposite of the atheroma were incised from within the vessel, thus creating an opening into the false lumen of the dissecting aneurysms through which bright arterial blood spurted upon a momentary release of the proximal clamp (Fig. 15). This operative maneuver, a purely accidental finding, known as the "fenestration" of the dissected intima, is performed to allow the blood flow to be rerouted into the normal lumen. Following closure of the arteriotomy, pulsations were restored in the extremity. The patient died on the sixth postoperative day of renal failure. Shaw emphasized the same principle, using the technique of fenestration of the intimal layer of the aneurysm in the abdominal aorta, with establishment of a double-barreled aorta. Following repair of the aortotomy good pulsations were restored in the aorta and peripheral arteries. As in the previous case, the patient died of renal insufficiency, on the ninth postoperative day. The first successful result of the surgical management of a dissecting aneurysm was reported the same year (1955) by DeBakey and associates (Fig. 16).[15] Since then, besides refinement in surgical techniques, medical management of arterial hypertension, associated with the condition, has added a new dimension to this problem.

SYNTHETIC GRAFTS

The shortcomings associated with tissue grafts became readily apparent soon after the introduction of both arterial homografts and autogenous vein grafts. It was only natural when in 1952, Voorhees, Jaretski, and Blakemore reported their observations on successful arterial replacements with synthetic fabric, that the prosthetic grafts generated an enthusiastic response.[55] In fact, this report ushered in a new phase in vascular surgery, and it altered, radically, some of the classic concepts concerning intravascular thrombosis. This finding of the relative nonthrombogenicity of such grafts reinforced what Dos Santos had already pointed out in 1946 about the myth of the intima being a prerequisite for vascular reconstruction.

Historically, this development was not entirely new. Blood vessel replacement with plastic tubes dates back to the beginnings of experimental vascular surgery, with Carrel leading the field. Glass and aluminum tubes were used by Tuffier in World War I.[54] More recently, many other inert materials were used either experimentally or clinically. Among these were vitallium tubes, polyethylene tubing, siliconized rubber, steel mesh tubes, and Ivalon. None of these proved acceptable. The development of prosthetic vessels constructed of synthetic porous materials subsequently proved to be the only suitable nonbiologic material for grafting purposes (Fig. 17).

The rationale for the use of plastic prostheses is based on some prelim-

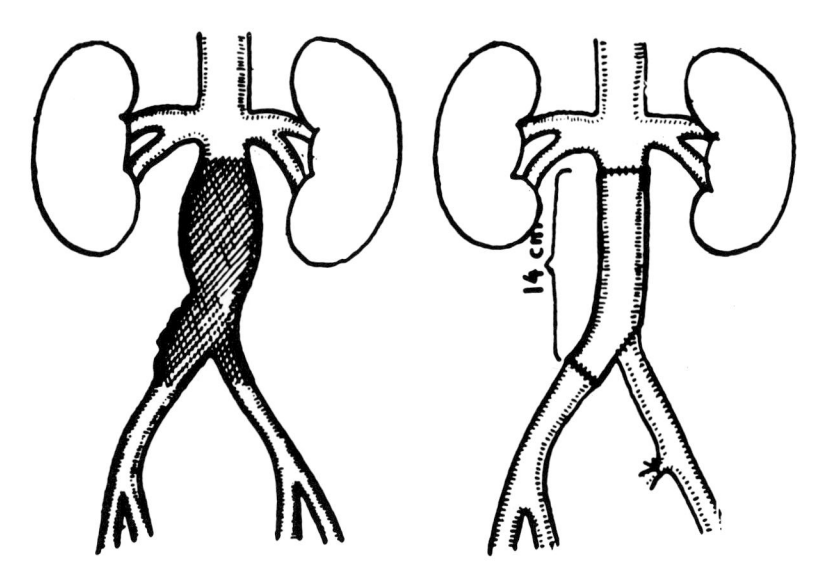

FIGURE 14. Drawing of the original article by Dubost et al published in 1951 in which they reported the first successful resection of an abdominal aortic aneurysm and insertion of a homograft (Mem Acad Chir 77:381, 1951).

inary observations made by Voorhees and associates who found that "a simple strand of silk suture traversing the chamber of the right ventricle of the heart of a dog in a few months became coated throughout its length by a glistening film, free of microscopic thrombi. As an outgrowth of this observation, it was conceived that if arterial defects were bridged by a prosthesis, constructed of fine mesh cloth, leaking blood through the walls of the prosthesis would be terminated by formation of fibrin plugs, and would allow the cloth tubes to conduct arterial flow."

Porous Vinyon "N" cloth tubes implanted in the abdominal aorta of 15 dogs resulted in over 75 percent patency. After two and one-half years of laboratory investigation, Blakemore and Voorhees[3] began the clinical use of this material in 1953. In 1954 they reported 18 cases of arteriosclerotic aneurysms (17 abdominal and 1 popliteal), treated by resection and replacement with Vinyon "N" cloth prostheses. They were gratified by the versatility and functional results obtained. A new milestone in vascular surgery had been achieved. The advances in this field, and the development of synthetic grafts, are now history.

CONCLUDING REMARKS

The basic early developments upon which vascular technology was established may be traced, among others, to three major stages of break-

ACUTE DISSECTING AORTIC ANEURYSM

Treatment by Fenestration of the Internal Wall of the Aneurysm

ROBERT S. SHAW, M.D.

BOSTON

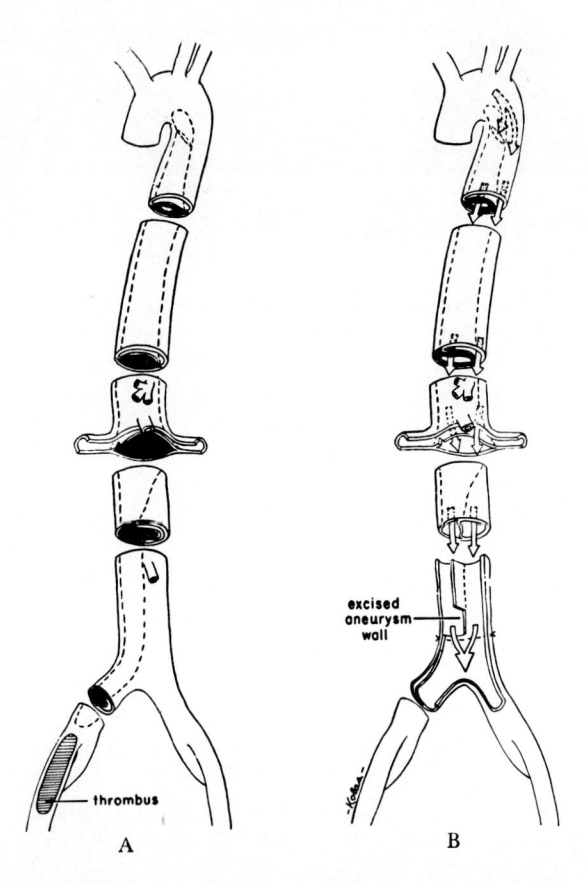

FIGURE 15. Diagram of treatment by fenestration of the internal wall of the aneurysm by Shaw. [Status of the aorta before (A) and after the fenestration operation (B).] (Reprinted by permission of The New England Journal of Medicine. 25:331, 1955.)

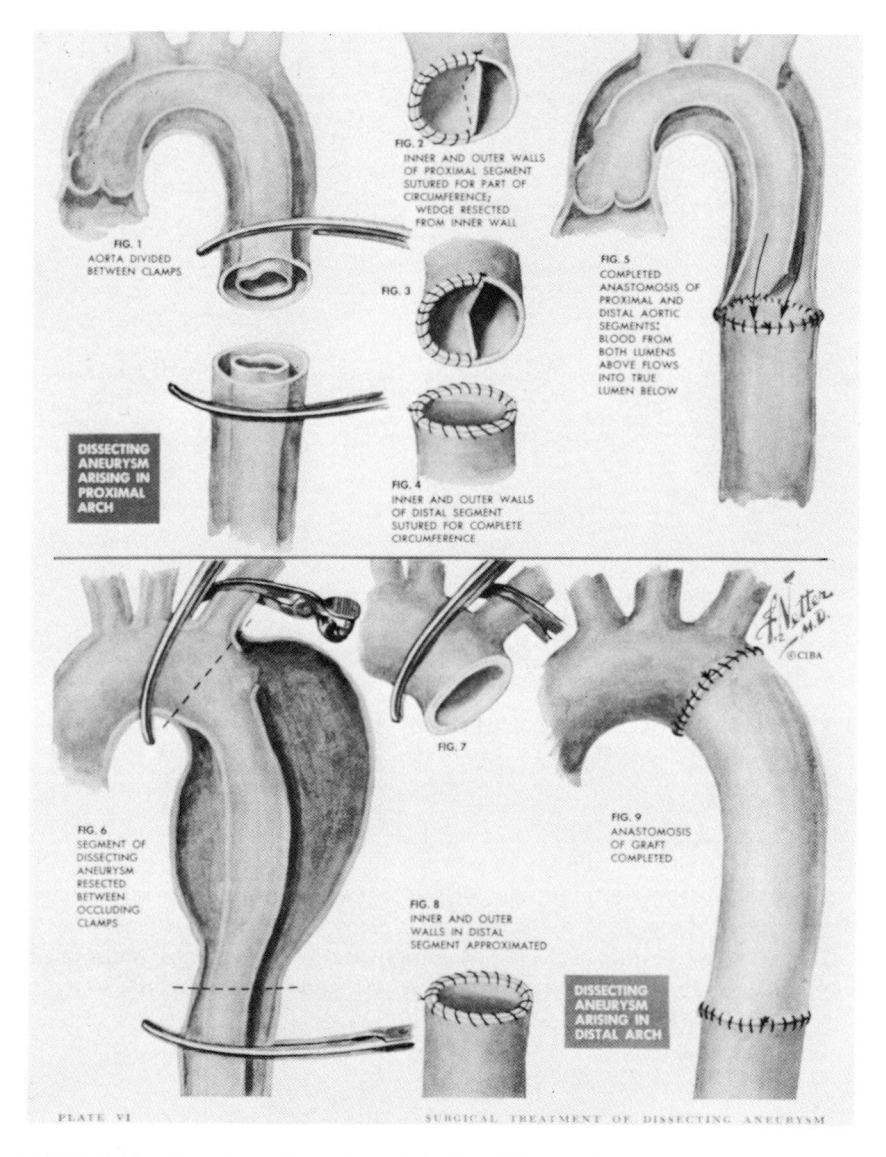

FIGURE 16. Drawings from the original article on "Surgery of the Aorta" by DeBakey et al which appeared in 1956.[15]

throughs: technique of blood vessel anastomosis, thromboendarterectomy of occluded arteries, and prosthetic grafts. By eliminating or neutralizing the thrombogenic factors, these technical achievements not only paved the way to the triumphs of present-day vascular surgery, but also generated new concepts about the endothelial-blood interface.

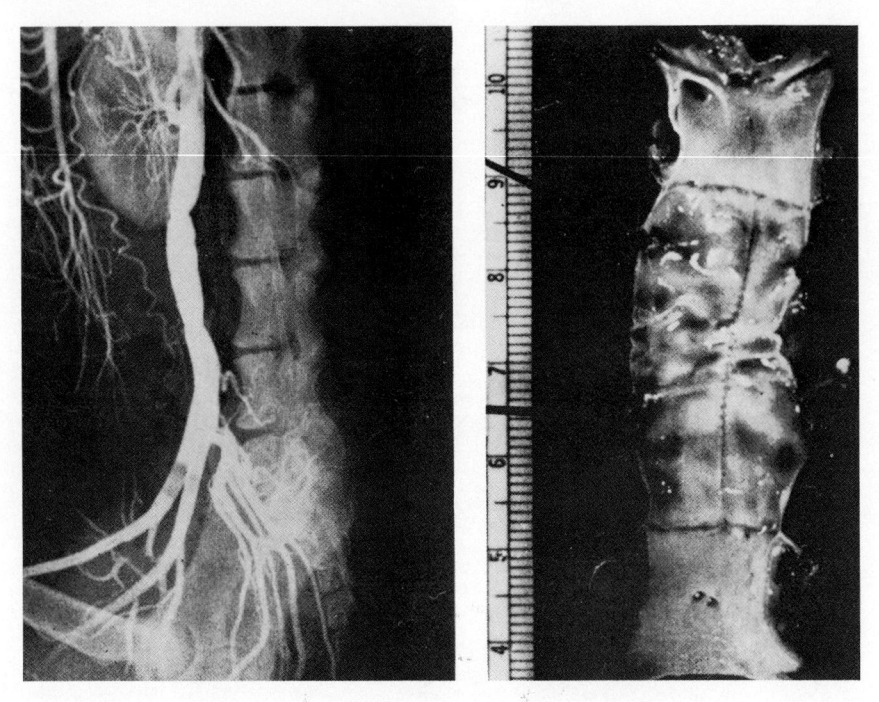

FIGURE 17. From the original article by Voorhees et al.[55]

Thus, Dos Santos, by establishing arterial patency after a thromboendarterectomy, in spite of the denuded media, concluded that the integrity of the intima was a "myth," as a prerequisite for achieving a successful arterial disobstruction. Similar results obtained with prosthetic grafts further reinforced such a concept.

While early results of biologic or prosthetic grafts implantation are generally gratifying, the late failures represent a real trial to the vascular surgeon. In this connection, one of the major problems in our current pursuit of newer and better grafts is the biomedical research of the graft-blood interface and related subjects.

Today, after three decades, arterial grafts—the centerpiece of vascular surgery—still offer a number of challenges. The search for the so-called ideal graft ever since the introduction of Vinyon "N" has never ceased. Combined massive efforts have been invested in this endeavor by an array of multidisciplinary investigators in the biologic, physicochemical, surgical, and industrial areas. To this day an "ideal" graft seems to have eluded us. Or did it? And if so, why?

It is not my intent to undertake here even briefly an analysis of the multiple factors regarding the biologic behavior of grafts and their interplay with those of the host. Suffice it only to restate the known fact that the results of arterial grafting do not depend only on the type of vascular substitutes, but to a great extent on the location and size of the arterial involvement, the degree and progression of the host arterial lesions, and of course, as well as upon meticulous surgical technique.

Excluding the use of grafts for replacement of large- or medium-sized arteries, which fare generally well, the real focus remains on the smaller arteries. The failures of grafts used for these vessels are usually attributed to two major factors: 1) intimal hyperplasia, proximal and distal to the anastomosis,[17,35] and 2) loss of compliance of the graft. Contributing heavily to these morphologic alterations, and ultimately to the graft failure, are a number of intrinsic and extrinsic host factors (hemodynamic, atherogenic, thrombogenic, occlusive arterial patterns of the inflow or of outflow tracts).[31,51]

A better understanding of the major factors in graft failures and their management are the important challenges that we face today. An entirely satisfactory long-term solution may not be yet on the horizon because of the many intrinsic host factors. The latter will probably be more difficult to solve than the problem of an "ideal" graft.

To put it succinctly: Do not place your trust only in the graft—examine carefully the host factors into which it is implanted. They may be decisive.

REFERENCES

1. Bernheim BM: Surgery of the Vascular System. Philadelphia, Lippincott, 1913
2. Bernheim BM: The ideal operation for aneurysms of the extremity, Report of a case. Bull Johns Hopkins Hospital 27:93, 1916
3. Blakemore A, Voorhees AB Jr: The use of tubes constructed from Vinyon "N" cloth in bridging arterial defects: experimental and clinical. Ann Surg 140:324, 1954
4. Blalock A, Taussig HB: The surgical treatment of malformations of the heart where there is a pulmonary atresia. JAMA 128:189, 1945
5. Carrel A: La technique operatoire des anastomoses vasculaires et la transplantation des visceres. Lyon Med 98:859, 1902
6. Carrel A, Guthrie CC: Results of the biterminal transplantation of veins. Am J Med Sci 132:415, 1906
7. Carrel A, Guthrie CC: Uniterminal and biterminal venous transplantation. Surg Gynecol Obstet 2:266, 1906
8. Carrel A: The surgery of blood vessels. Bull. Johns Hopkins Hosp 18:18, 1907
9. Carrel A: Latent life of arteries. J Exper Med 12:460, 1910

10. Carrel A: Permanent intubation of the thoracic aorta. J Exp Med 16:17, 1912
11. Carrel A: Resultats eloignes de la transplantation des veines sur les arteres. Rev de Chir 41:987, 1910
12. Carrel A, Guthrie CC: Anastomosis of blood vessels by the patching method and transplantation of the kidney. JAMA 47:1648, 1906
13. Child CG: Eck's fistula. Surg Gynecol Obstet 96:375, 1953
14. Crafoord C, Nylin G: Congenital coarctation of the aorta and its surgical treatment. J Thorac Surg 14:346, 1945
15. DeBakey ME, Cooley DA, Creech O Jr: Surgical considerations of dissecting aneurysm of the aorta. Ann Surg 142:586, 1955
16. Delbet P: Chirurgie arterielle et veineuse, les modernes acquisitions. Paris, J.B. Bailliere et Fils, 104, 1906
17. DeWeese JA: Anastomotic intimal hyperplasia. In Sawyer PN, Kaplitt MJ (eds): Vascular Grafts. New York, Appleton-Century-Crofts, 1978, p 147
18. Dorfler J: Uber Arteriennaht. Beitr Z Chir 25:781, 1899
19. Dos Santos JC: Sur la desobstruction des thromboses arterielles anciennes. Mem Acad Chir (Paris) 73:409, 1947
20. Dos Santos JC: Leriche Memorial Lecture. From embolectomy to endarterectomy or the fall of a myth. J Cardiovasc Surg 17:113, 1976
21. Edwards WS: Alexis Carrel, Visionary Surgeon. Springfield, Ill., Thomas, 1974, p 38
22. Edwards WS: Arterial grafts. Arch Surg 113:1225, 1978
23. Goyanes J: Nuevos trabajos de chirurgia vascular, substitucion plastica de las arterias por las venas o arterioplastia venosa, applicada como nuevo metodo. El Siglo Med 53:446, 561, 1906
24. Gross RE: A surgical approach for ligation of a patent ductus arteriosus. N Engl J Med 220:510, 1939
25. Gross RE, Hurwitt ES, Bill AH Jr, Peirce EC II: Preliminary observations of the use of human arterial grafts in the treatment of certain cardiovascular defects. N Engl J Med 239:578, 1948
26. Gross RE: Treatment of certain aortic coarctations by homologous grafts, a report of 19 cases. Ann Surg 134:753, 1951
27. Gurin DJ, Blumer W, Derby R: Dissecting aneurysm of aorta, diagnosis and operative relief of acute arterial obstruction due to this cause. NY State J Med 35:1200, 1935
28. Guthrie CC: In Harbison SP, Fisher B (eds): Blood Vessel Surgery and its Applications. Pittsburgh, The University of Pittsburgh Press, 1959, p 360
29. Haimovici H, Maier N: Experimental evaluation of arterial homografts. In Wesolowski SA, Dennis C (eds): Fundamentals of Vascular Grafting. New York, McGraw-Hill, 1963, p 212
30. Haimovici H: History of arterial grafting. J Cardiovasc Surg 4:152, 1963
31. Haimovici H: Patterns of arteriosclerotic lesions of the lower extremity. Arch Surg 95:918, 1967
32. Haimovici H: History of vascular surgery. In Haimovici H: Vascular Surgery, Principles and Techniques. New York, McGraw-Hill, 1976, p 2

33. Halsted WS: An experimental study of circumscribed dilatation of an artery immediately distal to a partially occluding band, and its bearing on the dilatation of the subclavian artery observed in certain cases of cervical rib. J Exper Med 24:271, 1916
34. Herzog M: Annapurna, First Conquest of an 8,000 Meter Peak. New York, Dutton, 1953
35. Imparato AM, Baumann FG, Pearson J et al: Electron microscopic studies of experimentally produced fibromuscular arterial lesions. Surg Gynecol Obstet 139:497, 1974
36. Jaboulay M, Briau E: Recherches experimentales sur la suture et la greffe arterielle. Lyon Med 81:97, 1896
37. Jassinowsky A: Die Arteriennhat, eine Experimentelle Studie. Inaug Diss Dorpat, 1889
38. Jeger E: Die Chirurgie der Blutgefasse und des Herzens. Berlin, A. Hirschwald, 1913
39. Jianu I: Trombectomia arteriala pentru un caz de gangrena uscata a piciorului. Bucarest, Soc de Chirurgie, 27:11, 1912
40. Kunlin J: Le traitement de l'arterite obliterante par la greffe veineuse. Arch Mal Coeur 42:371, 1949
41. Leriche R: Des obliterations arterielles hautes (obliterations de la terminaison de l'aorte) comme causes des insuffisances circulatoires des membres inferieurs. Bull Mem Soc Chir (Paris) 49:1404, 1923
42. Lexer E: Die ideale Operation des Arteriellen und des Arteriovenosen Aneurysma. Arch F Klin Chir 83:459, 1907
43. Matas R: Traumatic aneurysm of the left brachial artery, failure of direct and indirect pressure; ligation of the artery immediately above tumor, return of pulsation on the tenth day; ligation immediately below tumor; failure to arrest pulsation; incision and partial excision of sac; recovery. New York Med News 53:462, 1888
44. Matas R: Surgery of the vascular system. In Keen WW, DaCosta JC (eds): Keen's Surgery, Its Principles and Practice. Philadelphia, Saunders, 1909
45. Matas R: Personal experiences in vascular surgery. Ann Surg 112:802, 1940
46. Merton RK: On the Shoulders of Giants. New York, Harbinger Book, Harcourt Brace & World Co., 1965
47. Moseley J: Alexis Carrel, the man unknown. JAMA 224:1119, 1980
48. Murphy JB: Resection of arteries and veins injured in continuing end-to-end suture; experimental and clinical research. Med Rec 51:73, 1897
49. Oudot J: La greffe vasculaire dans les thromboses du carrefour aortique. Presse Med 59:234, 1951
50. Oudot J: Necrology. Mondor H: Presse Med 61:1181, 1953
51. Pearse HE: Experimental studies on the gradual occlusion of large arteries. Ann Surg 112:923, 1940
52. Shaw RS: Acute dissecting aortic aneurysms treated by fenestration of the internal wall of the aneurysm. N Engl J Med 25:331, 1955
53. Stich R, Makkas M, Dowman CE: Beitrage zur Gefasschirurgie, cirkulare Arterienaht und Gefasstransplantionen. Beitr Klin Chir 53:113, 1907

54. Tuffier M: De l'intubation arterielle dans les plaies des grosses arteres. Bull Acad Natl Med 74:455, 1915
55. Voorhees AB Jr, Jaretzki A III, Blakemore AH: The use of tubes constructed from Vinyon "N" cloth in bridging arterial defects. Ann Surg 135:332, 1952

Part One

New Techniques in Diagnosis and Management

TWO

Echography and Computed Tomography in the Diagnosis and Evaluation of Abdominal Aortic Aneurysms

Eugene F. Bernstein, Ronald D. Harris, and George R. Leopold

In view of the limitations of the physical examination and conventional radiographs, and the fact that both aortography and radionuclide aortic scans document only the lumen size and do not indicate the thickness of laminated clot and atheromatous material, other noninvasive and accurate means of diagnosis and sizing of abdominal aortic aneurysms have become the routine diagnostic modalities for this condition. Both ultrasound and computed tomography (CT) scanning fulfill all necessary requirements for such techniques and permit routine documentation of the presence or absence of an abdominal aneurysm, an accurate depiction of its configuration and location, and good estimates of its size.

The applications of echography and CT are quite similar in the investigation of the aorta in both normal and pathologic states. Both methods are accurate in identifying those patients with an aneurysm and properly diagnosing those in whom clinical suspicion of aneurysm is raised but who prove to have aortic ectasia and tortuosity, an overlying abdominal mass, or a normal aorta. Both techniques are safe, fast, noninvasive, and can be performed easily on an outpatient basis without discomfort to the patient. The fine detail obtained by these imaging modalities also may provide added information about other structures important to the surgeon at the time of operation, including the position and state of the renal vessels, vena cava, and associated vascular anomalies, such as retroaortic or circumaortic renal veins.

ULTRASOUND

The use of a reflected beam of ultrasound to identify and characterize clinical pathology has been developed during the past two decades, including the use of the A-mode, B-mode scan, B-mode real-time, and M-mode ultrasonic modalities. In each of these techniques, a crystal is oscillated by electrical energy, producing sound at frequencies exceeding 2 million cycles per second (cps), with each burst of ultrasound lasting approximately 1 μsec. This ultrasonic beam is directed at the tissues to be studied and is reflected when it contacts any change in tissue density or tissue interface with a different acoustic impedance. The reflected waves then may be displayed on an oscilloscopic screen in a variety of ways.

In the A-mode presentation, the reflected echoes are demonstrated as vertical deflections from a horizontal baseline, which represents the time for the echo to travel to the target and return to the receiver, and permits measuring the depth of acoustically different tissue planes from the transducer (Fig. 1). By moving the transducer in a plane of

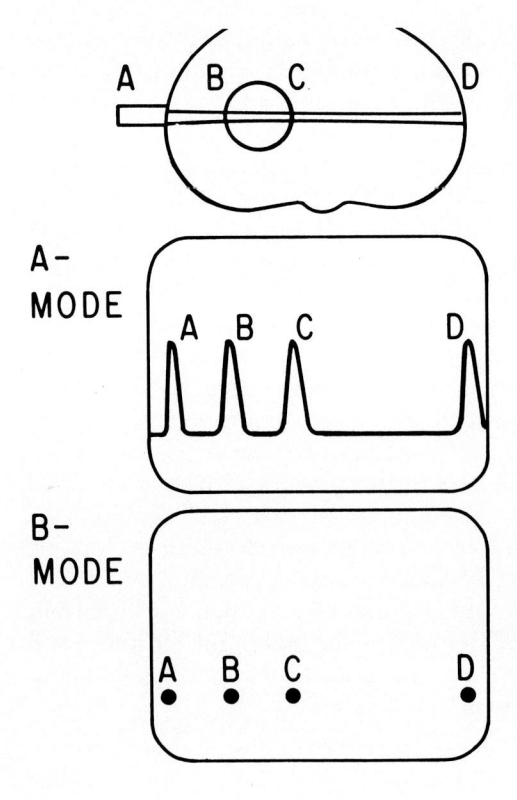

FIGURE 1. Scheme of A-mode echography, which represents each reflecting surface as a spike on the oscilloscope, the height of which is proportional to the acoustic density difference between the two materials at the interface. In the B-mode each such interface between different layers is represented as a dot, the brightness of which is proportional to the density difference. It is comparable to looking down onto the top of the A-mode spikes. Each of these techniques provides a one-dimensional output of the distance between layers traversed by the sound beam. (From Bernstein EF: Ultrasound techniques in the diagnosis and evaluation of abdominal aortic aneurysms. In Bernstein EF(ed): Noninvasive Diagnostic Techniques in Vascular Disease. St. Louis, Mosby, 1978.)

section and representing echos on the oscilloscope in accordance with the transducer position, a two-dimensional impression of the interior of the body may be obtained by what is referred to as B-mode, or ultrasonic, scanning (Fig. 2). Combining the A-mode and B-scan techniques has been useful, utilizing the B-scan to identify and characterize the shape of the aneurysm, particularly in the longitudinal echogram, with identification of the maximum diameters in both AP and transverse planes by the A-mode technique (Figs. 3 and 4).[11] Our current experience with this approach exceeds 400 cases at the University of California, San Diego, and we have increasingly more confidence in the sensitivity and accuracy of the method.[2,3,11]

ACCURACY OF B-MODE ULTRASOUND

Earlier studies of abdominal aneurysms with ultrasound, involving both A- and B-mode investigations to obtain three-dimensional data and accurate sizing, demonstrated the ability of the technique to adequately visualize such lesions in a routine manner. The diagnostic capability of ultrasound was first compared with surgery in 1971, and indicated that B-scanning accurately diagnosed 79 of 80 cases of abdominal aneurysms.[13] More recently, Maloney and associates[12] measured the AP and transverse diameter of abdominal aortic aneurysms at surgery and com-

FIGURE 2. B-scan is obtained by rotating the B-mode transducer to obtain many B-mode reflections and storing them on an oscilloscope screen. This permits building up a detailed two-dimensional image in any plane or section. (From Bernstein EF: Ultrasound techniques in the diagnosis and evaluation of abdominal aortic aneurysms. In Bernstein EF(ed): Noninvasive Diagnostic Techniques in Vascular Disease. St. Louis, Mosby, 1978.)

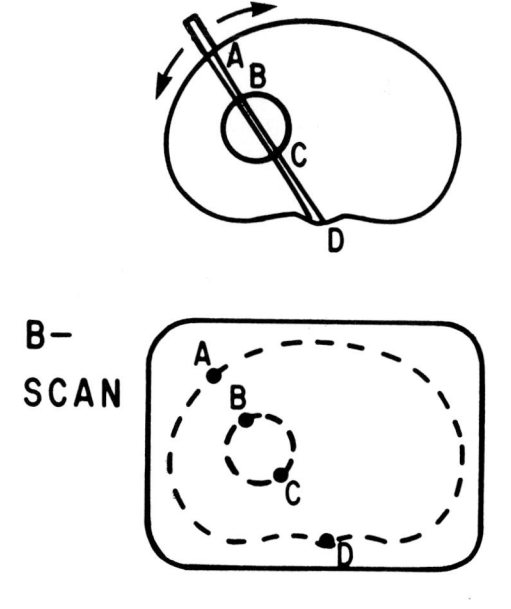

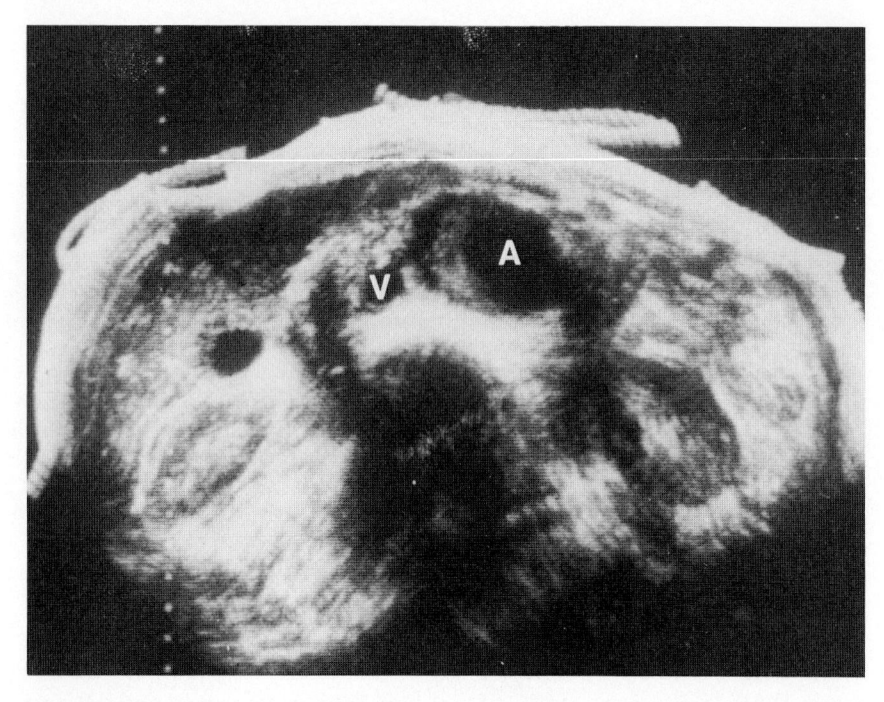

FIGURE 3. B-scan echogram in transverse plane demonstrating an abdominal aortic aneurysm (A) and the inferior vena cava (V).

pared them with AP and lateral x-rays and B-mode ultrasonic images. In only 72 percent of patients was the lateral x-ray suggestive of the diagnosis, and size measurements were possible from x-rays in only 55 percent of the cases. On the other hand, B-mode ultrasound accurately made the diagnosis and permitted size measurements in each instance. In both the AP and transverse planes, the ultrasonic estimates of size averaged within 4 mm of the surgical measurement. In those 55 percent of the patients in whom measurements could be obtained from the plain x-ray films, there was an average of 8.7 mm of variance from the intraoperative data in the AP dimension, and 15 mm in the transverse plane. Thus, ultrasound not only is a better diagnostic technique than the plain x-ray, but also is more precise in sizing abdominal aortic aneurysms in both the AP and transverse dimension. A similar study was recently published by Hertzer and Bevan,[10] in which the physical examination overestimated the aneurysm size by an average of 1 cm, as did the lateral x-ray. The B-mode ultrasonic measurements were identical with the operative measurements in 34 percent of patients and within 0.5 cm in 75 percent. The mean diameter of the aneurysms measured by ultrasound was within 2 mm of that measured directly at operation.

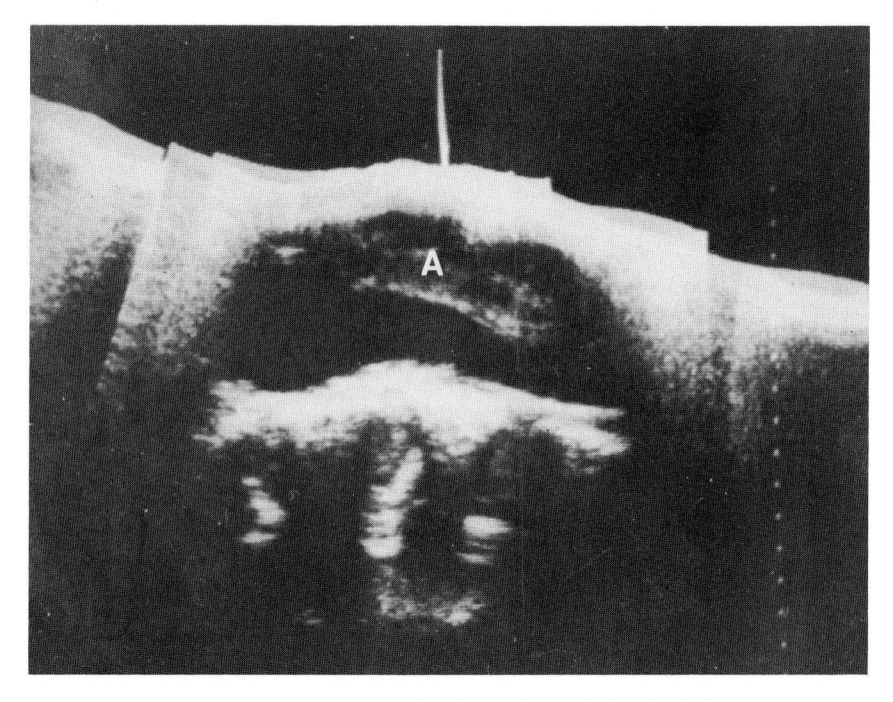

FIGURE 4. Sagittal plane B-scan echo through an abdominal aortic aneurysm (A) with sizing scale.

Finally, the reproducibility of B-mode ultrasonic measurements has been demonstrated in our own experience in which over 100 patients have been followed rather than operated upon, because they represented poor-risk patients with small asymptomatic lesions.[2,3] These patients have had repeated studies, some over periods up to 6 years. Studies performed at 3-month intervals rarely varied by more than 2 or 3 mm, and produced such consistent data that growth rates could be accurately defined.

ABDOMINAL ANEURYSM GROWTH RATES

In a group of poor-risk patients with asymptomatic abdominal aortic aneurysms measuring less than 6 cm in largest transverse diameter, a policy of continued observations with sequential B-mode echo scans at 3-month intervals initially provided data concerning small aneurysm growth rate in 49 patients.[2] The mean aneurysm growth rate was 0.4 cm per year in those patients observed for at least 1 year. In 10 patients, however, no evidence of growth occurred over periods of observation extending to 42 months, whereas in others there was sudden, unexpected, and rapid growth within a very short time, often without the development of symptoms. The growth of small aneurysms was not correlated with patient age or blood pressure.

This growth rate information appears valuable in evaluating the risk of elective surgery in a poor-risk patient with an asymptomatic abdominal aneurysm measuring less than 6 cm. It suggests that the average aneurysm takes 7½ years to grow from 3 to 6 cm and permits weighing the mortality of elective surgery in a given case against the known likelihood of rupture at a particular aneurysm size. It has been our policy to observe such high-risk patients until the aneurysm reaches a size of 6 cm or symptoms develop. In contrast, in standard risk patients early elective surgery is indicated for aneurysms of any size.

These data have recently been updated to include a total of 117 patients followed for 181 patient years. In those cases followed 12 months or longer, the available data remain consistent with the previous study, although the growth rates are somewhat less than the previously reported figure. Those aneurysms diagnosed between 3 and 5.9 cm in diameter grow at 0.26 cm per year, based on 159 patient years of observation. Those few aneurysms that have been studied at sizes larger than 6 cm indicate a definitely increased growth rate, as would be expected by the law of LaPlace.

COMPUTED TOMOGRAPHY

CT scanning is based on an array of highly sensitive x-ray detectors that are in precise alignment with an x-ray tube. The x-ray beam is tightly collimated into a shape that matches the configuration of the detectors. As each x-ray beam passes through anatomic structures, the intensity of the beam is altered by tissue absorption in the beam's path. The detectors convert this information into electrical signals that are precisely digitized for each sampling interval or until the scan is completed. A computer calculates the precise x-ray absorption value for each specific pixel point within the scanned section, and these values represent a mathematical picture of the patient's anatomy. The data may be manipulated for optimal evaluation and reproduction. Newer scanners complete a procedure in 2 to 5 seconds and have a skin surface radiation dose of as low as 0.1 rad per section.

To study abdominal aortic aneurysms, most authors suggest palpation of the maximal part of the abdominal mass and then scanning 3 cm above and 3 cm below this point at 2-cm intervals.[1] The patient is then given intravenous radiographic contrast material either by a bolus injection of 50 to 100 ml of a high iodine content substance (Renografin 76 or Conray 400), or by an infusion of 300 ml of a 25 to 30 percent radiographic contrast medium. Scans are then repeated following the contrast injection.

Another technique is to scan from the xiphoid to below the umbilicus at 2-cm intervals to gain information about other intra-abdominal organs, the proximal aorta, and the renal, visceral, and iliac arteries. Contrast material is then administered and the scans repeated, occasionally overlapping at 1-cm intervals. The administration of contrast material also helps to identify problems of renal excretion and ureteral obstruction. In an emergency, a primary contrast exam may be performed, which will clearly define the aortic lumen, thrombus within the aneurysm, and the outer wall of the aneurysm within 30 to 40 minutes. The procedure without, and then with, contrast takes about 60 minutes.

In the early CT experience, scans were done without intravenous contrast material, and, although aneurysms could be recognized, the wall of the aorta was indistinguishable from the lumen unless the wall was calcified. Thrombi were indistinguishable from flowing blood. Each scan took approximately 4 minutes and the skin radiation dose approximated 8 rads.[1] With the newer scanners and techniques, the aortic diameter is easily and accurately measured even if not calcified, and aneurysms may be distinguished from other intra-abdominal masses or hematomas and aortic tortuosity.[5,6,8] Aneurysms of the iliac arteries and dilatation of the proximal abdominal aorta are also readily detectable. In a few instances, CT may be diagnostic when ultrasound is not effective because of patient obesity, barium retention, or excessive intestinal gas. Obese patients are easily scanned because the fat acts as a contrast against which the soft tissues stand out (Fig. 5). Gas also does not interfere with the CT scans, especially if the patient is given an intravenous injection of 1 mg of glucagon to inhibit bowel motility. Barium may produce some artifacts but does not significantly degrade the scans. One very important source of CT artifacts is the presence of metallic surgical clips, since small detailed areas are obscured by streaks from the metal.

Size estimates of the aneurysms have been quite accurate on CT when correlated with findings at surgery.[4,12] They do not vary more than 4 mm, and in a series of 23 patients, the measurements were identical in 17 cases.

One of the great advances in CT scanning has occurred with the use of intravenous radiographic contrast material (RCM). Exams with RCM have allowed detailed evaluation of the lumen size, and the position and amount of thrombus present in all patients studied. The different phases of clot formation can be sharply defined regardless of the degree of organization.[7,8] A newer clot close to the lumen is less dense than the older clot close to the outer wall, as confirmed by serial sectioning of pathologic specimens.[7] In most cases, the majority of thrombus lies

38 Critical Problems in Vascular Surgery

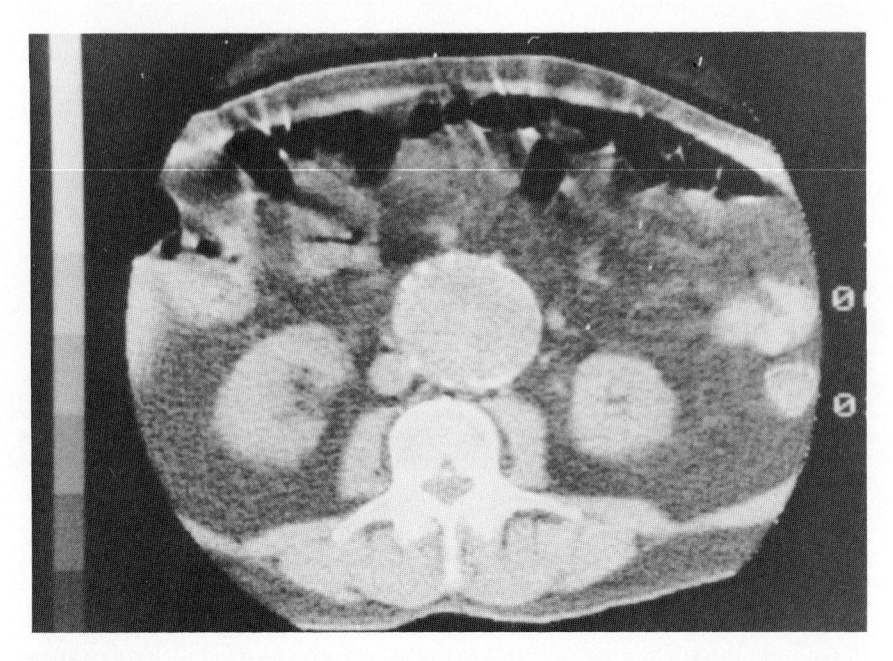

FIGURE 5. A scan from a patient with a large amount of body fat shows how the fat acts as a contrast substance against which the organs stand out. Here the aneurysm dwarfs the inferior vena cava. CT scans are read with the patient's right on the viewer's left, as if looking up at the section from the patient's feet. (From Bernstein EF, Harris RD, Leopold GR: Ultrasound and CT scanning in the noninvasive evaluation of abdominal aortic aneurysms. In Bergan JJ, Yao JST(eds): Surgery of the Aorta and Its Body Branches. New York, Grune & Stratton, 1980.)

anterior to the lumen that is in turn located symmetrically somewhat posterior to the center (Fig. 6). The clot can also be further evaluated after contrast enhancement. Clot liquefication or clot dissection can be identified by the presence of an eccentric lumen. Often a tail of contrast is seen close to the lateral wall, which indicates clot dehiscence or dissection.

Although not a common problem in abdominal aortic aneurysms, dissections of the aortic wall may be seen on CT scans as a separation of the wall and development of two lumens. Additional information regarding whether both lumens contain flowing blood is available from the RCM studies.

Retroperitoneal hematomas secondary to leaking or rupturing aneurysms also can be assessed by CT, especially with contrast enhanced scans. Extravascular blood is a high-density substance, which disrupts the normal anatomic configurations in the retroperitoneum.[5,7] After

RCM, the clot has a characteristic lower density than surrounding structures that normally "blush" with the contrast (Fig. 7). The hematoma may also have some rim enhancement (Fig. 7B) because of an inflammatory response around the hematoma to the presence of the blood. These findings are considerably better seen on CT than echo.[5]

A new and important role for CT is the postoperative evaluation of patients undergoing aortic reconstruction. Repeat scans permit following the resolution of periprosthetic hematomas. Both aortoprosthesis disruption and false-aneurysm formation can be diagnosed, even when accompanied by an attendant paralytic ileus that would render echo ineffective. Early postoperative changes associated with graft infection include the loss of periaortic fat, inflammatory rim enhancement around an abscess, and the identification of pockets of gas due to pyogenic organisms. These gas pockets are usually multiple and characteristically located posterior to the lumen (Fig. 8). RCM enhancement demonstrates that these gas

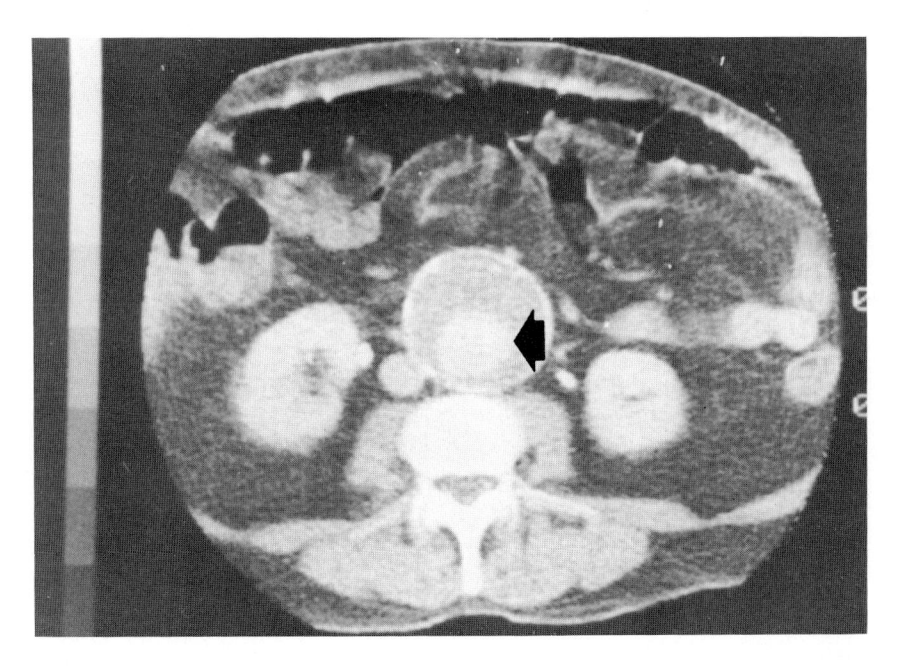

FIGURE 6. Following intravenous contrast material, the lumen of the aorta is seen to enhance with flowing blood (arrow). The thrombus is easily differentiated and is typically located anterior and lateral to the lumen. (From Bernstein EF, Harris RD, Leopold GR: Ultrasound and CT scanning in the noninvasive evaluation of abdominal aortic aneurysms. In Bergan JJ, Yao JST(eds): Surgery of the Aorta and Its Body Branches. New York, Grune & Stratton, 1980.)

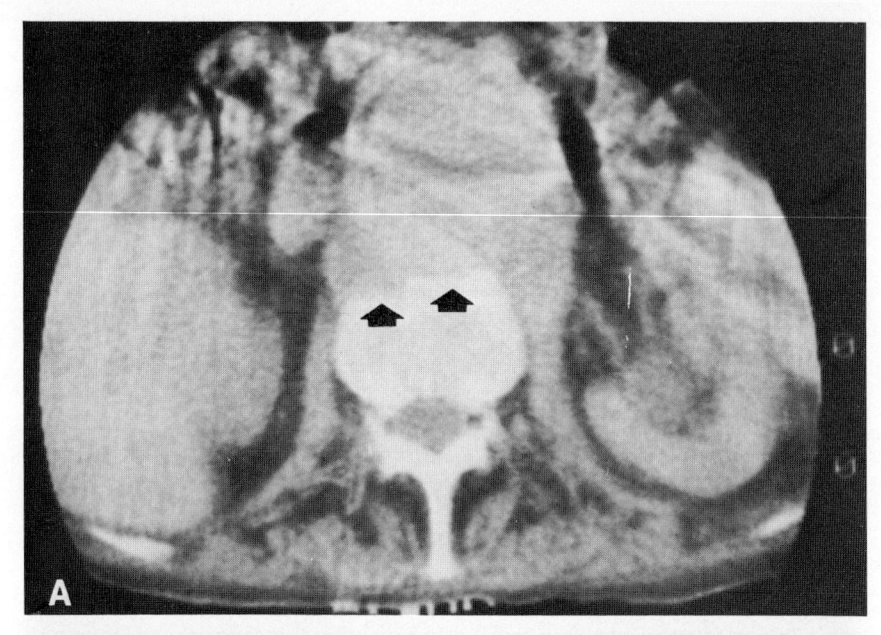

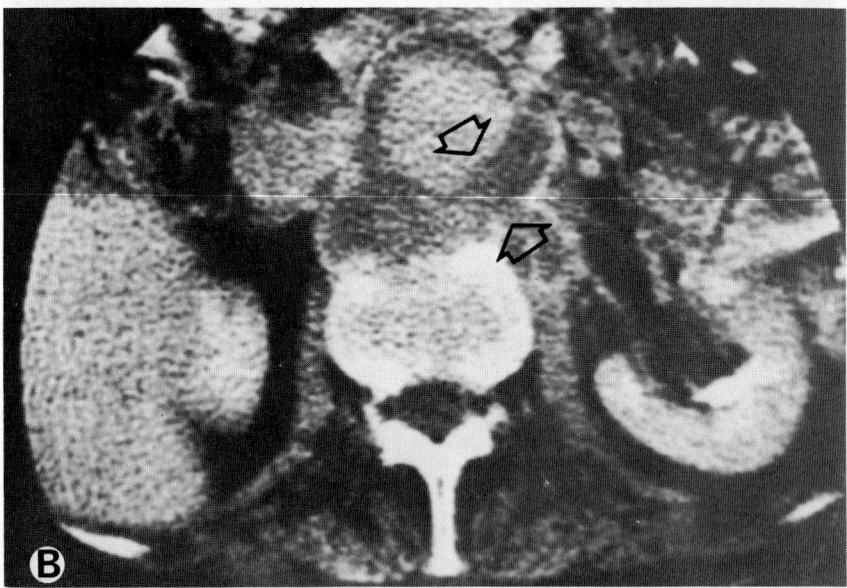

FIGURE 7. A retroperitoneal hematoma surrounds a leaking aortic prosthesis. **A.** The high density blood obscures the normal anatomic configurations of the aorta and anterior psoas muscle margins. Vertebral body erosions are also noted (arrow heads). The bleeding was due to an aortoprosthetic graft disruption. **B.** Contrast enhancement clearly delineates the aortic lumen, and the limits of the periprosthetic hematoma (white arrows). (From Bernstein EF, Harris RD, Leopold GR: Ultrasound and CT scanning in the noninvasive evaluation of abdominal aortic aneurysms. In Bergan JJ, Yao JST(eds): Surgery of the Aorta and Its Body Branches. New York, Grune & Stratton, 1980.)

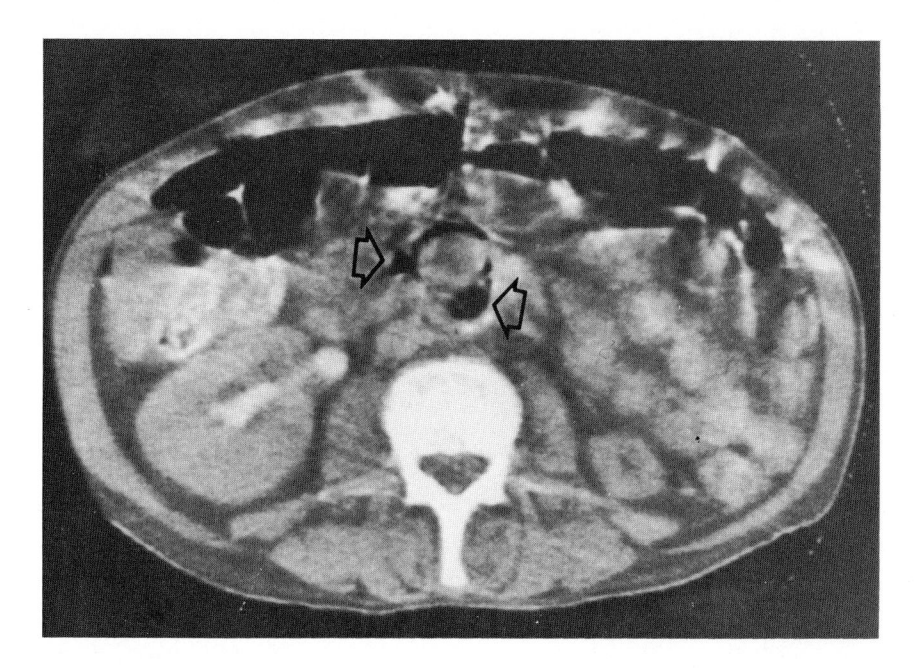

FIGURE 8. This patient became febrile after aortic graft surgery. The scan shows collections of gas that appear as a black area posterior to the lumen of the aorta (arrows). These gas pockets are felt to be pathognomonic for a pyogenic infection. (From Bernstein EF, Harris RD, Leopold GR: Ultrasound and CT scanning in the noninvasive evaluation of abdominal aortic aneurysms. In Bergan JJ, Yao JST(eds): Surgery of the Aorta and Its Body Branches. New York, Grune & Stratton, 1980.)

pockets are indeed extraluminal.[8,9] Gas in normal patients is often seen anteriorly and as a single collection up to 10 days postoperatively, compared to the posteriorly located and persistent multiple gas bubbles of an abscess.[9]

COMPARATIVE ANALYSIS OF ULTRASOUND AND CT SCANNING (Table 1)

Both echography and CT scanning are quite accurate in diagnosing 99 to 100 percent of abdominal aneurysms and generally correlate within 3 to 4 mm of the findings at surgery.[4,6,7,10-12,14] The occasional errors seen with echography may be a result of increased wall thickness with old organized thrombus, leading to difficulty in acoustically separating the aortic wall from surrounding tissue and to differences in equipment and its application, or skill in interpretation. Through the use of ultrasound the presence of thrombus within an aneurysm can frequently

Table 1. Comparison of Ultrasound and CT in the Diagnosis and Evaluation of Abdominal Aortic Aneurysms

	Ultrasound	CT
Examining modality	High frequency sound (1–20 mHz)	X-ray
Accuracy in aneurysm diagnosis	Excellent	Excellent
Accuracy in aneurysm size estimates	±3 mm	Not fully documented, but probably ± 3 mm
Radiation dose (skin surface)/slice	None	0.1–2 rad
Time for examination	10–60 min	30–60 min
Cost of examination	$75–150	$75–300
Dependence upon technician skill	Great	Modest
Dependence upon interpretive skill	Great	Straightforward
Limitations	Intestinal gas, barium, obesity; cannot distinguish clot from flowing blood	Motion; only cross-section images generally available now; metallic clips distort image

be detected, although the various phases of clot organization may not be as accurately distinguished as with CT. The clinical importance of this distinction, however, remains uncertain at this time.

Large amounts of intestinal gas are a problem for ultrasound, and the worst cases occur in patients with paralytic bowel ileus. The presence of an abdominal aneurysm may push aside the overlapping bowel, however, so that the diagnosis can still be made in most instances. Radiodense contrasts in the bowel, such as barium, also serve as an obstacle to ultrasound, but usually do not interfere with aneurysm diagnosis. Finally, in some obese patients, the body size is too great to permit adequate penetration of the sound beam for an accurate anatomic examination.

On the positive side, echography has at least two major advantages over CT: it is possible to scan in a longitudinal plane, and that the energy used is nonionizing. The CT limitation to transverse scanning increases the likelihood that CT will yield a false positive diagnosis of aneurysm when an ectatic aorta swings transversely. Whether such errors are common is still not known, however. This advantage of ultrasound in permitting longitudinal scans will be equalized by newer CT software packages that allow both longitudinal and coronal reconstruction images of the abdomen, but these are available in less than 1 percent of installations in the United States at the present time.

Finally, real-time ultrasonography represents an additional modality for the study of aortic wall motion, which eliminates the need for highly skilled technical specialists, and permits the recognition of aortic dissection.

One of the problems with the older CT scanners was the time required for each study. With the newer machines, however, the entire procedure can be accomplished within 30 to 60 minutes, which compares with the 10 to 60 minutes required for ultrasonic examinations. Radiation dosage has also been a CT drawback, but with the newer scanners, the skin dose has been significantly reduced to 0.1 to 2 rads per slice, and the patient dosage is no greater than that received from a GI series.

Metallic hemostatic surgical clips produce serious CT image artifacts, especially when they are located adjacent to moving structures such as a pulsatile aorta. Because of their dependence on postoperative CT scans, most neurosurgeons have ceased using such clips for hemostasis; vascular surgeons may be forced to do the same if postoperative CT scanning becomes progressively more valuable.

SUMMARY

Improving ultrasonic and CT scanning technology should permit the risk-free and accurate diagnosis of abdominal aneurysms on a routine basis in an outpatient setting. The identification of patients without aneurysmal disease but with aortic ectasia or tortuosity and other intra-abdominal masses will save such patients from needless angiography. The clear detection of unsuspected aneurysms will permit early elective aneurysm resection in other patients and should decrease the eventual mortality from this disease. In addition, the improved delineation of smaller anatomic details that appears to be possible with the newer techniques may permit localizing such para-aneurysmal structures as the renal arteries, the left renal vein, anomalous venous structures, and other items of importance to the vascular surgeon. The CT scan appears particularly useful in assessing graft complications in the postoperative period. Finally, the increasing trend toward mass screening centers for the diagnosis of asymptomatic disease may provide an opportunity to use ultrasound and CT screening to detect the presence of aneurysmal disease in asymptomatic patients. In the long run, availability, reproducibility, cost, and technical proficiency will be the final determinants in the choice of which of these two diagnostic modalities is best for examining patients with abdominal aortic aneurysms.

REFERENCES

1. Axelbaum SP, Schellinger D, Gomes MN, et al: Computed tomographic evaluation of aortic aneurysms. Am J Roentgenol 127:75, 1976
2. Bernstein EF, Dilley RB, Goldberger LE, Gosink BB, Leopold GR: Growth rates of small abdominal aortic aneurysms. Surgery 80:765, 1976
3. Bernstein EF: Ultrasound techniques in the diagnosis and evaluation of abdominal aortic aneurysms. In Berstein EF(ed): Noninvasive Diagnostic Techniques in Vascular Disease. St. Louis, Mosby, 1978, pp 330–338
4. Brewster DC, Darling C, Raines JK: Assessment of abdominal aortic aneurysm size. Circulation 56 (Suppl II):164, 1977.
5. Carter BL, Wechsler RJ: Computed tomography of the retroperitoneum and abdominal wall. Semin Roentgenol 13:201, 211, 1978
6. Gomes MN: Acta scanning in the diagnosis of abdominal aortic aneurysms. Comput Tomogr 1:51, 1977
7. Gomes MN, Hakkal HG, Schellinger D: Ultrasonography and CT scanning: A comparative study of abdominal aortic aneurysms. Comput Tomogr 2:99, 1978
8. Haaga J, Reich NE: Computed Tomography of Abdominal Abnormalities. St. Louis, Mosby, 1978, p. 163–169
9. Haaga JR, Baldwin GN, Reich NE, et al: CT detection of infected synthetic grafts: Preliminary report of a new sign. Am J Roentgenol 131:317, 1978
10. Hertzer NR, Beven EG: Ultrasound measurement and elective aneurysmectomy. JAMA 240:1966, 1978
11. Leopold GR, Goldberger LE, Bernstein EF: Ultrasonic detection and evaluation of abdominal aortic aneurysms. Surgery 72:939, 1972
12. Maloney JD, Pairolero PC, Smith BF Jr, et al: Ultrasound evaluation of abdominal aortic aneurysms. Circulation 56 (Suppl II):1180, 1977
13. Nusbaum JW, Freimanis AK, Thomford NR: Echography in the diagnosis of abdominal aortic aneurysm. Arch Surg 102:385, 1971
14. Raskin MM, Cunningham JB: Comparison of computed tomography and ultrasound for abdominal aortic aneurysms: A preliminary study. J Comput Tomogr 2:21, 1978

THREE

Diagnosis of Deep Vein Thrombosis of the Lower Extremities

Michael A. Bettmann and Edwin W. Salzman

Deep vein thrombosis (DVT) of the lower extremities presents a difficult clinical problem. It is a common disease particularly in patients undergoing open urologic or hip surgery and those at prolonged bed rest. The accuracy of the clinical diagnosis of DVT, however, is no greater than 30 to 50 percent.[12,14] The error lies, in part, in the fact that many cases of DVT are asymptomatic even when the thrombosis is extensive, as has become apparent from prospective studies utilizing ^{125}I-labeled fibrinogen. Second, DVT is mimicked by several other processes, including lymphatic obstruction, deep muscle hematoma, ruptured Baker's cyst, chronic venous disease, cellulitis, and even superficial venous thrombosis. The clinical diagnosis, therefore, lacks both sensitivity and specificity.

In general deep vein thrombosis, once diagnosed, must be treated because of the sequellae of pulmonary embolism and chronic venous disease. Systemic anticoagulation is effective in decreasing the incidence of these problems, but this therapy is not without significant morbidity and mortality.[21] The disease must be diagnosed accurately, although no currently available diagnostic modality is ideal. This chapter will examine the advantages and drawbacks of the currently available techniques and will attempt to place them in functional perspective.

CONTRAST PHLEBOGRAPHY

Phlebography is the most accurate technique available for the diagnosis of established thrombi. Methods in use range from those in which both legs are studied simultaneously with the patient supine and a fixed amount of contrast injected to study of a single leg by injection of contrast into the marrow cavity at the ankle (intraosseous phlebography). Probably the most popular and rational technique is that described by Rabinov and Paulin.[22] Because of the presenting symptoms or findings of noninvasive studies, there is only need to study one leg at a time. The patient is elevated 45° with the head up. The weight is supported primarily by the contralateral foot, which avoids incomplete filling secondary to muscular contraction. Contrast is infused via a small bore needle (usually 23 gauge) in a distal dorsal pedal vein, and venous filling is monitored fluoroscopically. The muscular veins, which in essence are part of the deep vein system, fill from the superficial system, so tourniquets are not used. After enough contrast material has been infused to fill the entire venous system to the midthigh, overhead films are exposed while contrast infusion continues. In this fashion, there is good visualization of the entire venous system from the foot to the external iliac vein or higher (Fig. 1). If questions remain after the films are exposed, reinjection is undertaken with repositioning of the needle, placement of tourniquets or a blood pressure cuff at the ankle level, or additional patient elevation.

The diagnosis of acute deep vein thrombosis can be made only by visualization of an intraluminal filling defect (Fig. 2). Other findings proposed as criteria, such as abrupt termination of the column of contrast, diversion of flow or collateral filling, are not necessarily secondary to acute thrombosis. They may be due to faulty needle position, muscle contraction, or chronic venous disease, and therefore are not sufficient to mandate systemic anticoagulation with its attendant risks. With fastidious technique, careful perusal of the radiographs, and a low threshold for repeat injection, it is very rare that a contrast phlebogram cannot be interpreted as definitively positive or negative for DVT.

Compared to other techniques, phlebography (venography) is very accurate. It is available in any well equipped radiology department. Objective results are produced that allow review and comparison with prior or subsequent studies, and the technique is generally safe.

Phlebography is a relatively expensive modality, however, and requires a level of technical expertise to perform and interpret and is not easily repeated. Further, side effects can occur, such as contrast extravasation which is usually heralded by pain. With cessation of the contrast infusion and local care, significant sequellae are rare.[3] Some discomfort, usually a cramp-like pain, occurs in about 70 percent of patients when routine contrast agents (288 mg I/ml) are used, but when dilute contrast is employed (i.e., 200 mg I/ml) this discomfort occurs in only about 30 percent of patients.[3] The postphlebography syndrome of pain, swelling, and erythema in the low calf beginning 2 to 12 hours after the study occurs in about 25 percent of patients studied with routine, hypertonic

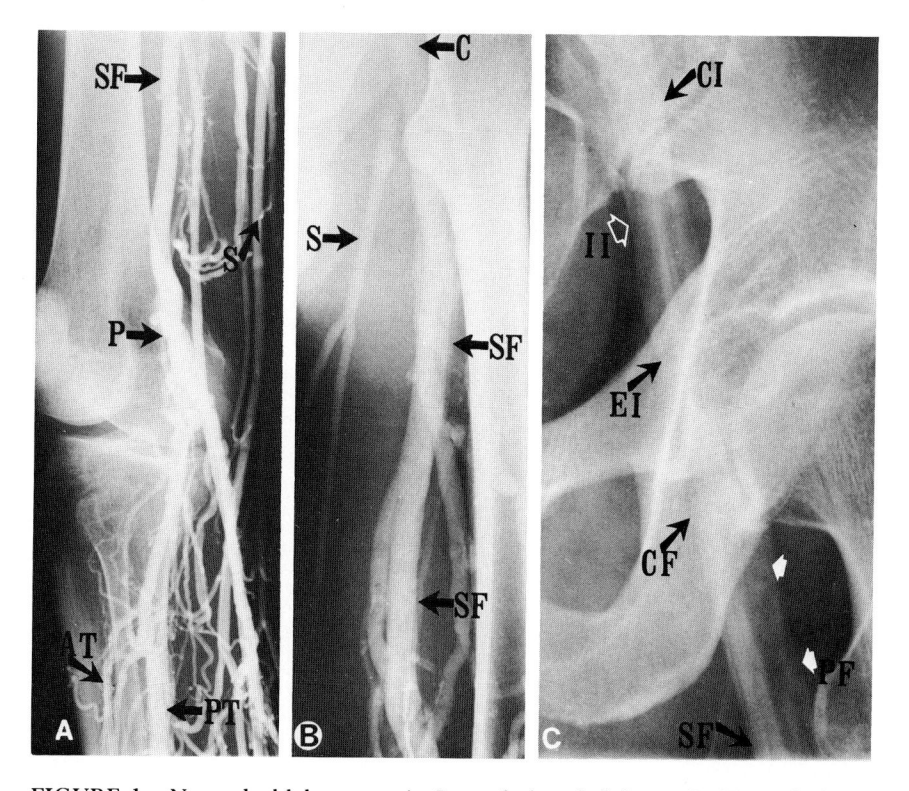

FIGURE 1. Normal phlebogram. **A.** Lateral view, left knee. **B.** Frontal view, thigh. **C.** Frontal view, pelvis. Note flow defects due to emptying of unopacified blood from profunda femoris and internal iliac veins. AT, paired anterior tibial veins. PT, common posterior tibial-peroneal trunk. P, popliteal vein. SF, superficial femoral vein. S, greater saphenous vein. CF, common femoral vein. PF, profunda femoris vein. EI, external iliac vein. II, internal iliac vein. CI, common iliac vein.

contrast agents, but the incidence drops to 7.5 percent when the contrast is diluted to three-quarter strength.[3] Most disturbingly, thrombi may form subsequent to phlebography and probably secondary to it. The stated incidence of this problem has varied over a wide range. A recent study by the authors[5] indicated that thrombosis following phlebography with routine contrast agent occurred in 26 percent of patients (13 percent superficial and 13 percent DVT). When dilute contrast agent was used, this decreased to 9 percent overall with a 3 percent incidence of deep vein thrombosis. Essentially all of these thrombi were small and confined to veins below the knee.

The most promising developments in regard to contrast phlebography are new nonisotonic contrast agents. In addition to be nearly isotonic to blood at high iodine concentrations (plasma = 300 mOsm; nonionic

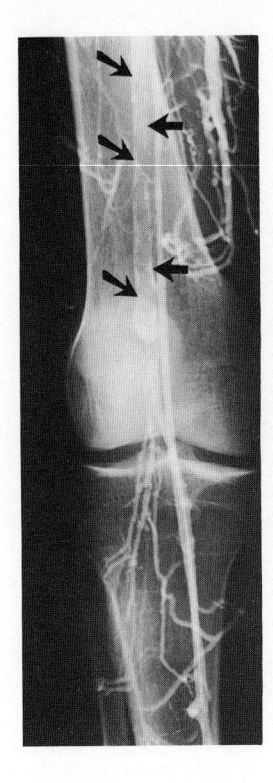

FIGURE 2. Positive phlebogram. Large thrombus in superficial femoral vein, with cephalad propagation. There is filling of only muscular and greater saphenous veins below the knee, suggesting occlusive thrombi of unknown age.

agents = 400–450 mOsm; standard agents = 1100–1500 mOsm/liter), these newer contrast agents are less hyperviscous than standard contrast agents. In initial studies, two such agents appeared to cause less discomfort when used intra-arterially and fewer sequellae when used for phlebography.[1]

The key role that contrast phlebography plays is as the ultimate standard for determining whether or not deep vein thrombosis is present. As this method is somewhat complex and expensive, it is not ideal as a screening test. Phlebography is indicated in patients suspected of having deep vein thrombosis, either on clinical grounds or on the basis of noninvasive studies.

^{125}I-FIBRINOGEN POINT COUNT SCANNING

This technique was originated in the early 1960s and was refined by Flanc, Kakkar, and Clarke.[10] It is most widely used for surveillance of patients at risk of developing deep vein thrombosis. ^{125}I emits low energy gamma photons (35 keV) that are not suitable for imaging because of inadequate tissue penetration but can be counted with a scintillation detector. ^{125}I can be stably bound to fibrinogen and injected intravenously. The usual dose is 100 μCi, administered after thyroid uptake is blocked by 100 mg sodium iodide given orally. The duration of usefulness of a single injection of labeled fibrinogen is about 7 days, a function of the half-life of ^{125}I (60 days) and the biologic half-life of fibrinogen (about 3 days). If scanning is to be continued, the compound can be reinjected when the count density falls.

"Scanning," actually point counting, is carried out at 1-or 2-day intervals, beginning 8 to 24 hours after injection. Counting is first done over the heart for a fixed time period, and counts are then obtained for the same length of time over seven or more marked points on each leg. The scan is regarded as positive if there is a 15 percent (using a 4-inch collimator[10]) or 20 percent (using a 2-inch collimator[6]) increase in counts, expressed as a percentage of precordial counts, at one site compared to the same site on the other leg, adjacent sites on the same leg, or the same site on a previous examination. Because transiently positive readings may occur, the test is repeated 24 hours after the initial positive scan to increase specificity.

There are obvious advantages to this test over other available modalities. It is simple, relatively safe, inexpensive, and readily available; it allows prospective evaluation of patients at risk, e.g., those at prolonged bed rest. The results are objective and scanning can easily be repeated. The disadvantages are that results cannot be obtained for at least 12 to 14 hours after injection of the isotope; because anticoagulant therapy during that interval will block fibrinogen accumulation in thrombus as fibrin, it must be withheld. Because of the low photon energy and the relatively high blood pool background, scanning is not generally accurate above the midthigh. Also, uptake of isotope in any area of fibrin accumulation occurs, not just in actively forming thrombus. This limits the usefulness of the technique in patients with pelvic, hip, or lower extremity surgery as well as in patients with cellulitis or trauma. Conversely, if thrombi are more than a few days old, fibrinogen accumulation may no longer be occurring.

The accuracy of this test ranges from 70 to 90 percent compared to contrast phlebography, depending on the patient population. These figures may be slightly misleading, as it has been shown that fibrinogen deposition occurs in areas of endothelial damage before thrombi can be visualized phlebographically and after embolization has occurred[15]; that is, when a patient has a positive fibrinogen scan and a negative phlebogram, the fibrinogen scan may be truly, rather than falsely, positive.

Modifications of this test have been suggested to increase its accuracy and achieve more rapid results, but their efficacy is not yet established. Labeling fibrinogen with ^{131}I or ^{123}I has also been attempted, since both of these isotopes have higher energy photons than ^{125}I and thus can be imaged using a gamma camera. Neither has proved advantageous. ^{131}I is readily available but emits harmful beta, as well as gamma, photons, limiting the dose, and it has not proven superior in accuracy to ^{125}I. ^{123}I has a half-life of only 13.3 hours; in limited clinical studies it has shown promise.[9]

^{125}I-fibrinogen scanning is a well investigated and accurate technique, with some significant limitations. It is the most useful screening test currently available for prospective use in high-risk patients.

IMPEDANCE PLETHYSMOGRAPHY

This technique was originated by Mullick et al[19] using the principle of Ohm's Law: $R = V/I$, where R is impedance (electrical resistance), I is current, and V is voltage drop. Blood is a good conductor of electrical current; thus, at a constant voltage, as blood volume (or venous capacitance) increases, resistance decreases and current increases. Blood volume and venous capacitance in the lower extremities increases with obstruction to outflow and falls as this obstruction is released. Using either maximal inspiration or a blood pressure cuff to cause a relative obstruction, normal patients demonstrate a typical pattern of increasing current with time, and a rapid falloff following release of the deep breath or cuff. In patients with occlusive thrombi in the major deep veins, particularly above the knee, both the rise in current and the rate of falloff are delayed. The use of a large cuff, foot elevation, and slight flexion of the knee increase the accuracy of this technique. A 15-cm wide cuff inflated to 45 cm of water is now standard—inflation is generally held for 2 minutes. Accuracy is further increased by the use of sequential 2-minute inflations. For each inflation-deflation cycle, the fall in impedance (i.e., decreased resistance secondary to increased venous capacitance) is plotted against the rise in impedance (decreased capacitance) in the first 3 seconds after release of the cuff. A discriminant line can then be constructed, allowing one to distinguish a normal response from deep vein thrombosis (Fig. 3).[13]

The advantages of impedance plethysmography (IPG) are that it is totally noninvasive, inexpensive, rapid, relatively objective and reviewable, and easily repeated. Some expertise is needed to perform the study, but this is easily learned. There are several drawbacks to this modality, some inherent and some not. Patient cooperation is necessary, since

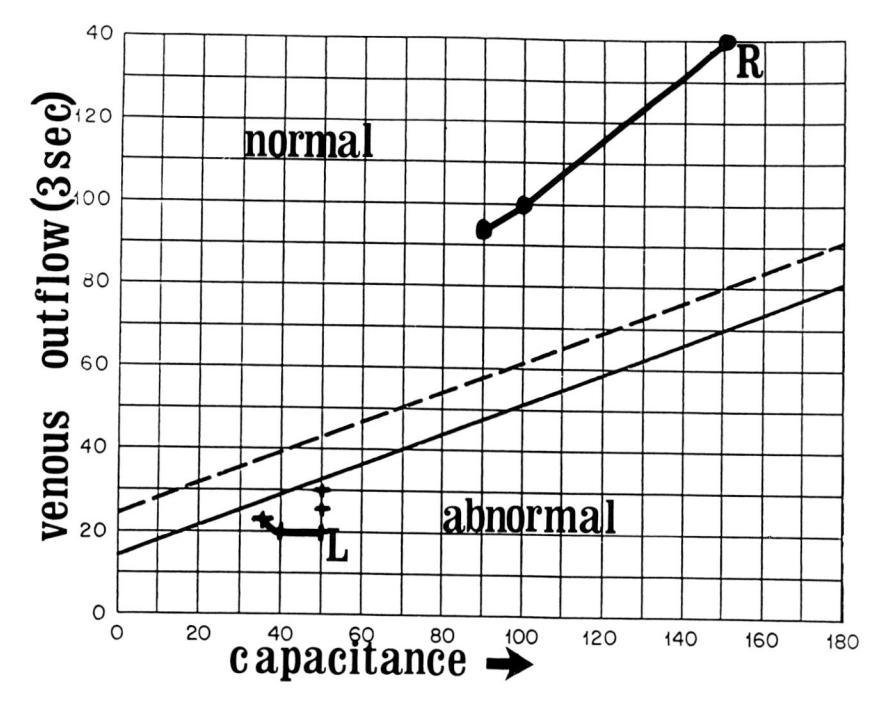

FIGURE 3. Impedance plethysmography. Results of tracings of three cycles from the right leg are normal (top). Results of five cycles from left leg are abnormal, indicating occlusive thigh thrombosis.

muscle contraction may alter venous capacitance. Because alteration in venous flow from any cause may lead to an abnormal study, impedance plethysmography is of limited use in patients with congestive heart failure, lower limb edema, or chronic venous disease. Finally, because this technique depends on alterations of venous filling and emptying secondary to thrombosis, small or nonocclusive thrombi, particularly if below the knee, may not be demonstrable. The significance of such thrombi is still the subject of debate, but it is clear that, at least in many cases, small, nonocclusive thrombi in the deep veins of the calf propagate and embolize.[14] IPG has been claimed 70 to 97 percent accurate in comparison to contrast phlebography, with greater accuracy in symptomatic patients as well as in those with thrombi above the knee level.[13] Hull and Hirsh,[13] in addition to using a multiple-cycle approach, have used an electromyograph to ensure adequate relaxation and eliminate the possible inaccuracy due to patient muscle contraction.

Cranley[8] has investigated the use of phleborheography, a variation that utilizes several cuffs placed from the ankle to the abdomen. Volume changes are recorded by one cuff in response to rapid inflation of an adjacent one. In Cranley's hands, this technique has been highly accurate. Respiratory variations in thigh volume are obliterated by acute DVT but begin to return at 2 weeks. It is claimed that 75 percent of thrombi below the knee were diagnosed. Thus this technique may be slightly more accurate than impedance plethysmography, but it is possessed of the same basic advantages and disadvantages.

Impedance and volume plethysmography are most valuable in evaluating symptomatic patients. Their value is limited as a prospective screening modality and in high-risk patients suspected of DVT who may have small, nonocclusive, or distal thrombosis.

DOPPLER ULTRASOUND

This technique uses the Doppler principle: A sound wave encountering a stationary object will be reflected back without a change in frequency; if the object encountered is moving, however, the frequency of the sound wave will be altered in a fashion linearly related to the velocity of the object. A five MHz piezoelectric crystal generates the ultrasound waves, and the difference in frequency of the incident and reflected waves is recorded by a second crystal mounted adjacent to the first and is converted to an auditory signal that reflects both the direction and the velocity of flow.

The usual approach is that of Strandness.[23] The femoral artery is located in the groin and then the femoral vein is identified. After respiratory alterations in femoral vein flow are evaluated, the more distal aspect of each leg is examined point by point. Compression of the leg distal to any point normally causes increased flow past the transducer, and a "wooshing" sound is heard. Absence of this sound or its alteration in comparison to the same point on the other leg or absence of phasic changes in the sound in the iliofemoral region are indicative of deep vein thrombosis.

Doppler ultrasound is simple, rapid (about 5 minutes per examination), noninvasive, and inexpensive (simple models are available for about $400). The study can be repeated at will and can be of value in patients with congestive heart failure or a lower leg cast. No objective record is available for review, however, and although the technique is very simple, experience and expertise are necessary for adequate interpretation. The results are of necessity somewhat more subjective than those obtained with other modalities. The major disadvantage of Doppler ultrasound is the same as that of impedance plethysmography: reliability is greatest with occlusive thrombi of proximal deep veins. The test, therefore, may not be of great value as a prospective screening procedure. The overall accuracy in symptomatic patients varies in different reports between 62 and 94 percent.

In summary, Doppler ultrasound, as a method for diagnosis, is restricted in its applicability, both because of its limitations for prospective screening of patients at risk and because of its requirement for subjective interpretation. There is little justification (except for perhaps very experienced investigators) for relying on this modality alone.

THERMOGRAPHY

Based on the clinical observation that the skin of the leg of a patient with deep vein thrombosis is warmer than normal, infrared camera recordings of skin temperature can be used to make the diagnosis of DVT. In the presence of deep vein thrombosis there is increased temperature in the muscle groups drained by the involved veins as well as alteration in the normal thermographic pattern because of redirection of venous drainage. Each thermographic study requires 10 to 20 minutes. The legs are uncovered to allow equilibration to ambient temperature, and they are elevated slightly to prevent stasis. Images obtained on a Polaroid camera demonstrate cooler areas as black and warmer areas as white. A 1.5 C elevation in temperature is usually considered diagnostic of DVT. Using this criterion, thermography is about 90 percent accurate compared with contrast phlebography in symptomatic patients but is less accurate when used prospectively in patients at risk of developing DVT.[2]

The advantages of thermography are that it is totally noninvasive and painless, requires little patient cooperation, and can be repeated as desired; objective results are produced. The disadvantages are that the equipment is expensive, proximal venous thrombosis (e.g., nonocclusive external iliac thrombosis) may be missed, and the modality is not reliable in inflammatory conditions that may be confused with DVT, such as cellulitis, acute arthritis, or ruptured Baker's cyst. This technique is promising, but it has not yet received sufficient evaluation to allow definition of its eventual role in the diagnosis of DVT.

RADIONUCLIDE PHLEBOGRAPHY

This is a method with tremendous theoretical advantages: it is simple, rapid, safe, and inexpensive. To garner these advantages, however, advances are necessary in the radiopharmaceuticals. To date, most investigators have used ^{99m}Tc, which is an excellent isotope for gamma camera

54 Critical Problems in Vascular Surgery

imaging (the half life is 6.04 hours and the principal gamma photon is 140 keV), either as free pertechnitate or complexed with macroaggregated albumin or human albumin microspheres. As these latter two are normally used for perfusion lung scanning, isotope phlebography may be used as a part of the lung scan without additional patient dose.

Generally the isotope is injected in divided doses via a small vein in each foot. Dynamic imaging demonstrates flow patterns, and subsequent static images, for reasons that are not clear, may demonstrate isotope sequestration on thrombi. The accuracy of radionuclide phlebography using this approach in small series has ranged from 75 to 96 percent.[24]

This approach has the assets of relative ease, simplicity, safety, and objectivity, and the theoretical advantage of being available routinely as an adjunct to lung scanning. Further, although as yet unproven, radionuclide phlebography should be of use in the diagnosis of iliac or inferior vena cava thrombosis. Because the volume of the isotope is small, it is unlikely that minor alterations in venous flow or small thrombi will be demonstrated. The procedure is frequently time consuming, as it is difficult to place small needles stably in distal dorsal pedal veins and multiple injections and images are frequently needed. Perhaps the major disadvantage of the technique is that it has not been prospectively evaluated in a large group of patients, so its sensitivity, its most vulnerable factor, remains in doubt.

THROMBUS SCINTIGRAPHY

Many radiopharmaceuticals have been investigated for use in identification of both forming and stable thrombi. The most carefully evaluated to date is ^{125}I-fibrinogen, which has been discussed previously. Many of the other preparations have been reviewed elsewhere in detail,[4,16] and only the promising ones will be considered here.

^{99m}Tc-fibrinogen has only recently been made by a process that does not denature the protein, but it has not yet been evaluated in a clinical trial. Platelet labeling with ^{111}indium, using a lipid-soluble complex with 8-hydroxyquinoline, leads to platelets with a half-life comparable to ^{51}Cr-labeled platelets, and little sequestration. In limited studies in both animals and humans, ^{111}In-labeled platelets were accurate in localizing fresh venous and arterial thrombi, but the accuracy appeared to fall off rapidly if thrombi were greater than 24 hours old.[11,17] Because the half-life of ^{111}indium is 2.8 days, ^{111}indium-labeled platelets might be used to monitor prospective patients at risk, as ^{125}I-fibrinogen is currently used, but with the advantages that the former can be imaged and may be accurate above the low-thigh level.

Much effort has been expended in labeling thrombolytic compounds. To date, clinical success has been very limited with all of these agents, including plasminogen, streptokinase-activated plasmin, streptokinase, and urokinase. A recent study[20] compared ^{99m}Tc-labeled porcine plasmin to contrast phlebography and a modified ^{125}I-fibrinogen procedure and showed 94 percent sensitivity and 56 percent specificity at 30 minutes, figures comparable to those of the ^{125}I-fibrinogen test at 24 to 48 hours. This procedure clearly needs further clinical assessment before its role can be determined.

PEDAL VENOUS PRESSURE

In theory, supine pedal venous pressure measurement should give an indication of gross alterations in venous flow. In practice, these measurements have not been shown to have value in the diagnosis of deep vein thrombosis.[18]

LABORATORY DIAGNOSTIC METHODS

Laboratory studies have been investigated most extensively in reference to pulmonary embolism, but they may also be useful in patients suspected of having deep vein thrombosis. Fibrin-fibrinogen degradation products are elevated in patients with DVT, but only transiently and not to as great a level as in patients with pulmonary embolism. Further, levels are elevated by many other unrelated processes, such as neoplasia, surgery, and collagen-vascular diseases. A recent study of the accuracy of tests of fibrin metabolism as screening tests for pulmonary embolism showed that fibrin-fibrinogen degradation products, while not very sensitive, were 84 percent specific. Soluble fibrin complexes were 92 percent sensitive. Thus, the use of these two determinations together may be of value. Because plasma fibrinopeptide A, a specific fibrinogen breakdown product, may be elevated in patients with DVT, pulmonary embolism, malignancy, or recent surgery, its determination is not sufficiently specific and is somewhat cumbersome to perform. Possibly a more promising test, particularly in symptomatic individuals, is the radioimmunoassay of fibrinogen-fibrin fragment E.[7] Levels have been shown to be higher in symptomatic patients with DVT than in those without.

SUMMARY

Because of its frequency and inaccuracy of clinical diagnosis, as well as because of the morbidity associated with the untreated disease and with the treatment itself, the accurate diagnosis of deep vein thrombosis is an important clinical problem. The diagnosis can be considered in two sets of patients: first, in symptomatic patients suspected of having DVT and second, patients in high-risk groups requiring prospective screening. In symptomatic individuals, a strong argument can be made for the routine use of contrast phlebography that, despite its drawbacks, is accurate and generally available. Combinations of noninvasive studies, such as ^{125}I-fibrinogen and impedance plethysmography, have been utilized, but in many cases noninvasive studies require confirmation by contrast phlebography. For screening purposes, ^{125}I-fibrinogen scanning is a well investigated, established, and sensitive technique. It is most useful for evaluation of the calves, and may be used in conjunction with impedance plethysmography or other noninvasive studies for evaluation of the thighs. The use of other radionuclide tests, such as ^{111}indium-labeled autologous platelets, and serum studies, such as the radioimmunoassay of fibrinogen-fibrin fragment E, are promising but require further evaluation.

REFERENCES

1. Albrechtsson U, Olsson CG: Thrombosis after phlebography: A comparison of two contrast media. Cardiovasc Radiol 2:9, 1979
2. Bergvist D, Hallböök T: Thermography for diagnosis of deep vein thrombosis and screening of postoperative venous thrombosis. Thrombos Hemost 42:28, 1979
3. Bettmann MA, Paulin S: Leg phlebography: The incidence, nature and modification of undesirable side effects. Radiology 122(1):101, 1977
4. Bettmann MA, Salzman EW: Recent advances in the diagnosis of deep vein thrombosis and pulmonary embolism. In Poller L (ed): Recent Advances in Blood Coagulation. London, Churchill Livingstone, 1980
5. Bettmann MA, Salzman EW, Rosenthal D, et al: Reduction of venous thrombosis complicating phlebography. Am J Roentgenol 134:1169, 1980
6. Browse NL: The ^{125}I-fibrinogen test. Arch Surg 140:160, 1972
7. Bynum LJ, Crotty CM, Wilson JE III: Diagnostic value of tests of fibrin metabolism in patients predisposed to pulmonary embolism. Arch Intern Med 139:283, 1979
8. Cranley JJ: Phleborrheography. In Cranley JJ (ed): Vascular Surgery Vol. II. Hagerstown, Md., Harper & Row, 1975, pp 79–95
9. DeNardo SJ, DeNardo GL: Iodine-123-fibrinogen scintigraphy. Semin Nucl Med 7 (3):245, 1977
10. Flanc C, Kakkar VV, Clarke MB: The detection of venous thrombosis of the legs using ^{125}I-labeled fibrinogen. Br J Surg 55:742, 1968
11. Grossman ZD, Wistow BW, McAfee JG, et al: Platelets labeled with oxine complexes of Tc-99m and In-111. Part 2. Localization of experimentally induced vascular lesions. J Nucl Med 19:488, 1978
12. Harris WH, Salzman EW, Athanasoulis CA, et al: Comparison of ^{125}I-fibrinogen count scanning with phlebography for detection of venous thrombi after elective hip surgery. N Engl J Med 292:665, 1975

13. Hull R, Hirsh J: Diagnosis of venous thromosis. In Salzman EW, Hirsh J, Coleman R (eds): Textbook of Thrombosis and Hemostasis. Philadelphia, Lippincott, 1980
14. Kakkar VV, Flanc C, Howe CT, Clarke MB: Natural history of postoperative deep vein thrombosis. Lancet 2:230, 1969
15. Kerrigan GNW, Buchanan MR, Cade JF, Regoeczi E, Hirsh J: Investigation of the mechanism of false positive ^{125}I-labeled fibrinogen scans. Br J Haematol 26:469, 1974
16. Krohn KA, Knight LC: Radiopharmaceuticals for thrombus detection: Selection, preparation and critical evaluation. Semin Nucl Med 7:219, 1977
17. McIlmoyle G, Davis HH, Welch MJ, et al: Scintigraphic diagnosis of experimental pulmonary embolism with In-111-labeled platelets. J Nucl Med 18:910, 1977
18. Martin EC, Cohen L, Sawyer PN, Gordon OH: Supine pedal venous pressure measurement in patients with venous disease. Radiology 131:75, 1979
19. Mullick SC, Wheeler HB, Songster GP: Diagnosis of deep venous thrombosis by measurement of electrical impedance. Am J Surg 119:417, 1970
20. Olsson CG, Albrechtsson U, Darte L, Persson RBR: ^{99m}Tc Plasmin for rapid detection of deep vein thrombosis. In press, 1980
21. Porter J, Hershel J: Drug-related deaths among medical inpatients. JAMA 237:879, 1977
22. Rabinov K, Paulin S: Roentgen diagnosis of venous thrombosis. Arch Surgery 104:133, 1972
23. Strandness DE Jr, Schultz RD, Sumner DS, Rushmer RF: Ultrasonic flow detection: A useful technique in the evaluation of peripheral vascular disease. Am J Surg 113:311, 1967
24. Webber MM: Labeled albumin aggregates for detection of clots. Semin Nucl Med 7:253, 1977

FOUR
Transcatheter Therapeutic Embolization

James Chang and Barry T. Katzen

Angiography is of proven value in the identification and localization of vascular abnormalities including sites of bleeding, trauma, occlusive disease, malformations and fistulas, and neoplasms. With time, increased experience, and more sophisticated catheterization techniques, the same catheters so helpful in the diagnosis of vascular abnormalities could also be applied and adapted for therapy. Initially, transcatheter therapy was limited to the local infusion of vasoconstrictors for treating gastrointestinal hemorrhage. Pharmacoangiography was not always successful, however; thus, occlusive therapy came into being. Since the initial report by Rosch[13] in 1972 of successful clinical application of transcatheter embolic therapy in a patient with right gastroepiploic arterial bleeding, there have been many reports of successful uses of occlusive therapy. Every conceivable organ system accessible by catheterization techniques has benefitted from transcatheter therapeutic embolization.

MATERIALS AND TECHNIQUES

A large variety of embolic materials and delivery systems have been developed and used.[1] The primary factors that determine what material is to be used are: 1) the length of time occlusion is desired, that is,

We wish to thank Ms. Denise Valeggia for her dedicated assistance in the preparation of this manuscript and its photographic material.

whether temporary or permanent occlusion is needed; 2) the location, size, type, and number of vessels to be embolized; 3) the venous drainage pattern; 4) the collateral flow pattern; 5) the vulnerability of surrounding normal tissue; 6) the difficulty in catheterizing and gaining access to the particular vessels; 7) whether it is to be the definitive therapeutic procedure or a preoperative adjunct to facilitate surgery; and 8) the clinical condition of the patient.

The materials used are of three types: 1) particulate matter, such as clot, tissue, gelatin sponge, polyvinyl alcohol, and microspheres; 2) mechanical devices, such as spring coils[1,9] and detachable balloons[5,15]; and 3) tissue adhesives, such as silicone rubber and isobutyl 2-cyanoacrylate.

Because autologous clot was readily available and would not cause any tissue reaction, it was the very first substance used. It was difficult to manipulate, however, with respect to sizing and delivery via a catheter, because it tended to fragment and was difficult to control during embolization. Other disadvantages included difficulty in obtaining satisfactory clot in patients with clotting deficiencies or multiple transfusions. Clot also was unpredictable with respect to the duration of the occlusion. Generally, clot will lyse within a few hours. This can be an advantage only when occlusions of short duration are desired to achieve hemostasis but not cause tissue loss, as is occasionally the case with renal embolization. Fragments of muscle, fat, and dura tissues have been used. The handling characteristics of these are also imperfect and offer no significant advantage over other available synthetic materials.

Gelatin sponge (Gelfoam) is probably the most commonly used of the embolic materials and forms a lattice on which clot is subsequently deposited. Its advantages are that it is readily available and easy to size, shape, and deliver. Gelfoam is a semipermanent occlusive agent. It will be phagocytized and absorbed in weeks to months with resultant recanalization of the vessel. We have seen circumstances, however, where permanent occlusions have been achieved. Conversely, recanalization of vessels has also been observed.

Microfibrillar collagen (Avitene), an absorbable hemostatic agent, has also been used for embolization purposes. It is injected in a viscous liquid form that solidifies on contact with blood. The time required for setting is slightly longer than with some of the permanent tissue adhesives.

Polyvinyl alcohol (Ivalon) is similar to Gelfoam and has the property of being compressible in the dry form. Ivalon has the additional characteristic, however, of expanding in size many times once in contact with solution. The obvious advantage is that a much larger embolus can ultimately be delivered by a conventional-sized catheter. The disadvantage is that occasionally the material will expand in the catheter and occlude it. Microspheres (metallic, silicone, or silastic) are also permanent agents. A significant disadvantage arises, however, because catheters with a relatively large diameter are required to deliver these noncompressible emboli. Mechanical devices are primarily comprised of spring wire coils (Gianturco coils, with or without attached cotton or wool tails) and balloon catheters with ejectable balloon tips. These devices offer permanent vessel occlusion, and are designed for problems requiring larger diameter, more proximal occlusions or lesions such as arteriovenous shunts. Their ingenious design permits occlusions of vessels up to 8 mm in diameter while using conventional catheter sizes.

The tissue adhesives also offer a means of permanent vessel occlusion. Both silicone rubber and cyanoacrylate set relatively quickly, however, so rapid injection is important. There have been reports where catheters became adherent to the vessel wall. Tissue adhesions are particularly useful in lesions, such as arteriovenous malformations, where it is essential to obliterate permanently the entire vascular bed as well as the feeding vessels. The flow of the adhesive into these lesions can be controlled with the aid of balloon catheters that can slow or block the flow in the feeder arteries in order to permit the adhesive to set.

Intra-arterial electrocoagulation has also been used both experimentally and clinically to cause vessel occlusion.[17] The risk of perforation and longer time required to induce thrombosis, together with the need for exact placement of the anode at the site of occlusion, make this modality unacceptable in its present state.

APPLICATIONS

The variety of applications of transcatheter therapeutic embolization are as long as the list of embolic materials available.[2-16,18] A partial list of some of the locations and diseases amenable to embolic therapy include:

1. Gastrointestinal tract: ulcers, Mallory Weiss tears, varices, diverticular bleeding, and neoplasms
2. Solid visceral organs (liver, kidney, spleen): benign and malignant primary and secondary neoplasms, posttraumatic (including biopsy related) bleeding, arteriovenous malformations and fistulas, arterial aneurysms,[7,11] and such miscellaneous conditions as hypersplenism[14] and hypertension with or without severe proteinuria secondary to chronic end-stage renal disease

3. Pelvis: posttraumatic hemorrhage, neoplasms (especially of bladder, colonic, and uterine origins), postoperative hemorrhage (e.g., hips), arteriovenous malformations and fistulas, aneurysms,[12] and ureteral fistulas
4. Extremities: arteriovenous malformations and fistulas, pseudoaneurysms,[3] and bone neoplasms both primary and secondary
5. Central nervous system[1,2,5]: arteriovenous malformations and fistulas (including spinal), aneurysms, vascular tumors, and spine metastasis
6. Cardiopulmonary: pulmonary arteriovenous malformations, bronchial arterial hemorrhage secondary to neoplasms, cystic fibrosis or bronchiectasis, and patent ductus arteriosus
7. Head and neck[16]: arteriovenous malformations and fistulas, and neoplasms (juvenile angiofibromas, hemangiomas, glomus tumors, and parathyroid adenomas)

The gastrointestinal tract has certainly been the most common site for the application of embolic therapy. Except in extreme life-threatening situations, a trial of vasoconstrictors before occlusive therapy is recommended. Frequently, vasoconstrictors will be adequate and the arterial system can be left intact, in the event that future surgical intervention is needed. In addition to treating the obvious arterial sources of bleeding, recent work has been performed in the embolic occlusion of varices.[18] Obviously, this in no way alters the hemodynamics of the basic underlying disease. Reports indicate, however, that embolic therapy may provide time to adequately prepare the patient for shunt surgery and consequently reduce morbidity and mortality. The procedure is performed through the percutaneous transhepatic route with direct entry into the portal venous system. Occlusions of the coronary and short gastric veins are performed using various combinations of Gelfoam, sclerosing agents such as hypertonic glucose, tissue adhesives, and mechanical coils.

Bleeding secondary to pelvic trauma has long been a difficult clinical situation to manage. There is often massive blood loss, and even at operation the sites of bleeding were usually not identified. Because of the extremely rich collateral circulation from adjacent arteries, ligation of the hypogastric artery has met with little success. The leading cause of death in pelvic fractures remains hemorrhage, even though the bleeding sites are relatively small. Vasoconstrictors are of little help in this situation because the patient is often hypovolemic and already maximally vasoconstricted. In the past, the general inability of surgical intervention to control bleeding has prompted some to advocate conservative treatment with large volume blood replacement. This view may no longer be correct in view of the poor results with conservative therapy, however, and the availability of good diagnostic angiography and its natural complement, therapeutic embolization. Early angiography with diagnosis and treatment of bleeding sites may avoid the hepatic, renal, pulmonary, and other complications of massive transfusions and large hematomas. Embolization permits the nonsurgical occlusion of vessels as close to the bleeding site as possible. Also, it permits instantaneous treatment of secondary bleeding from collaterals, especially from the opposite hypogastric system. High mortality can still result because these patients generally have multisystem injuries that can further complicate the problems of pelvic injury. Matalon[10] reported 28 cases of pelvic trauma in which 20 active bleeding sites were demonstrated. Of these 20, 18 were embolized, and 17 showed evidence of good clinical control of bleeding. Two cases were not embolized because one went to surgery and the second had a technical problem that prevented embolization. Of these 18 patients undergoing embolization, 9 died, 7 reportedly because of associated injuries, one because of extra-pelvic fracture and one secondary to hypotension. The average transfusion before the diagnostic angiogram was 32 units. After embolization, over the next 48 hours, the average blood requirement was 4 units in the 18 cases.

The most common causes of posttraumatic bleeding in the pelvis are disruption of the anterior division of the internal iliac artery (most often the obturator and pudendal branches) and the lateral sacral branches of the posterior division. Venous bleeding is not uncommon, but this is more difficult to diagnose and treat via catheter techniques. Venous bleeding, however, is also more likely to be tamponaded by the secondary pressure from the hematoma that arterial bleeding sites. Following successful embolization, evaluation of the contralateral arterial supplies is essential to exclude secondary collateral bleeding.

Traumatic hemobilia has also been treated successfully. Before embolization became available, the surgical alternative was resection and packing or possibly surgical hepatic artery ligation. The more distal occlusion possible with embolization can allow minimum loss of tissue with satisfactory control of bleeding and reduced morbidity.

Treatment of renal hemorrhage is one of the more rewarding areas of therapeutic embolization, largely because surgery often results in partial or total nephrectomy. Therapeutic embolization minimizes tissue loss, often producing only a small cortical infarct. Again, because a diagnostic angiogram is being performed, it is a relatively simple matter to embolize the bleeding branch at the time of the diagnostic study. Thus far, we are not aware of any reports of hypertension secondary to renal ischemia resulting from the embolization procedure. Chuang[4] has followed his series from 4 months to 2 years with no evidence of hypertension observed, and was able to avoid nephrectomy in five out of seven cases. Although the treatment of hematuria secondary to renal trauma is generally conservative, there is a tendency for more aggressive operative approaches in patients with penetrating trauma. Arteriovenous fistulas are not infrequent. Although some will heal spontaneously, most cases associated with penetrating trauma such as stab wounds will not. Aggressive attempts at achieving hemostasis via catheter techniques are justified to avoid major loss of renal tissue. Even if surgery is subsequently required, control of bleeding converts an emergency procedure to an elective one. It is important, with respect to placing coils or balloons in arteriovenous fistulas, that the embolic device be placed on the arterial side.

Treatment of aneurysms by transcatheter embolization has recently attracted interest.[7,11,12] Surgical treatment for intrahepatic arterial aneurysms can be difficult. Hepatic arterial aneurysms are associated with significant mortality and morbidity. The etiology of these lesions may be secondary to blunt or penetrating trauma, sepsis, malignancy, granulomatous disease, atherosclerotic disease, polyarteritis, or congenital abnormalities. In the presence of cirrhosis and decreased portal blood flow, proximal hepatic artery ligation itself can result in significant mortality. Recently, Kadir[7] has reported the successful treatment of four intrahepatic arterial aneurysms by embolization techniques. Likewise, Prost[11] has reported successful treatment of splenic artery aneurysm via the embolization route. Aneurysms of the peripheral vascular system can, in some instances, also be treated by transcatheter occlusion and extra-anatomic bypass.[12]

RESULTS

In our experience with 103 attempts at embolization in a variety of organ systems, the procedure was successful in 90 cases (87 percent). Success is gauged by cessation of hemorrhage in patients with bleeding problems or obliteration of lesions such as arteriovenous malformations and fistulas. In the gastrointestinal tract (Table 1), the majority of the failures were in the attempted occlusions of varices via the transhepatic portal venous route. This lower success rate is not surprising since the portal hypertension had not been altered, and the only attempt made was to divert flow from the bleeding site to provide time to stabilize the patient for eventual shunt surgery. Two of twenty left gastric embolizations were not successful because of bleeding from collaterals. The failure of the small bowel embolization will be discussed in the section on complications.

In the cases of posttraumatic hemorrhage and arteriovenous fistulas (Table 2; Figs. 1–4), 25 out of 27 cases were treated successfully (92 percent). Of the 11 cases of pelvic posttraumatic hemorrhage (Figs. 5 and 6), 10 were successfully treated. Of these 10, however, three died subsequently because of multisystem injury (one from prolonged hypotension). Embolization in the extremities resulted in one failure secondary to retrograde bleeding from radial and ulnar collaterals that ultimately required surgery. Antegrade flow in the bleeding interosseous artery had been successfully stopped. Two traumatic arteriovenous fistulas of the external carotid circulation were occluded successfully (Fig. 7). The main feeder vessels were the superficial temporal and posterior auricular branches, respectively. A chronic lumbar pseudoaneurysm that caused considerable morbidity and a prolonged clinical course was also embolized satisfactorily (Fig. 2).

In the miscellaneous category (Table 3), the largest group is composed of neoplasms, most of which are hypernephromas that were embolized to facilitate surgical excision. Three out of 10 cases, however, were palliative in patients who were not considered operative candidates. Chronic bleeding from uterine malignancies and bladder carcinomas have been embolized successfully.

Arteriovenous malformations from multiple sites have also been successfully treated by embolic techniques (Figs. 8–10). Combinations of embolic materials were used, which included Avitene, Gelfoam, mechanical coils, and Ivalon. Early in our experience, the lesions were treated with Gelfoam primarily because of its availability and our own familiarity with the properties of Gelfoam. Thus far we have not had any patients return with recurrence of lesions. Such recurrences, however, are known to happen (Veith and Sprayregen, personal communication). In the event of recurrences, repeat embolizations could be performed with more permanent agents, such as tissue adhesives. Embolic therapy is indicated for arteriovenous malformations and fistulas when 1) the patient refuses or is not able to tolerate surgery; 2) previous surgery has failed; 3) in the chronic or diffuse type where surgery is likely to fail; or 4) possibly to facilitate operation in inaccessible areas such as the pelvis. With respect to item 2, it should be noted that, if the proximal feeding vessels have been ligated, it is often extremely difficult to embolize arteriovenous fistulas and malformations. Therefore, the point could be made that all these lesions, unless clearly and easily resectable, be initially treated by embolization techniques. If the embolization is unsuccessful, surgery can then still be attempted.

Pulmonary arteriovenous malformation can be difficult to manage clinically, particularly when there are multiple lesions. The majority of pulmonary arteriovenous malformations are asymptomatic; however, com-

66 Critical Problems in Vascular Surgery

Table 1. Gastrointestinal Results

Source of Hemorrhage	No. of Cases	Hemostasis
Stomach	20	18 (90%)
Duodenum	9	9 (100%)
Gastroesophageal junction	5	5 (100%)
Varices	12	7 (58%)
Small bowel	2	1 (50%)
	48	40

Table 2. Results of Posttraumatic Hemorrhage and Arteriovenous Fistulas

Source of Hemorrhage	No. of Cases	Hemostasis
Pelvis	11	10 (91%)
Kidney	6	6 (100%)
Extremity	3	2 (67%)
Liver	2	2 (100%)
Spleen	2	2 (100%)
External carotid arteriovenous fistulas	2	2 (100%)
Retroperitoneal	1	1 (100%)
	27	25

Table 3. Miscellaneous Results

Abnormality	No. of Cases	Successful Control
Arteriovenous malformation		
Facial	5	4 (80%)
Extremity	3	3 (100%)
Pulmonary	1	1 (100%)
Neoplasm		
Renal		
hypernephroma	10	10 (100%)
angiomyolipoma	1	1 (100%)
Pelvic		
uterine	2	2 (100%)
bladder	1	1 (100%)
Hepatoma	1	1 (100%)
Bronchial hemorrhage	3	1 (33%)
Second-degree hypertension to end-stage renal disease	1	1 (100%)
	28	25

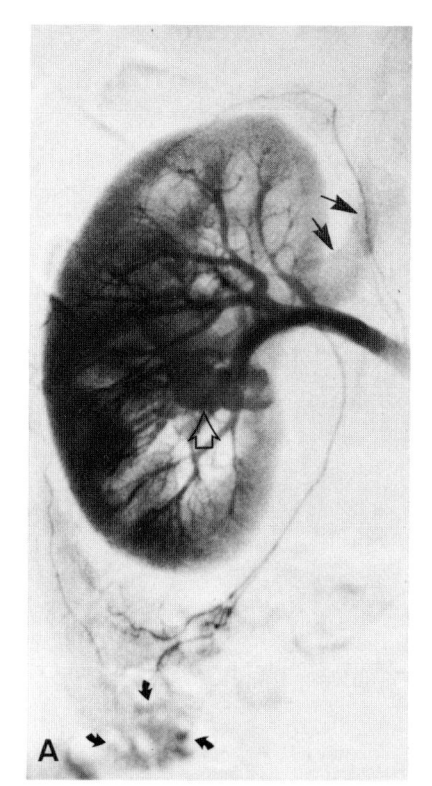

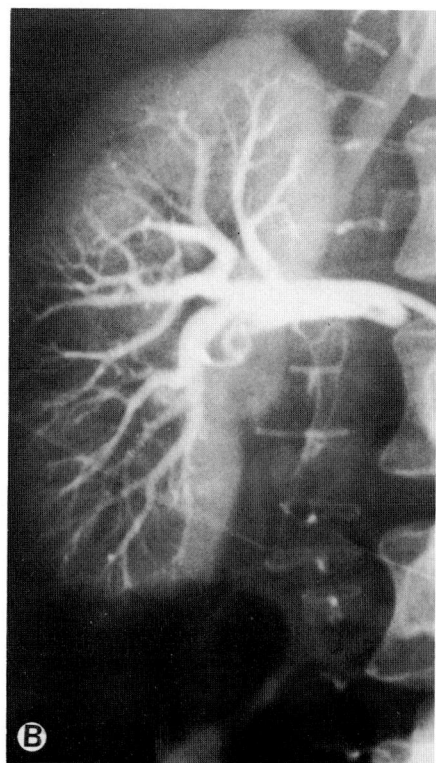

FIGURE 1. A 37-year-old man with multiple stab wounds to the right flank and gross hematuria. The blood pressure was 70 mm Hg palpable. **A.** Selective renal arteriogram reveals large pseudoaneurysm (open arrow) with arteriovenous shunting as evidenced by visualization of the renal vein and inferior vena cava (arrows). Displacement of the inferior capsular artery from the kidney together with evidence of extravasation of contrast material from the capsular artery (curved arrows) is noted. **B.** The pseudoaneurysm is no longer visualized in postembolization. A Gianturco coil is in place at the origin of a inferior polar branch. No early venous visualization is seen from the capsular artery that was embolized with Gelfoam.

plications or death can result in 20 percent of these lesions if untreated. If a single lesion is present, surgical resection is probably still the treatment of choice. In the face of diffuse disease where resection is not possible, however, embolic therapy should be considered.

Facial arteriovenous malformations and hemangiomas can also be treated via embolic techniques.[1,2,8] It is essential that all small feeders

68 Critical Problems in Vascular Surgery

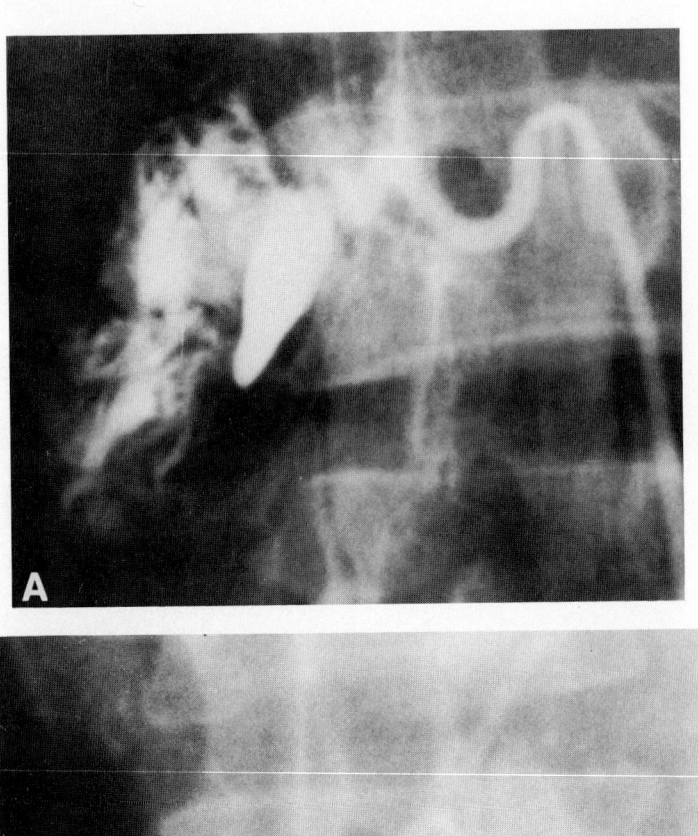

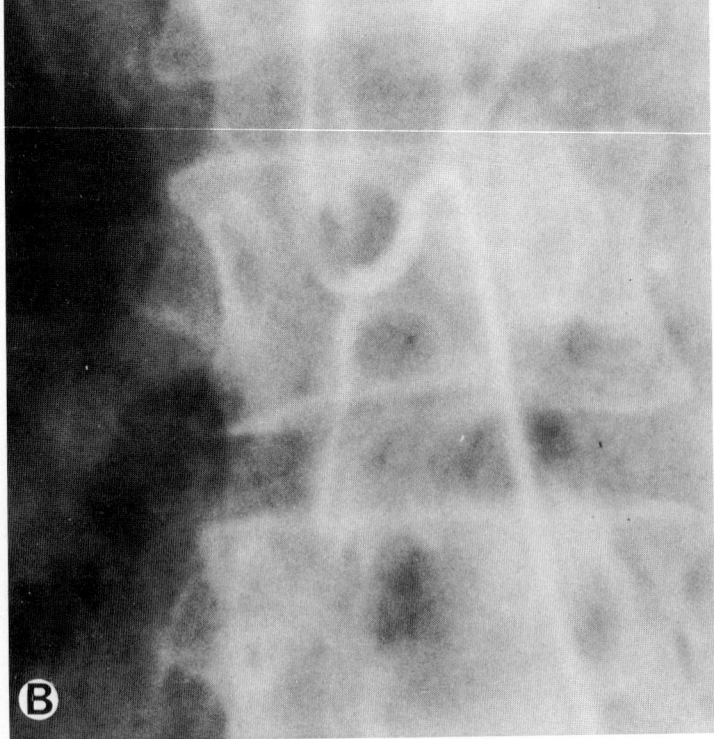

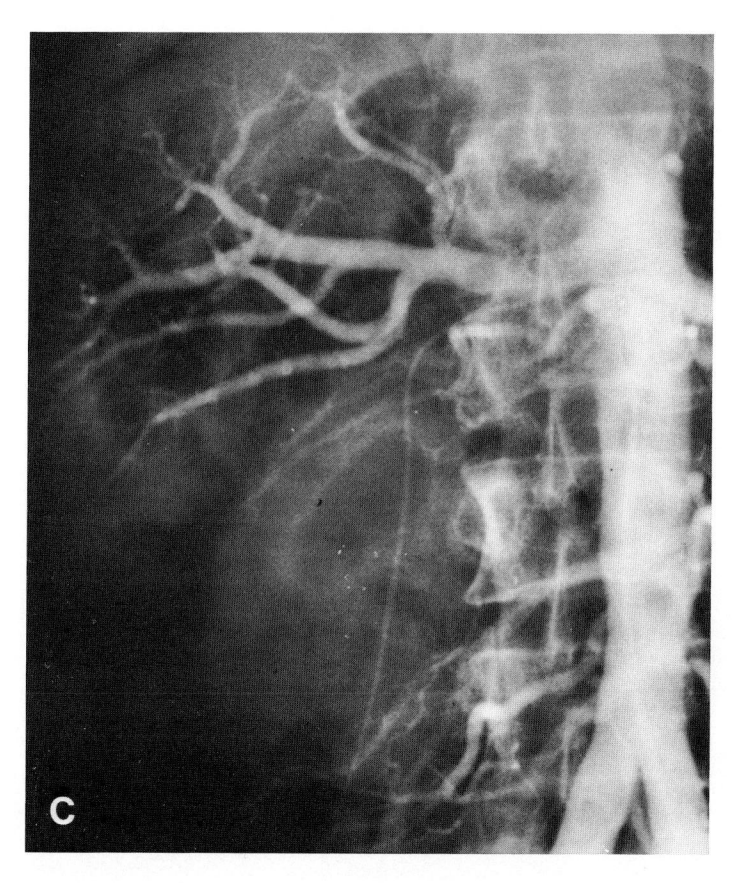

FIGURE 2. A 39-year-old man with a stab wound to the right back followed by a protracted course including two surgical procedures for evacuation of hematoma. Angiography was performed 6 months after the initial trauma because of severe back pain and decreasing hematocrit. **A.** Selective lumbar artery injection reveals a large artery. **B.** Following embolization with Gelfoam, the Gelfoam plug is seen as a defect in the contrast column. **C.** Follow up angiogram at 6 months fails to reveal evidence of bleeding.

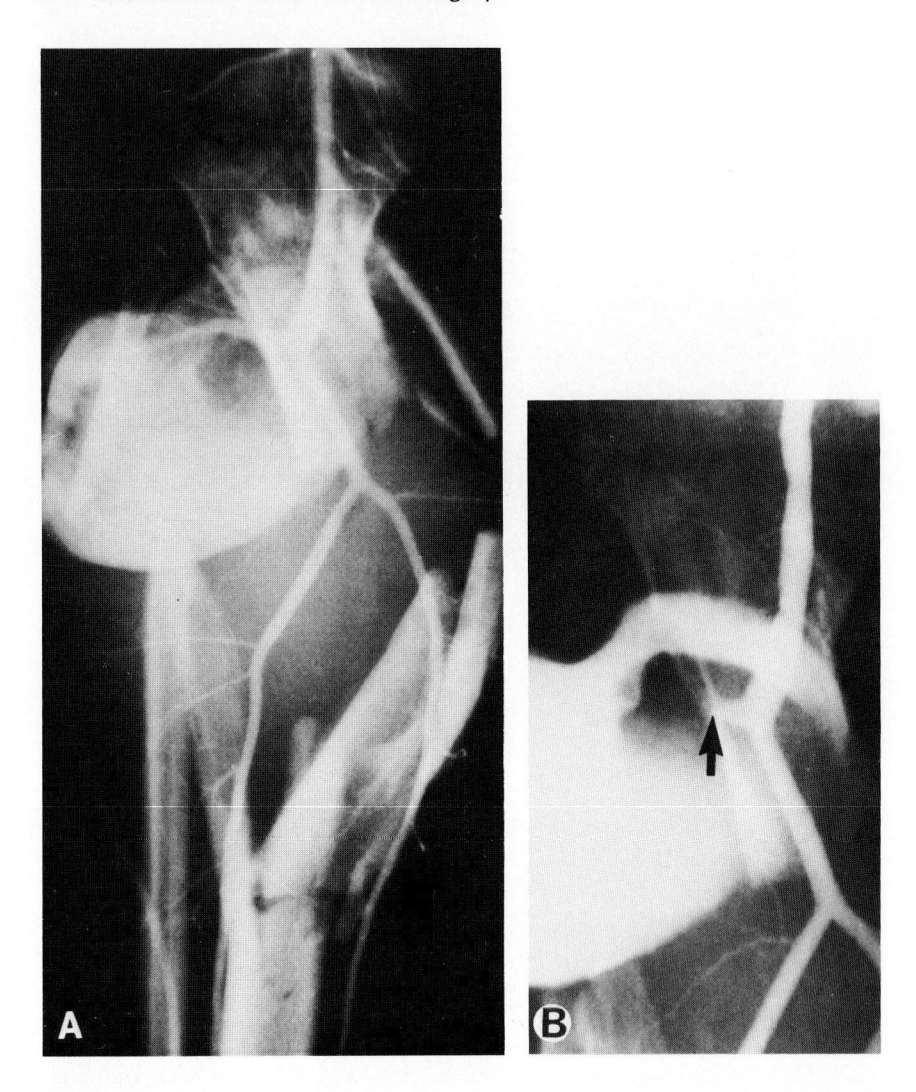

FIGURE 3. A 55-year-old woman with multiple fractures of the lower extremity. After a long protracted hospital course with gradual distraction of the fracture fragments she came to angiography on the 67th hospital day. **A.** A large pseudoaneurysm emanating from the anterior tibial artery is seen. **B.** Following successful embolization with Gelfoam, the anterior tibial artery is noted to be occluded (arrow). Because of the size of the pseudoaneurysm together with the distraction of the fracture fragments, however, operative evacuation was necessary. If angiography was performed earlier, it is possible that surgery could have been obviated, her hospital course shortened, and morbidity decreased.

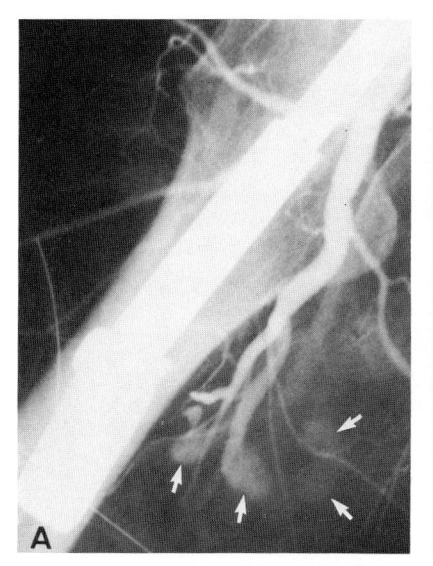

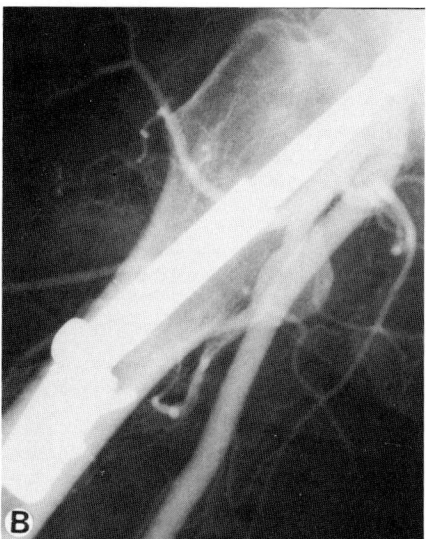

FIGURE 4. A 62-year-old man, 6 weeks after hip pinning with evidence of hemorrhage. At surgery several branches of the profunda femoris artery were ligated. He continued to bleed, however, requiring an additional 8 units of blood. **A.** Angiogram reveals multiple collections of extravasated contrast from profunda branches. **B.** These were embolized and follow-up common femoral angiogram at one week shows no further evidence for bleeding. (Courtesy of Dr. Seymour Sprayregan.)

be embolized to prevent recurrence. Radical surgical resection leaves obvious marked cosmetic deformities. Before embolization and in addition to surgery, radiation therapy, sclerosing agents, and systemic steroids have all been used to treat these lesions with limited success.

COMPLICATIONS

Most complications arise from the inadvertent passage of embolic material into other than desired vessels.* Although we feel that the vast majority result from technical failure, inexperience, and poor catheter placement, complications will occasionally occur even in the most experienced hands. Much has been written with respect to the use of balloon

*In 103 patients, the following three complications resulted: infarcted gastrojejunostomy, reflux of embolic material with secondary bowel ischemia, and transient unilateral fascial weakness.

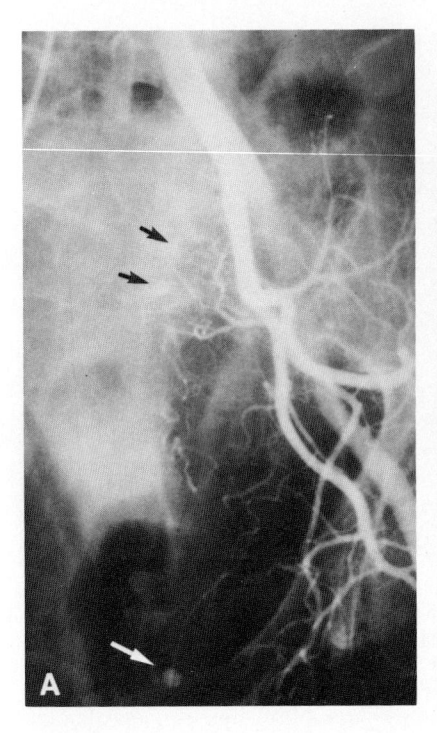

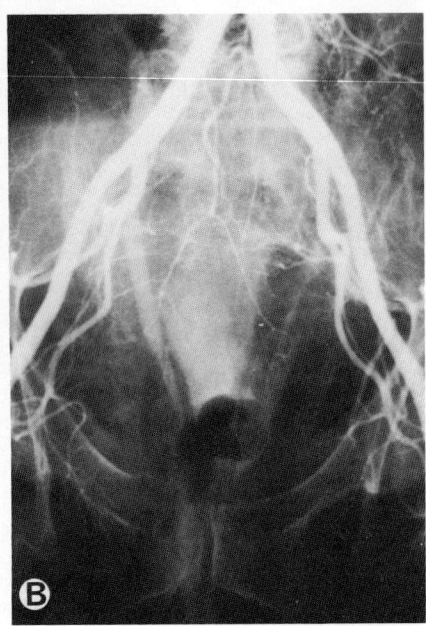

FIGURE 5. A 60-year-old with pelvic fractures. **A.** Selective injection of the left hypogastric artery reveals multiple sites of extravasation (arrows) emanating from both the anterior and posterior divisions. Note the displacement of the bladder by the pelvic hematoma. **B.** Following embolization with Gelfoam, repeat angiogram fails to reveal evidence of bleeding. Note the entire hypogastric artery is not occluded. Patient was admitted with blood pressure if 90/50 mm Hg, received a total of 8 units of blood, and did well following the embolization.

catheters to prevent reflux of embolic material. Our personal belief is that, while it is true that emboli will not reflux if the arterial orifice is occluded, it is also true that the emboli will not be carried peripherally when there is no blood flow. In fact, the emboli will probably remain near the catheter tip until the balloon is deflated and blood flow is restored. At that time, there may be turbulence and an increased risk of reflux; in contrast, a well-placed catheter with surrounding normal arterial blood flow allows one to constantly monitor the progress of the embolization. In our experience we have had one case of inadvertent embolization to the superior mesenteric arterial branches while attempting to occlude an anomolous hepatic artery arising from the superior mesenteric artery. The procedure was performed by an inexperienced angiographer and the complication was clearly a technical failure.

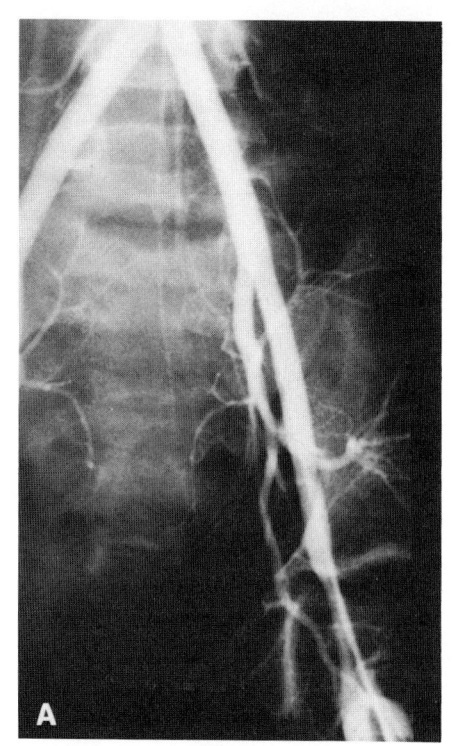

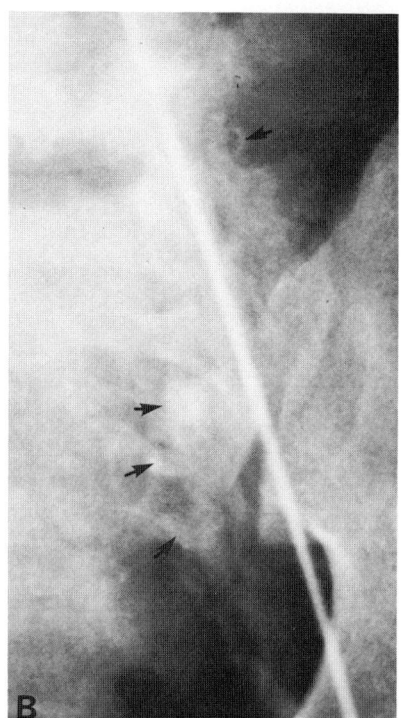

FIGURE 6. An 8-year-old girl with multiple trauma sustained following a fall from the fourth floor. She required 11 units of blood. An angiogram was performed (**A.** arterial phase; **B.** late venous phase) revealing multiple areas of extravasation along the left sacroiliac joint. During the course of the study the patient had a respiratory arrest. **C.** It was elected, therefore, to immediately insert a Gianturco coil (arrow) in the proximal left hypogastric artery that resulted in immediate cessation of bleeding. No further transfusions were required.

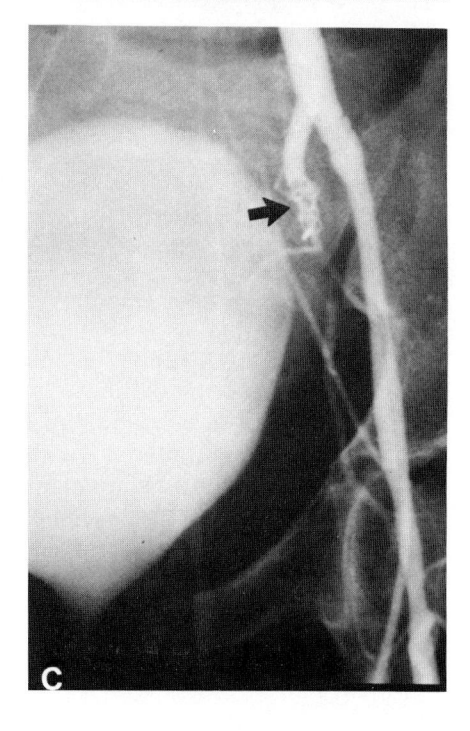

74 Critical Problems in Vascular Surgery

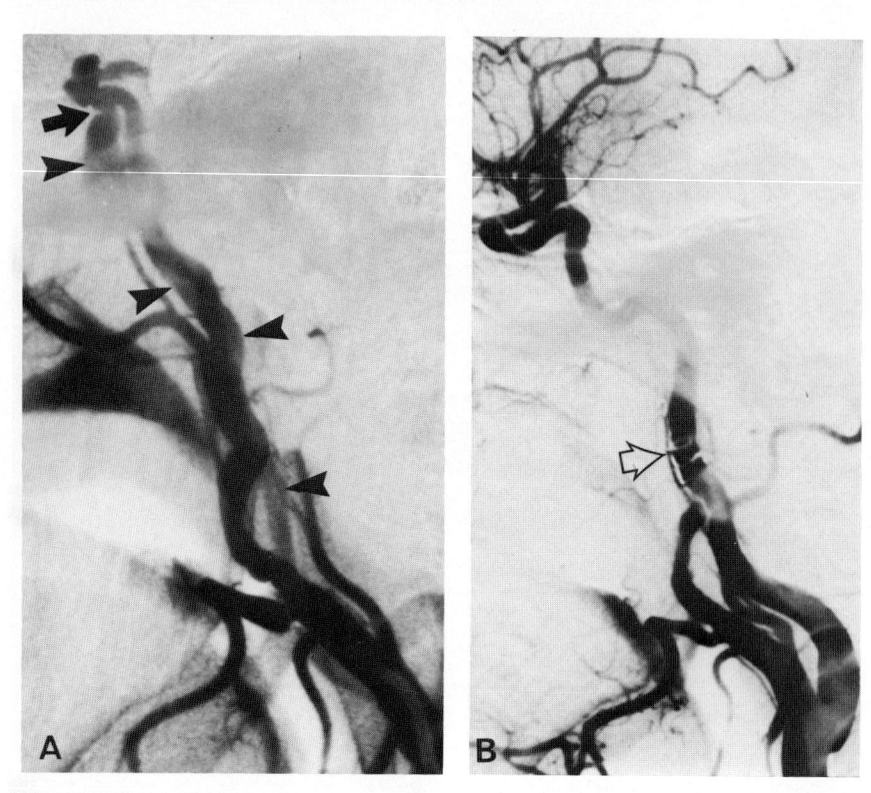

FIGURE 7. A 39-year-old man with trauma to the left side of the head 6 months before admission, resulting in a loud noise in his ear. **A.** Selective injection of the external carotid artery reveals a large arteriovenous fistula (large arrow) with evidence of rapid venous filling (small arrows). Initially plugs of Gelfoam and Ivalon were used. **B.** The embolization was completed by insertion of Gianturco coil at the origin of the superficial temporal artery (open arrow) with complete obliteration of the arteriovenous fistula. There was complete clearing of the noise in the left ear.

Other complications that have been recorded relate to infection and abscess formation in the embolized arterial bed. Angiography is generally performed in what is at best a partially sterile fashion. This creates no problems when dealing with a normal intact vascular system. In embolization, however, where we are deliberately decreasing or eliminating blood flow, there is significant potential for developing infection. Therefore, if more rigid aseptic technique is observed these complications can possibly be decreased. Gas formation in an embolized organ may not necessarily indicate abscess formation. We have had one such occurrence

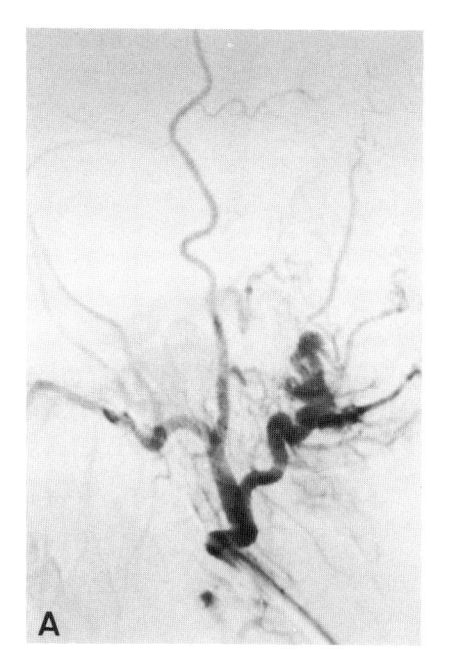

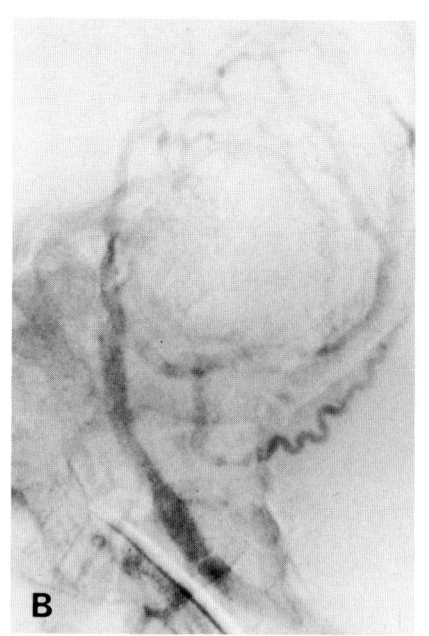

FIGURE 8. A 44-year-old woman with progressively enlarging arteriovenous malformation behind the left ear associated with buzzing noises. **A.** Initial external carotid arteriogram revealed arteriovenous malformation, fed from both the posterior auricular and superficial temporal branches. **B.** The large draining veins are shown. **C.** Following embolization with Gelfoam and Ivalon, there is complete occlusion of the arteriovenous malformation. Patient's symptoms were completely relieved.

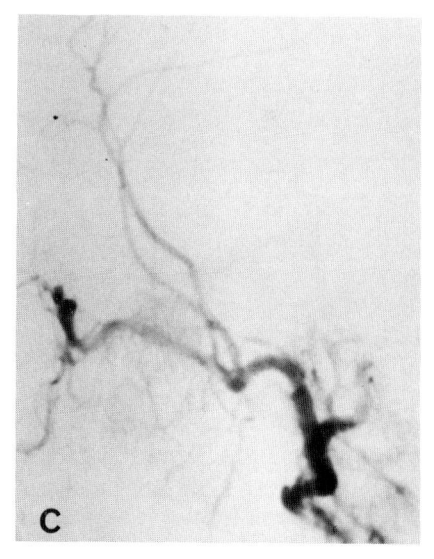

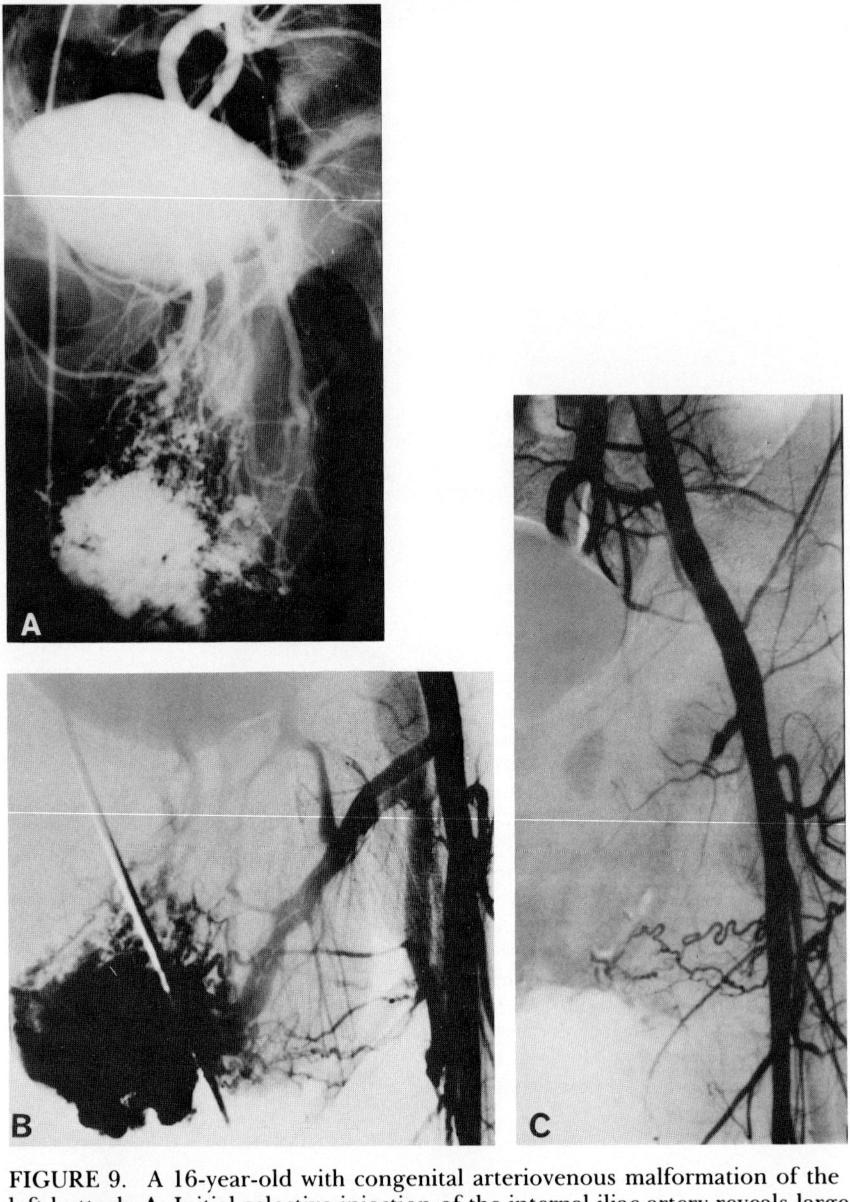

FIGURE 9. A 16-year-old with congenital arteriovenous malformation of the left buttock. **A.** Initial selective injection of the internal iliac artery reveals large feeding branches from the anterior division. **B.** In addition, large feeding branches were also noted from the profunda femoris artery. **C.** Following selective embolization of both the hypogastric and profunda branches the common iliac arteriogram reveals the arteriovenous malformation (AVM). Aviten introduced through the balloon catheter was used to obliterate the bed of the AVM. In addition, the cross-pubic collateral branches were initially embolized with Gelfoam so that the AVM would not be supplied from the contralaterial side. A few small profunda branches persist and may hypertrophy, at which time they will also be embolized.

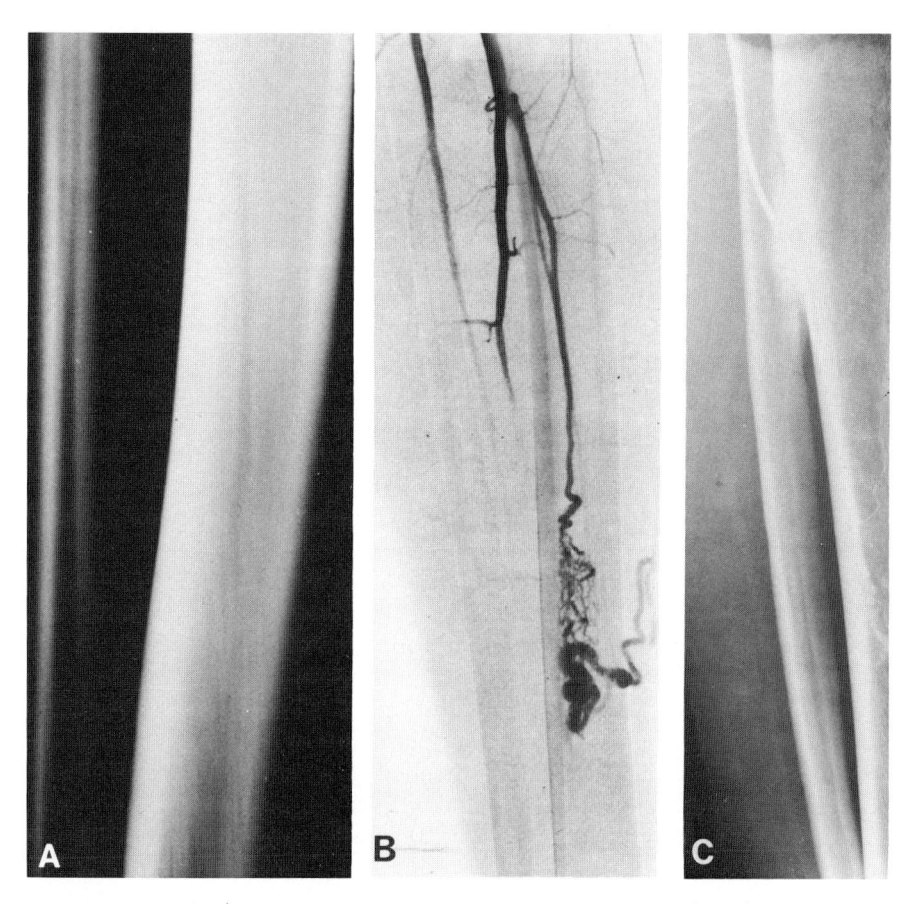

FIGURE 10. A 28-year-old with a lump on the anterior aspect of the tibia that eventually became painful and pulsatile. **A.** Plain film reveals a large nutrient canal. **B.** Angiography demonstrated the presence of an intraosseous arteriovenous malformation that was embolized with Gelfoam. The patient continued to have severe pain. **C.** Follow-up angiogram after 6 months demonstrated a decrease in size of the AVM with some arterial supply from periosteal branches. There was considerable clinical improvement, however, after embolization.

following embolization of an inoperable renal carcinoma. The gas was seen approximately one week after embolization without clinical or laboratory evidence for infection. This has been reported elsewhere, and it is postulated that the gas may be secondary to oxygen release by the infarcted tissue.

The last major group of complications relate to ischemia and infarction. There have been a few documented cases of infarction of stomach, small bowel, and gallbladder secondary to embolic therapy. In most of these cases, embolization has been combined with surgery or the administration of vasoconstrictors. These combinations of therapy are more likely to cause complications than is the embolization alone. In these situations, the potential for collateral circulation has been either eliminated or drastically compromised and infarction or severe ischemia is more likely to occur. We have encountered an infarcted gastrojejunostomy secondary to embolization of two jejunal branches for a bleeding marginal ulcer that was not well controlled by vasopressin. The patient did well initially, but bleeding recurred probably because of collateral circulation. At that time vasopressin therapy was reinstituted and infarction of the anastomosis occurred. This was resected with good clinical results.

The probability of complications is also dependent on the organ system; for example, the potential for complication is far greater in the central nervous system than in the liver. In a cooperative study (New York University, the University of Pittsburgh, and the University of Oregon) of 146 cerebral embolizations, the overall rate of significant complications was 7.5 percent (5 percent resulted in permanent neurologic deficits). Another significant complication in our series occurred in a patient who had a traumatic anteriovenous fistula involving the superficial temporal artery that was successfully embolized (Fig. 7). The patient had complained of an extremely loud, unbearable rushing sound in his ear. All symptoms disappeared after embolization. A portion of the internal maxillary artery on the ipsilateral side was also occluded, however, and the patient developed a transient facial weakness that cleared totally before discharge.

Additional reported complications of therapeutic embolizations include pulmonary emboli secondary to occlusion of arteriovenous fistulas or malformations, catheters becoming adherent to the intima while using tissue adhesives, spontaneous rupture of the spleen following splenic embolization, rupture of pseudoaneurysms in patients with chronic pancreatitis, distal embolization with need for limited amputation secondary to reflux of emboli, and colonic stricture secondary to embolic therapy for diverticular bleeding.

In summary, in order to minimize the potential for complications, one must carefully evaluate the organ or vessel to be occluded with respect to its size, potential for collaterals, and the type of embolic material to be used before any attempt at embolization. The risk of embolization must be carefully weighed against the potential risks of other types of therapy or no therapy at all. Also, additional data must still be collected on the long-term effects of various embolic materials in the vascular system.

DISCUSSION

It is clear that transcatheter therapeutic embolization has wide ranging applications. Vascular abnormalities can be treated on either a temporary or permanent basis. Embolization can be used either as the definitive therapy or as an adjunct to surgical intervention. The procedures are relatively simple but require meticulous and expert catheterization techniques. Just as all vascular surgeons are not competent to do microsurgery, neither are all angiographers capable of doing embolic work. These sophisticated procedures should be left to angiographers who have had extensive experience in conventional angiography. Superselective catheterization techniques are essential in the performance of embolic therapy. It is absolutely imperative that the catheter be placed as close to the site of abnormality as possible, thereby minimizing tissue loss and the potential for reflux of emboli, and at the same time maximizing the probability of a successful embolization. Occasionally, for technical reasons, a catheter may not be placed as distally as desired. Under these circumstances, if clinically indicated, smaller emboli can be initially introduced. Not infrequently, these emboli will gravitate toward the site of abnormality, which could be due to altered hemodynamics. A "sump effect" has been postulated, particularly in cases of hemorrhage. This has yet to be verified experimentally.

The angiographer has the advantage of constant and instantaneous visual feedback of the hemodynamics and, more importantly, of any alterations in the hemodynamics that may occur during the course of an embolization. The role of collaterals can be quickly appreciated and dealt with (if necessary at the same time) rather than waiting for more gross clinical evidence to develop.

Because in the evaluation of vascular problems a diagnostic angiogram must be performed first, it would seem reasonable that any necessary and appropriate embolic therapy be done while the catheter is still in place and the anatomy clearly defined. Difficult lesions may be better done in stages, however, rather than attempting heroic measures. One should always bear in mind contrast limitations. No single technique or embolic material is suitable for all cases. Therefore, the angiographer must be familiar with and have available multiple delivery systems and embolic materials for immediate utilization and for appropriate application to the specific needs of a given case. The success of embolic procedures is dependent on several factors, among which are: 1) the clinical situation, 2) the type of vessels involved, 3) the particular organ system, and 4) skill of the angiographer.

Angiography should be performed early in traumatic lesions. Considerable savings in morbidity and hospitalization can result from early diagnosis and treatment. This point is well illustrated by the problems encountered in the patients shown in Figures 2 and 3.

The indications for transcatheter occlusive therapy are: 1) when pharmacologic therapy or surgery is not possible or is unsuccessful; 2) stabilization of the patient before definitive surgery, i.e., to convert an emergency surgical procedure to an elective one; 3) to facilitate surgery and decrease blood loss as a highly vascular neoplasms (occasionally, lesions deemed inoperable become manageable for embolization); 4) for problems such as traumatic renal and pelvic hemorrhage, embolization should be the definitive therapeutic procedure; 5) congenital vascular malformations, traumatic arteriovenous fistulas, and aneurysms of some visceral organs that are difficult to manage surgically; and 6) palliative therapy for primary and secondary neoplasms, such as metastases to bone and liver and inoperable renal carcinomas.

CONCLUSIONS

Transcatheter occlusive therapy is a well recognized modality for the nonsurgical control of hemorrhage and treatment of other vascular abnormalities. It has widespread applicability and proven value in a variety of clinical situations. It can be used as the definitive therapeutic modality or as a preoperative adjunct. In the hands of experienced angiographers, morbidity and complication rates are well within acceptable limits.

REFERENCES

1. Berenstein A, Kricheff II: Catheter and material selection for transarterial embolization: Technical considerations. Radiology 132:619, 1979
2. Brismar J, Cronqvist S: Therapeutic embolization in the external carotid artery region. Acta Radiologica Diag 19:715, 1978
3. Chang J, Katzen BT, Sullivan KP: Transcatheter Gelfoam embolization of post-traumatic bleeding pseudoaneurysms. Am J Roentgenol 131:645, 1978
4. Chuang VP, Reuter SR, Walter J, et al: Control of renal hemorrhage by selective arterial embolization. Am J Roentgenol 125:300, 1975
5. Debrun G, Lacour P, Caron J-P, et al: Detachable balloon and calibrated-leak balloon techniques in the treatment of cerebral vascular lesions. J Neurosurg 49:635, 1978
6. Goldstein HM, Wallace S, Anderson JH, et al: Transcatheter occlusion of abdominal tumors. Radiology 120:539, 1976
7. Kadir S, Athanasoulis CA, Ring EJ, Greenfield A: Transcatheter embolization of intrahepatic arterial aneurysms. Radiology 134:355, 1980

8. Katzen BT, Rossi P, Passariello R, Simonetti G: Transcatheter therapeutic arterial embolization. Radiology 120:523, 1976
9. Layne TA, Finck EJ, Boswell WD: Transcatheter occlusion of the arterial supply to arteriovenous fistulas with gianturco coils. Am J Roentgenol 131:1027, 1978
10. Matalon TSA, Athanasoulis CA, Margolies MN, et al: Hemorrhage with pelvic fractures: Efficacy of transcatheter embolization. Am J Roentgenol 133:859, 1979
11. Probst P, Castaneda-Zuniga WR, Gomes AS, et al: Nonsurgical treatment of splenic artery aneurysms. Radiology 128:619, 1978
12. Reuter SR, Carson SN: Thrombosis of a common iliac artery aneurysm by selective embolization and extraanatomic bypass. Am J Roentgenol 134:1248, 1980
13. Rosch J, Dotter CT, Brown MJ: Selective arterial embolization. Radiology 102:303, 1972
14. Spigos DG, Jonasson O, Mozes M, Capek V: Partial splenic embolization in the treatment of hypersplenism. Am J Roentgenol 132:777, 1979
15. Terry PB, Barth KH, Kaufman SL, White RI: Balloon embolization for treatment of pulmonary arteriovenous fistulas. N Engl J Med 302:1189, 1980
16. Thompson JN, Fierstien SB, Kohut RI: Embolization techniques in vascular tumors of the head and neck. Head & Neck Surg 2:25, 1979
17. Thompson WM, Johnsrude IS, Jackson DC, et al: Vessel occlusion with transcatheter electrocoagulation: Initial clinical experience. Radiology 133:335, 1979
18. Viamonte M, Pereiras R, Russell E, et al: Transhepatic obliteration of gastroesophageal varices: Results in acute and nonacute bleeders. Am J Roentgenol 129:237, 1977

FIVE

The Current Status of Percutaneous Transluminal Angioplasty

Seymour Sprayregen

HISTORICAL DEVELOPMENT AND TECHNIQUE

Dotter and Judkins[9] in 1964 first described a technique of percutaneous transluminal angioplasty (PTA). They believed that forceful dilatation of atherosclerotic lesions could compress the inelastic atherosclerotic core against the intact confining arterial wall resulting in dilatation of the lumen but not of the outer wall of the artery. Recently Castaneda et al[5] demonstrated intimal cracking and separation from the media following angioplasty. They proposed that the media is stretched during dilatation and carries with it the intima and atheromatous material, while the plaques remain essentially unchanged.

Several dilating techniques have been used. All procedures, however, are performed under local anesthesia and are controlled fluoroscopically. There are two basic methods for traversing a stenotic arterial segment. The most common technique uses a guide wire that is advanced through the stenotic or occluded segment. This is followed by a straight catheter or a deflated balloon catheter with subsequent balloon inflation. This technique is used for all lesions of the iliac, femoral, popliteal, and leg arteries and is the technique most frequently used for the renal arteries. In the other technique, a small balloon catheter (rather than guide wire) is initially passed through the narrowed arterial segment.

The author gratefully acknowledges the assistance of Dr. Frank Veith in the preparation of this manuscript.

This method was devised by Grüntzig[15] for coronary angioplasty and remains the technique of choice for coronary artery dilatation. It is rarely used for dilating arteries other than coronaries.

Dotter's original technique for dilating femoropopliteal lesions consisted of percutaneous antegrade puncture of the femoral artery and passage of a guide wire through the stenotic or occluded segment. An 8 French catheter was advanced over the guide wire and a 12 French catheter was passed over the 8 French catheter. One major disadvantage of this coaxial catheter technique is that there is a step effect where the larger catheter is advanced over the smaller. This may cause intimal and atheromatous tissue to be pushed forward as the larger catheter is advanced. Van Andel[37] developed a series of catheters with gradual tapering of the outer diameters to avoid this step effect.

Dotter's and Van Andel's[7] catheters are generally adequate for the femoropopliteal segment, but the 12 French catheter, which measures 4 mm in diameter, cannot produce adequate dilatation of most iliac arteries. Use of the 12 French catheter at times also made hemostasis difficult, especially if patients were anticoagulated following angioplasty. To overcome these difficulties balloon catheters were used by Zeitler,[51] Porstmann,[27] and Dotter.[11] Zeitler initially used Fogarty balloons; Porstmann, however, observing that latex balloons are soft and usually are deformed by the atheromatous lesions rather than compressing them, introduced a "corset" balloon catheter with the balloon encased within supporting struts in the catheter. Dotter devised a similar catheter.

The most recent technologic advance is the development by Grüntzig[17] of a catheter with a polyvinyl chloride balloon that can be inflated to a predetermined cylindrical shape. Balloons of various widths and lengths are available so that the angiographer can select the appropriate balloon for a particular lesion.

The balloons are distended with contrast material under fluoroscopic guidance to 4 to 6 atmospheres of pressure. Although pressure gauges are available to indicate what pressure is being generated in the balloon, distension is usually controlled according to the fluoroscopic appearance of the balloon deformity and the "feeling" of resistance experienced by the angiographer. The deflated balloon is placed at the level of the atherosclerotic lesion and then inflated.

Balloon catheters have been widely used for femoropopliteal as well as iliac lesions. A theoretical advantage of the balloon catheter over large diameter, nonballoon catheters is that pressure is exerted laterally without the shearing effect of longitudinal movement.

At present, nearly all iliac stenotic lesions are dilated with balloon catheters. The artery is distended to a diameter of 6 to 8 mm. Although femoropopliteal lesions are usually dilated with balloon catheters, many angiographers, including the author, use straight Teflon catheters as the catheter of choice for these lesions. The straight catheter is advantageous in this application because every area of the artery is dilated to the size of the catheter and the angiographer need not be concerned about failure to dilate a secondary lesion. These straight catheters are also easier to use, require less fluoroscopic exposure since it is not necessary to place a balloon at the correct arterial segment, and are much less expensive. For most femoropopliteal lesions, dilatation with a 10 French (3 mm) Teflon catheter is adequate. A 12 French (4 mm) catheter is available but is usually unnecessary for the femoropopliteal segment. The balloon most commonly used for the femoropopliteal segment distends to 4 mm.

Most authors perform angioplasty after administering heparin to the patient. We use 4000 to 5000 units of heparin intra-arterially or intravenously immediately prior to dilatation. Alternately, heparinization can be performed after the catheter has passed the stenosis or occlusion.[18]

Zeitler compared the efficacy of various drug regimens used in association with angioplasty for peripheral vascular disease and found that rethrombosis within 10 days occurred least frequently when aspirin was given for 2 days before and for at least 7 days following the procedure.[50] All authors agree that platelet inhibitors, such as aspirin, should be given before angioplasty. We have performed "urgent" or "emergency" angioplasties on several occasions, however, without the benefit of aspirin and have obtained good results.

Angiographers do not agree on the use of heparin and/or Coumadin after angioplasty. Zeitler[50] showed that heparinization after PTA for peripheral vascular disease increased the incidence of bleeding without increasing the patency rate, and we do not employ heparin after PTA for this reason. While the use of heparin appears to be the exception rather than the rule, several European authors report administering heparin up to 5 days after PTA.[38] The technique for coronary angioplasty as described by Grüntzig,[15] however, includes long-term anticoagulation with Coumadin.

PTA FOR PERIPHERAL VASCULAR DISEASE

The clinical indications for PTA are the same as those for surgery and include ischemic rest pain, nonhealing leg ulcers, and, on rare occasions, severe claudication. Angioplasty is also being performed in conjunction with peripheral vascular reconstruction. An example of the latter involves iliac angioplasty with the ipsilateral femoral artery then used as an inflow site for femorofemoral or femoropopliteal bypass. Angioplasty has also been used to dilate popliteal artery stenosis distal to a femoropopliteal bypass graft. This stenosis may be appreciated before or may develop following the bypass operation. We have also dilated a proximal popliteal stenosis to facilitate use of the distal popliteal artery as an inflow site for a popliteal to dorsalis pedal bypass when limited lengths of saphenous vein were available. PTA can also be used to dilate stenoses in vein grafts.[1]

The angiographic lesion most suitable for dilatation is a short-segment stenosis. Multiple stenoses, short-segment occlusions, and even long-segment occlusions, however, can often be recanalized.

Aortoiliac Segment

Determining the pressure gradient across an iliac stenosis is an important factor in evaluating the suitability for treatment of such lesions by angioplasty. In view of the limited significance of the lack of a gradient at rest, however, we will dilate iliac stenoses that narrow the artery by more than 50 percent even when no gradient is present if the ipsilateral femoral artery is to be used as a donor site for a bypass graft.

Table 1 lists iliac artery angioplasty success rates in various series. The term *primary success* is used to indicate patency of the artery one week after angioplasty. Primary success rates for iliac stenoses range from 77 to 92 percent. Figure 1 is an example of a typical successful iliac angioplasty.

Zeitler[43] in 1972 stated that recurrence may be expected during the first year in 5.5 and after 2 years in 12 percent of cases. In Grüntzig's[14] series reported in 1977, 87 percent of the initial successes were patent at 2 years. Schoop et al[30] in 1978 reported 5-year patency to be at least 50 percent of their initial successes. These authors found no differences in patency rates for iliac angioplasties between groups of anticoagulated and nonanticoagulated patients, or between groups of patients with patent or occluded superficial femoral arteries.[30] Recently PTA has been used for a total occlusion of the common iliac artery,[36] and the two dilatations of a stenotic aorta have been reported.[38] Recently PTA has been used for a total occlusion of the common iliac artery,[36] and two dilatations of a stenotic aorta have been reported.[38]

Femoropopliteal Segment

Table 2 summarizes the results of the major publications on femoropopliteal angioplasty. Reports of some of the larger series do not separate the results for stenoses and occlusions. Currently, one can expect approximately a 90 percent primary success rate for PTA performed for relief of stenosis of the femoropopliteal segment.

Table 1. Results of Iliac Angioplasty

Author	Type of Lesion	Number	Good Primary Results (%)	Long-Term Results
Dotter (1974)[12]	Stenosis	48	81	
Grüntzig (1977)[14]	Stenosis	54	92	87% of primary successes patent at 2 years
Schoop et al (1978)[30]	Stenosis	145	77	At least 50% of primary successes patent at 5 years
Zeitler (1978)[49]	Stenosis (1) Stenosis (2+)	220 42	78 81	
Cooperative study (1978)[21]	Stenosis	600	92	

Table 2. Results of Femoropopliteal Angioplasty

Author	Type of Lesion	Number	Good Primary Results (%)	Long-Term Results
Dotter et al (1968)[10]	Stenosis	41	71	
	Occlusion	112	29	
Brahme et al (1969)[4]	Stenosis	14	64	71% of primary successes patent at 1 year*
	Occlusion	92		
	<5 cm		80	
	5–15 cm		50	
	>20 cm		30	
Dotter (1973)[7]	Stenosis	237*	90	
	Occlusion			
	<2 cm		80	
	2–10 cm		30	
	>10 cm		10	
Wierny et al (1974)[43]	Stenosis plus occlusion	121*	76*	40% of primary successes patent at 2 to 7 years*

Zeitler (1975)[47]	Superficial femoral stenosis	116	84
	Occlusion		
	<10 cm	254	80
	>10 cm	120	56
	Popliteal Stenosis	12	50
	Occlusion	32	59
Grüntzig (1977)[14]	Stenosis plus occlusion	236*	84
Cooperative Study (1978)[19]	Stenosis	348	74*
	Occlusion	852	
Schmidtke et al (1978)[29]	Occlusion	79	

72% of primary successes patent at 2 years*

60% of primary successes patent at 2 years†

Occlusion length (cm)	5-year patency (%)
1–3	36
4–6	11.5
7–9	36
10–12	50
13–17	9

* Combined figures for both stenosis and occlusion.
† In this series, angiographic improvement was excellent in 47% and good in 33%; clinical improvement was excellent in 41% and good in 16%.

90 Critical Problems in Vascular Surgery

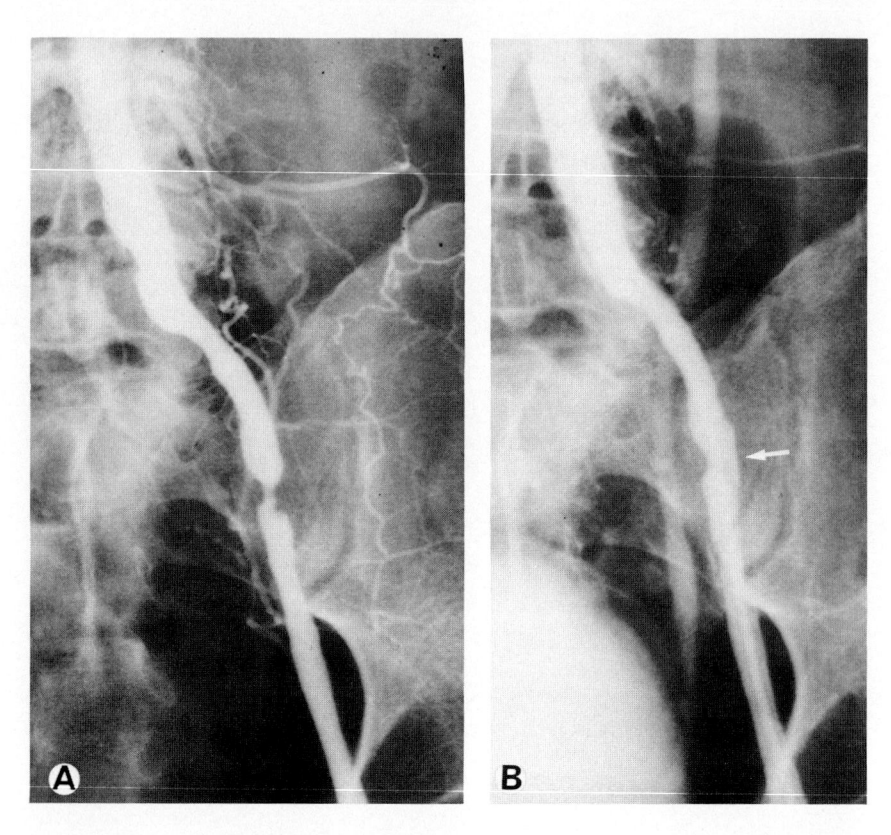

FIGURE 1. **A.** Marked stenosis of external iliac artery. **B.** After angioplasty, stenosis (arrow) and pressure gradient were corrected. Note small amount of subintimal contrast at lateral aspect of dilated segment.

The primary results obtained using PTA for occlusions of the femoropopliteal segment are seen to vary somewhat. Some authors report good results even with long-segment occlusions. Figure 2 shows the results of an angioplasty of femoropopliteal stenoses, and Figure 3 depicts recanalization of a localized occlusion of the superficial femoral artery.

Late results of angioplasty for femoropopliteal stenoses and occlusions are shown in Table 2. Schmidtke et al[29] reported that 26 percent of their primarily successfully treated occlusions remain patent at 5 years. These authors also noted that the reocclusion rate was approximately 40 percent during the first 2 years but slowed considerably after this. Schmidtke et al[29] also elucidated factors influencing long-term patency of recanalized femoropopliteal occlusions. Their 5-year patency rates of initial successes were inversely related to the length of the occlusions

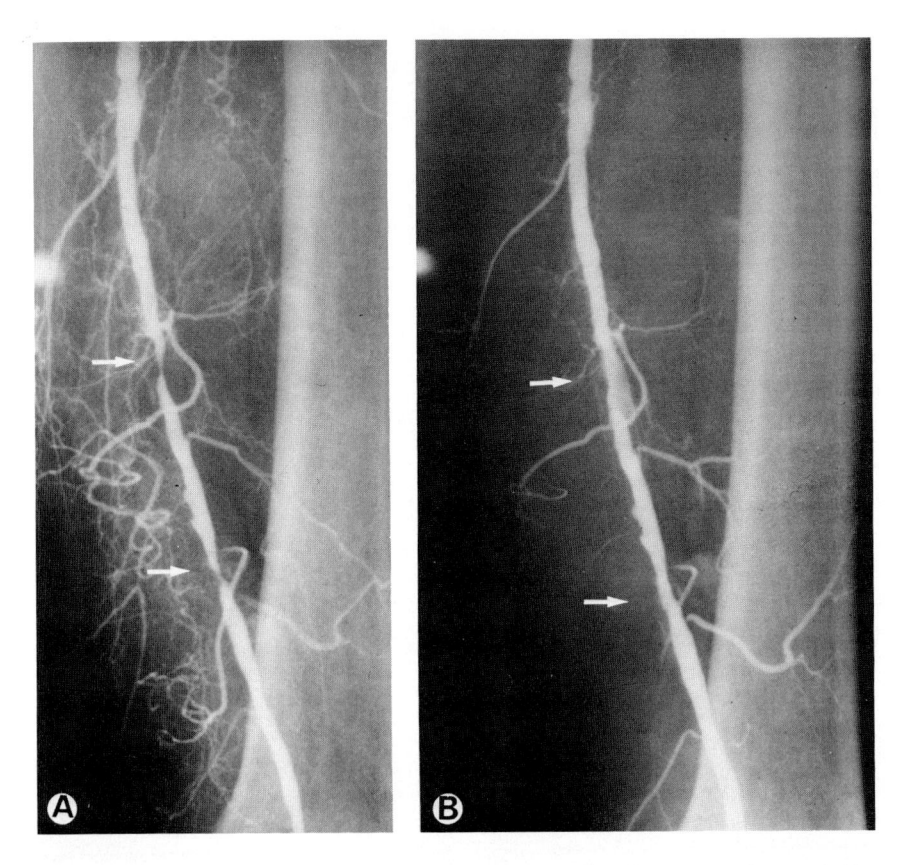

FIGURE 2. **A.** Two severe stenoses of femoropopliteal segment (arrows). **B.** After angioplasty, the lumen is widened (arrows). Subintimal contrast is present at the lateral aspect of the proximal stenosis.

(Table 2). Long-term anticoagulation was also found to be important. While the recurrence rate was similar in the first 6 months, 80 percent of recanalizations in the anticoagulated group remained patent at 30 months as opposed to 30 percent in the nonanticoagulated group. Wierny et al also showed a striking improvement in long-term patency in patients on anticoagulants: with long-term anticoagulation, 79 percent of primary successes remained patent as compared with 25 percent in the nonanticoagulated patients.[20]

Schmidtke et al found that another important factor in long-term patency was the site of occlusion.[29] At the end of 5 years, 16 of 60 cases (26.7 percent) of recanalized distal superficial femoral arteries were patent as compared with only 1 of 8 (12.5 percent) proximal superficial

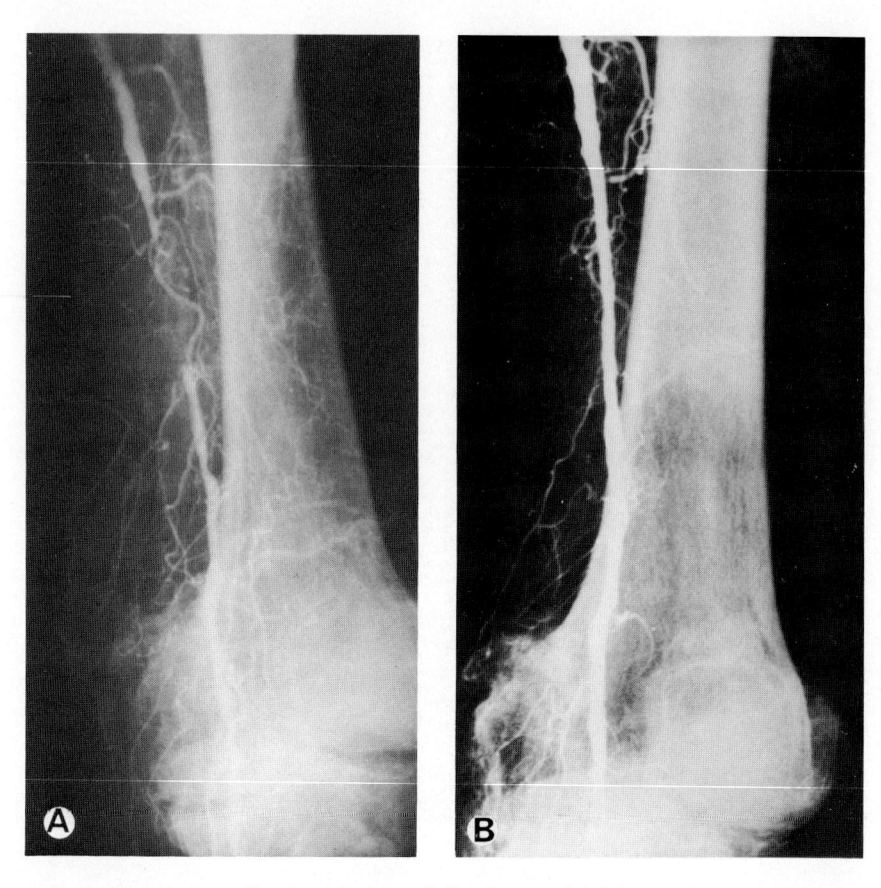

FIGURE 3. **A.** Localized occlusion of distal superficial femoral artery. **B.** After angioplasty, lumen is widely patent. The popliteal artery as well as the occluded superficial femoral artery was dilated.

femoral recanalizations. Three of 8 cases (37.5 percent) with popliteal occlusions were patent. Long-term results were also related to the post-dilatation angiographic appearance. The 5-year patency rate in patients without residual stenosis was 32 percent, while with those with minor and severe stenoses, the respective patency rates were 19 percent and 22 percent. Smoking habits after angioplasty influenced the ultimate result. Of those who stopped smoking, 45 percent were patent after 5 years as opposed to 19 percent for cigarette smokers and 14 percent for pipe or cigar smokers. Only one patient in the series was a nonsmoker. Factors that had no bearing on results were age and the presence or absence of hypertension. Also, the 5-year patency rate of initial successes was the same (25 percent) whether or not complications occurred.

Deep femoral stenoses and even occlusions can be successfully managed by the technique of PTA (Fig. 4). Motarjeme et al reported successful dilatation of all 12 deep femoral arteries for which percutaneous transluminal angioplasty was attempted.[26]

Szilagyi et al reported that fibrotic stenoses occurred in 8 percent of bypass grafts studied by routine postoperative angiography and fibrosis of valve cusps in 5 percent.[34] Alpert et al[1] reported successful balloon dilatation of 11 of 12 of these lesions for which PTA was attempted. Nine stenoses were located within 4 cm of an artery-to-vein anastomosis and presumably represented intimal hyperplasia, while the other three were in the midportion of the graft, presumably at a valve cusp.

Infrapopliteal PTA

Experience with infrapopliteal PTA is with lesions that are dilated with small (5–7 French) straight catheters. Balloons are usually not used because of the small size of these arteries. Dotter and Judkins[9] as early as 1964 showed three examples of PTA of the tibioperoneal trunk. In

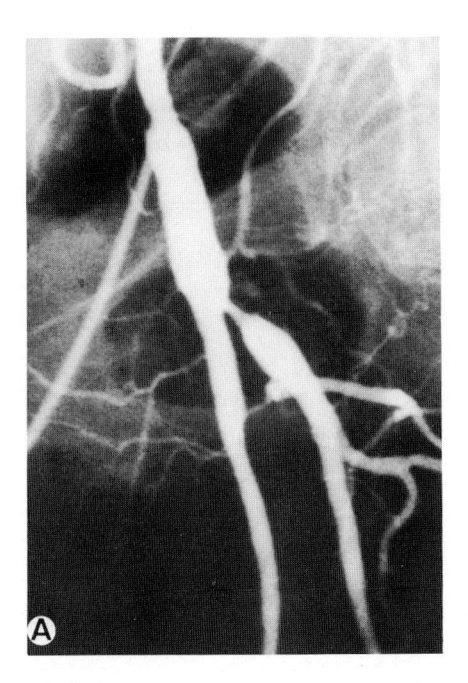

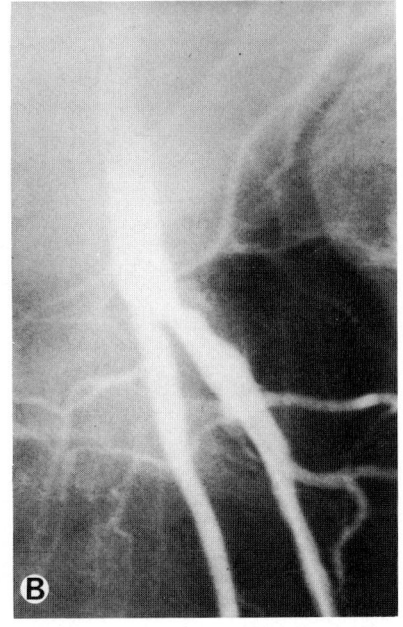

FIGURE 4. **A.** Marked narrowing of proximal profunda femoris artery. **B.** After angioplasty.

one case with severe stenosis of the tibioperoneal trunk and proximal peroneal artery, dilatation was achieved; however, the patient had severe pain after the procedure presumably due to thrombosis and amputation was performed. The other two patients had popliteal artery occlusions in continuity with tibioperoneal trunk occlusions. Both cases were successfully dilated with good clinical results. We attempted PTA of the infrapopliteal arteries in six patients.[33] Excellent dilatation as documented by angiography (Fig. 5) and Doppler segmental arterial pressure

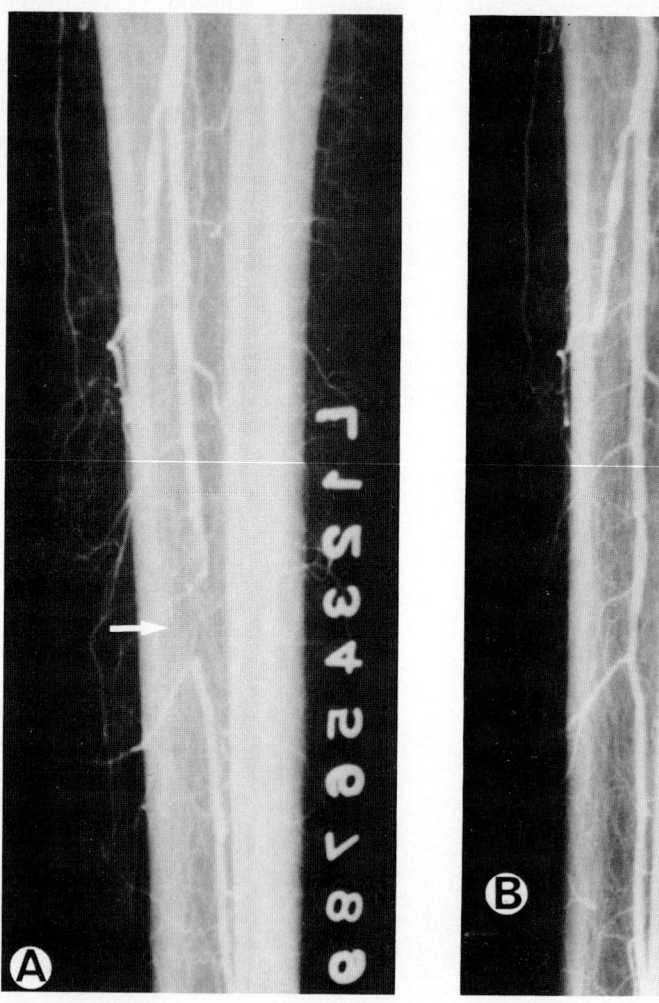

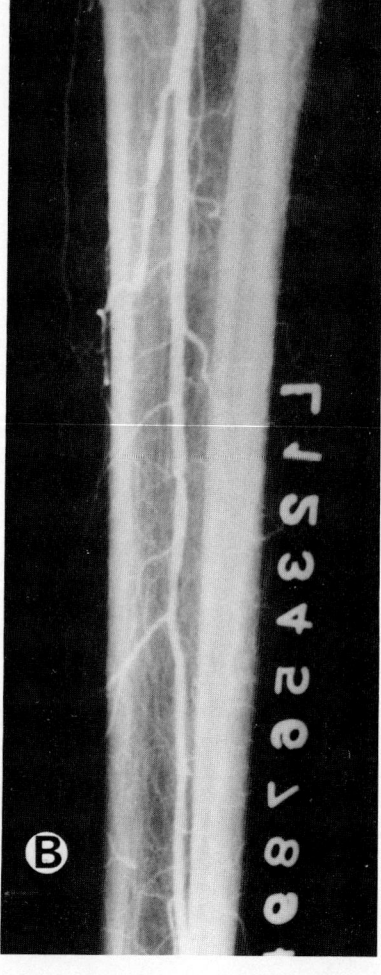

FIGURE 5. **A.** Localized occlusion of peroneal artery (arrow). **B.** Immediately after angioplasty artery is patent.

measurements was obtained in four cases and moderate and slight improvement in one case each. Two of the four patients with excellent results had prompt healing of toe amputations and are doing well at up to two years following angioplasty. Below knee amputation was necessary in the other two patients. Although the overall assessment of infrapopliteal angioplasty must await larger series, it is our impression to date that these procedures have been helpful in some patients and have not produced significant complications.

COMPLICATIONS

Puncture Site

Many authors stress that small or medium-sized hematomas are a frequent occurrence following PTA. Excessive bleeding at the puncture site is more common with the use of heparin during and after angioplasty. Bleeding, which can occur during or after the procedure, is most dangerous when a high puncture is performed and the bleeding is retroperitoneal rather than inguinal.[48] The risk of bleeding is much greater with hypertension. Zietler[48] states that women with slack subcutaneous connective tissue more often suffer posttreatment bleeding than men. Brahme et al[4] had five cases (of 116 procedures) that required blood transfusions. Zeitler[44,46] in series of 372 treatments and 508 treatments reported an overall incidence of hemorrhage of 1.75 percent. Grüntzig had four hematomas in 320 cases for an incidence of 1.3 percent.[14] In a cooperative study, the incidence of hemorrhage at various institutions ranged from 1.4 to 7.9 percent.[48] The incidence of false aneurysm in the cooperative study was 0.5 to 2 percent.[48]

Thrombosis may occur at the puncture site. In the cooperative study in two of the institutions that recorded this complication, thrombosis occurred in 0.32 percent (Zeitler) and 1 percent (Grüntzig).[48]

Periphery

Subintimal dissection of the guide wire is hardly completely avoidable especially with long occlusions. The proximal and/or distal end of an occlusion usually offers much more resistance than the thrombotic central core and are the sites of false routes. Once a false pathway has been formed, the tendency is for the guide wire to repeatedly enter it. In view of this, Dotter states that subintimal passage of the guide wire frequently heralds failure, and it may be necessary to have the procedure postponed for 6 weeks in order to allow the false route to heal by fibrosis.[37] Andresen and Gjemdal,[2] however, claim that it is only necessary to withdraw the guide wire a short distance and then to advance it again. In our experience, subintimal passage of the guide wire usually precludes a satisfactory result, at least temporarily. It should be emphasized that dissections of this kind rarely result in worsening of the patient's condition. Zietler, however, states that dissection by the guide wire can lead to thrombotic occlusion.[48] Zeitler also claims that complete perforation of the arterial wall by the guide wire can lead to a hematoma but usually has no practical consequences. Horvath et al report that through and through perforation of the arterial wall by the guide wire happens frequently and usually does not require any treatment.[23] Catheter perforation of the arterial wall is, of course, more serious and may result in bleeding that requires surgical correction. This is a more severe complication with an iliac than a peripheral artery. In the cooperative study, the incidence of perforation ranged from 0.2 to 2.9 percent.[48]

The most feared complication of angioplasty is thromboembolism. There are many factors that relate to thromboembolic complications including the preparation of the patient, the technique of the puncture, the length of the catheter, the duration of the procedure, the amount of heparin used, arterial spasm, coagulation abnormalities, severity of atherosclerosis, the size of the vessels, the degree of compression after catheter removal, smoking, and the existence of pancreatic carcinoma.[23] Horvath[23] reported that thromboembolic complications were much higher in smokers. Embolism occurs more often with the coaxial catheter system of Dotter[22] than with tapered catheters or balloon catheters.[14] Heparinization prior to angioplasty decreases formation of thrombus on the catheter and guide wire and in the vessel, where the intraluminal catheter hinders flow. The incidence of embolism is influenced by medication, type of instruments, and the experience of the angiographer.

Zeitler[48] reported a 3.1 percent incidence of peripheral embolization occurring in the performance of 922 iliac, femoral, and popliteal angioplasties. Grüntzig and Kumpe[18] reported a 5 percent incidence of distal embolization in a series of 303 angioplasties. The latter authors, however, stated that none of their patients had clinical sequellae or required surgery for embolization. Zeitler did not mention how many, if any, patients required surgery for embolization. He did, however, state that after a few days the emboli may disappear. This may be due to spontaneous thrombolysis and/or fragmentation. Dotter[8] stated that none of his 439 cases had significant downstream embolization. He mentioned that some of the minor symptoms, such as hyperesthesias that follow PTA, may be due to small emboli. He also stressed, however, that the benefit of opening up a major channel far outweighs the consequences of minor emboli. It is of interest to note that asymptomatic emboli occur from diagnostic as well as therapeutic catheterizations. A routine Doppler arterial pressure study of the extremities immediately following 106 diagnostic arteriograms (femoral, axillary, and translumbar) showed an incidence of thromboembolic complications of 4.8 percent.[3] None of the patients were symptomatic.

The complication of popliteal artery spasm due to irritation from the guide wire and catheter with subsequent thrombosis of the popliteal and leg arteries was described by Zeitler[48] and Horvath et al.[23] In 1973, Zeitler[45] reported that four of nine cases of popliteal recanalization showed clinical deterioration due to spasm and one required surgery. Grüntzig in 1977 encountered six cases with popliteal spasm among 320 angioplasties for an incidence of 2 percent[16]. In an attempt to decrease popliteal spasm, Zeitler injected 1 percent Xylocaine into the superficial femoral artery in 80 patients; severe spasm was not encountered and slight spasm was noted seven cases.[48] In a comparison group of 40 patients who did not receive Xylocaine treatment, severe spasm occurred in 4 and slight spasm in 12. We have not seen popliteal spasm with administration of 60 mg of papaverine and 40 mg of lidocaine intra-arterially immediately prior to guide wire and catheter manipulation in the popliteal and/or leg arteries.

RENAL ARTERY ANGIOPLASTY

Renal angioplasty can be performed via the femoral or left axillary artery. The left axillary artery is preferred if a pronounced caudal direction of the renal artery is present. This approach often allows easier passage of the guide wire and especially the catheter through the narrowed artery.

In renal as in peripheral angioplasty, opinion varies as to whether or not to heparinize patients after the procedure. It appears that good results can be obtained without heparin and we do not heparinize these patients. As with peripheral PTA, patients are placed on long-term salicylate therapy.

Renal artery angioplasty appears to have become the interventional treatment of choice for renovascular hypertension. Since Grüntzig et al reported the first case of successful balloon dilatation of an atherosclerotic renal artery stenosis in 1978,[21] many centers have had experience with this procedure. The largest series of renal angioplasties is that of Schwarten et al[31] who reported on the results of 76 procedures in 66 patients. The etiologies of the obstructing lesions were atherosclerosis in 55 patients, fibromuscular dysplasia in 7, atherosclerosis and fibromuscular dysplasia in 2, complications resulting from a Dacron bypass graft in 1, and neurofibromatosis with bilateral renal artery stenosis in 1. The reasons for angioplasty were hypertension in 54 and renal failure in 12 (5 with acute renal failure and 7 with progressive chronic disease). A success rate of 97.4 percent was achieved. Katzen et al[24] recently reported on renal angioplasty in 40 hypertensive patients. Excellent blood pressure responses were obtained in 35 of 40 patients and in 26 of 29 patients with atherosclerotic lesions. Tegtmeyer[35] reported that of 20 patients undergoing PTA for renal vascular hypertension, ten patients including two with transplant arterial stenosis, required no further treatment. Of these 10 patients, it was easier to control the blood pressure in six. Four stenoses in 3 patients were redilated and the redilatation was successful in 3. Weinberger et al performed renal artery PTA in 5 patients with stenosis of the renal artery of a solitary functioning kidney.[39] All 5 patients were hypertensive and had marked impairment of renal function. Blood pressure was improved in all 5 patients and renal function was improved in 3 following PTA. Figure 6 shows angioplasty of a severe left renal artery stenosis in a patient whose right renal artery was occluded.

COMPLICATIONS

Because there is a tendency for a great variation in blood pressure, especially hypotension, to occur after successful renal artery dilatation these patients must be observed very closely. Segmental renal infarction from thromboembolic phenomena appears to be a rather infrequent complication. The angiographer must be careful that the guide wire and catheter in the renal artery distal to the stenosis do not extend into a small branch and cause spasm and/or thrombosis. In the series of 40 patients reported by Katzen et al, complications included asymptomatic segmental renal infarction in two, transient oliguria in two, puncture site hematoma in one, and severe hypotension with symptoms of shock that responded to fluid and salt replacement in three patients.[24]

Angioplasty has the advantage over surgery in being a low-risk procedure. This is especially important in many of the older hypertensive patients in renal failure. Also, unsuccessful angioplasty usually does not result in significant damage to the kidney or renal artery and may be followed by bypass surgery.

Transplant Renal Artery Stenosis

In a recent study, significant hypertension occurred in 21 of 519 renal transplant recipients.[40] In 14 of these 21 patients, hypertension was due to transplant arterial stenosis. Transplant arterial stenosis should be suspected in the presence of severe hypertension occurring in the first year after transplantation. It can be associated with a decline in renal

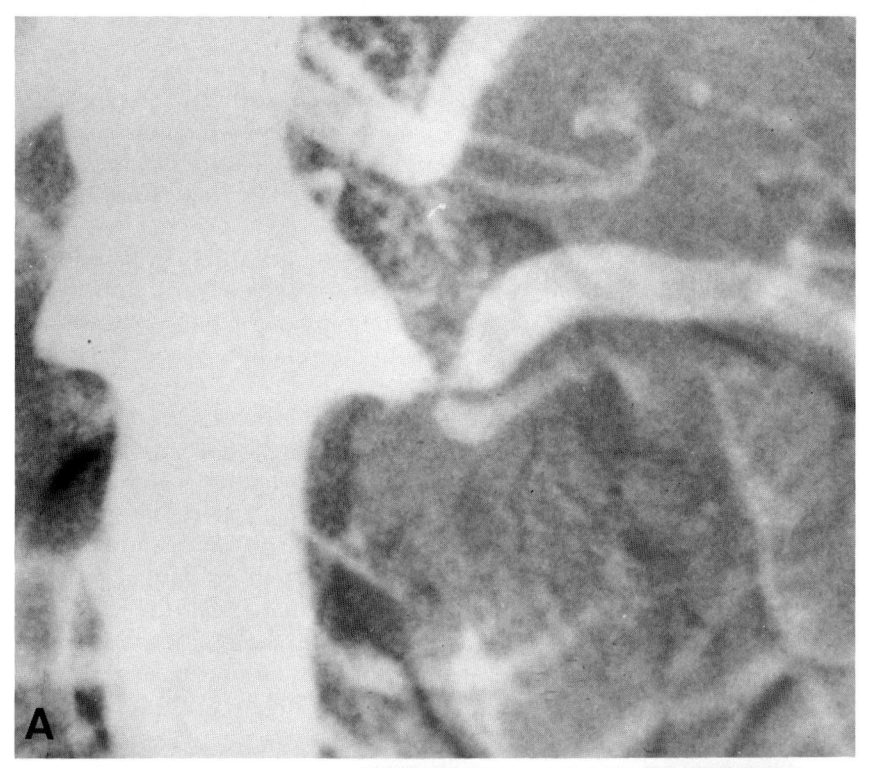

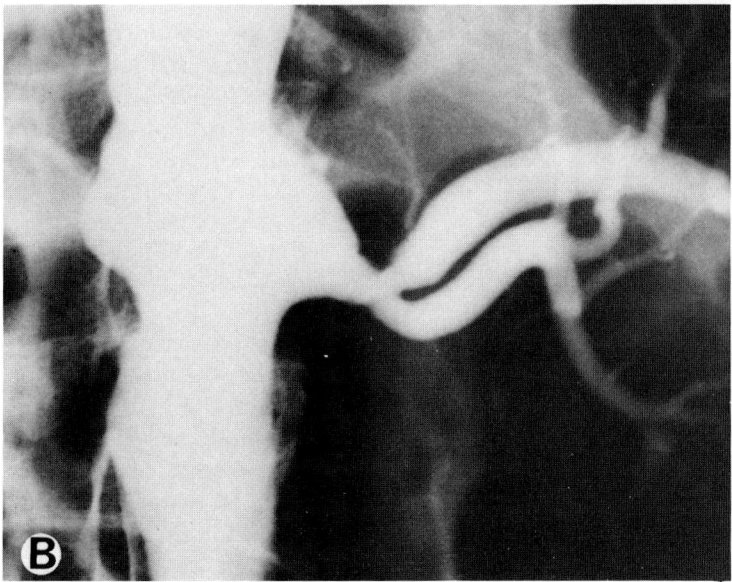

FIGURE 6. **A.** Severe arteriosclerotic narrowing of left renal artery. The right renal artery is occluded. **B.** After angioplasty of the left renal artery. The patient subsequently had a right iliac to right renal artery bypass and is normotensive on no medications at 1-year follow-up.

function. There are many etiologies postulated for renal arterial transplant narrowing, including trauma from perfusion or surgery, local reaction to sutures, faulty suture technique, kinking, rotation or extrinsic compression of the allograft artery, turbulent flow, rejection, and atherosclerosis.

The presence of a transplant renal artery stenosis can only be identified by arteriography; however not all transplant arterial stenoses are significant. It is essential at the time of arteriography to obtain pressure measurements across the stenosis to determine whether or not a gradient is present.

Angioplasty is an alternative to surgery, which can be difficult, for transplant renal artery stenosis. Successful angioplasty of arterial stenosis complicating renal transplantation is possible whether the anastomoses is to the hypogastric artery or the external iliac artery. The anatomic orientation of the transplant anastomosis will determine whether the axillary or femoral artery should be catheterized. Sniderman et al reported successful dilatation of 6 of 7 transplant renal artery stenoses complicating renal transplantation.[32] Prior to angioplasty, all patients were on multiple antihypertensive medications. Following successful angioplasty, the blood pressure fell from approximately 190/120 to 132/86 and remained at that level for up to 6 months with an average follow-up of 2.8 months on no or decreased antihypertensive medications. One of our cases of PTA of a renal transplant arterial stenosis is shown in Figure 7. Based on our experience, it appears that a transplant renal artery stenosis can be somewhat more difficult to dilate than atherosclerotic or fibromuscular stenoses. There also may be more of a tendency for transplant stenosis to recur. However, recurrence can sometimes be redilated.

CORONARY ANGIOPLASTY

We have had no personal experience with coronary angioplasty. The procedure is performed in a limited number of centers. The technique used is the coaxial balloon catheter system devised by Grüntzig.[15] The indications for coronary angioplasty are single lesions in the left anterior descending or right coronary artery and stenotic vein bypass grafts. Left main coronary artery disease and calcified plaques constitute contraindications for angioplasty.[20] It is now estimated that approximately 5 percent of patients undergoing coronary bypass operation are candidates for PTA.[25]

In 1973 Grüntzig[20] reported on attempted angioplasty on 53 coronary vessels in 50 patients. Successful dilatation was achieved in 29 of 46

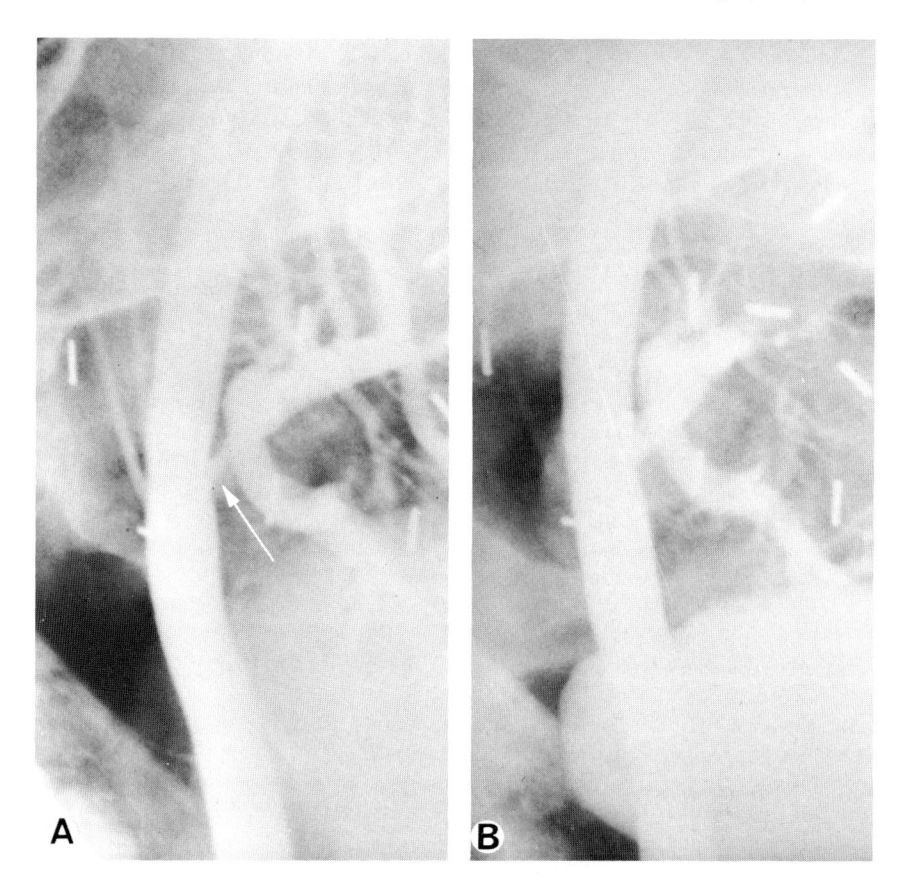

FIGURE 7. **A.** Marked narrowing of transplant arterial stenosis at and distal to anastamosis with external iliac artery (arrow). **B.** Dilatation of stenotic segment is noted after angioplasty.

(63 percent) coronary arteries and 5 of 7 (71 percent) saphenous vein bypass graft stenoses. Follow-up of 16 patients with good clinical results 6 to 9 months after dilatation showed patency of the dilated vessels in all patients.[20] Improvement in the caliber and vessel smoothness was noted in 13 of the 16 patients when the follow-up arteriograms were compared with the immediate postangioplasty angiograms. Six recurrences were observed by Grüntzig et al, all within 3 months of dilatation. Three of these recurrences were in saphenous vein bypass grafts. Wholey recently reported using straight (nonballoon) catheters to dilate stenotic saphenous vein grafts successfully in 7 of 10 cases.[39]

It must be stressed that coronary angioplasty can be performed only when there is a surgeon and operating room immediately available. Five patients in Grüntzig's series had complications requiring immediate operation. In two, an intimal dissection was produced at the stenosis, and in three, occlusion of the stenotic artery occurred after uneventful dilatation. It is generally considered that the mortality of coronary angioplasty is 1 percent and at best 5 percent of patients require emergency bypass.[28]

REFERENCES

1. Alpert JR, Ring EJ, Berkowitz HO, et al: Treatment of vein graft stenosis by balloon catheter dilatation. JAMA 242:2769, 1979
2. Andresen I, Gjemdal T: Transluminal behandlung ov arteriosclerosis obliterans T. Norske Laegeforen 87:1057, 1967
3. Barnes RW, Slaymaker EE, Hahn FJY: Thromboembolic complications of angiography for peripheral arterial disease; prospective assessment by Doppler ultrasound. Radiology 122:459, 1977
4. Brahme F, Swedenborg J, Tibell B: Evaluation of transluminal recanalisation of the femoral artery. Acta Chir Scand 135:679, 1979
5. Castaneda-Zuniga WR, Formanek A, Tadavarthy M, et al: The mechanism of balloon angioplasty. Radiology 135:565, 1980
6. Dotter CT: Arterial catheterization for diagnosis and therapy. Nippon Acta Radiol 25:495, 1965
7. Dotter CT: In Van Andel GJ: Percutaneous Transluminal Angioplasty. Amsterdam, Excerpta Medica, 1976, pp 80–81
8. Dotter CT: Transluminal angioplasty—pathologic basis. In Zeitler E, Grüntzig A, Schoop W (eds): Percutaneous Vascular Recanalization. New York, Springer-Verlag, 1978, pp 3–12
9. Dotter CT, Judkins MP: Transluminal treatment of arteriosclerotic obstruction. Circulation 30:654, 1964
10. Dotter CT, Judkins MP, Rosch J: Nichtoperative transluminal behandlung der arteriosklerotischero verschlussaffektionen. Fortsch Rontgenstr 109:125, 1968
11. Dotter CT, Frische LH, Judkins MP, Mueller R: The "nonsurgical" treatment of iliofemoral arteriosclerotic obstruction. Radiology 86:871, 1966
12. Dotter CT, Rosch J, Anderson JM, Antonovic R, Robinson M: Transluminal iliac artery dilatation. JAMA 230:117, 1974
13. Grollman JH, Del Vicario M, Mittal AK: Percutaneous transluminal abdominal aortic angioplasty. Am J Roentgenol 134:1053, 1980
14. Grüntzig A: Die perkutane transluminale rekanalisation chronisches arterienverschlusse mit einen neuen dilatationstechnik. Baden-Baden, Gerhard Witzstrack, 1977
15. Grüntzig A: Transluminal dilatation of coronary artery stenosis. Lancet 1:263, 1978
16. Grüntzig A: Der perkutane transluminale rekanalisation chronischer arterienverschlusse mit lines neuen dilatationstechnik. Baden-Baden, Gerhard Witzstrack, 1977 (English translation by Wipfelder R, Kumpe D, 1979)

17. Grüntzig A, Hopff H: Perkutane rekanalisation chronischer arterieller verschlusse miteinem neuen dilatation. Modification der Dotter-Technik. Dtsch Med Wschr 99:2502, 1974
18. Grüntzig A, Kumpe DA: Technique of percutaneous transluminal angioplasty with the Grüntzig balloon catheter. Am J Roentgenol 132:547, 1979
19. Grüntzig A, Zeitler E: Cooperative study of results of PTA in twelve different clinics. In Zeitler E, Grüntzig A, Schoop W (eds): Percutaneous Vascular Recanalization. New York, Springer-Verlag, 1978, pp 118–119
20. Grüntzig A, Senning A, Siegenthaler WE: Nonoperative dilatation of coronary artery stenosis. N Engl J Med 301:6, 1979
21. Grüntzig A, Kuhlman V, Vetter W, Lütolf V, Meier B, Siegenthaler W: Treatment of renovascular hypertension with percutaneous transluminal dilatation of a renal artery stenosis. Lancet 1:801, 1978
22. Hohn P, Wagner R, Zeitler E: Histologische befunde nach der katheterbehandlung arterieller obliterationen nach Dotter und ihre bedentung. Herz/Kreisl 7:13, 1975
23. Horvath I, Illes I, Varro J: Complications of the transluminal angioplasty excluding the puncture site. In Zeitler E, Grüntzig A, Schoop W (eds): Percutaneous Vascular Recanalization. New York, Springer-Verlag, 1978, pp 126–139
24. Katzen BT, Casarella WJ, Chang J: Nonoperative treatment of renovascular hypertension. Scientific exhibit at Radiological Society of North America meeting, Atlanta, Georgia, December 1980
25. Levy RI, Mock MB, William VL, Frommer PL: Percutaneous transluminal coronary angioplasty (editorial). N Engl J Med 301:101, 1979
26. Motarjeme A, Keifer JW, Zuska AJ: Percutaneous transluminal angioplasty of the deep femoral artery. Radiology 135:613, 1980
27. Porstmann W: Ein neuer korsett-ballonkatheter zur transluminalen rekanalisation nach Dotter unter besonderer berucksichtigung von obliteration an den beckenarterien. Radiol Diagn 14:239, 1973
28. Rapaport E: Percutaneous transluminal coronary angioplasty (editorial). Circulation 60:969, 1979
29. Schmidtke I, Zeitler E, Schoop W: Late results of percutaneous catheter treatment in occlusion of the femoropopliteal arteries. In Zeitler E, Grüntzig A, Schoop W (eds): Percutaneous Vascular Recanalization. New York, Springer-Verlag, 1978, p 96
30. Schoop W, Levy H, Cappius G, Mansjoer H, Zeitler E: Early and late results of percutaneous transluminal dilatation in iliac stenosis. In Zeitler E, Grüntzig A, Schoop W (eds): Percutaneous Vascular Recanalization. New York, Springer-Verlag, 1978, pp 111–117
31. Schwarten DE, Yune HY, Klatte EC, Grim CE, Weinberger MH: Clinical experience with percutaneous transluminal angioplasty of stenotic renal arteries. Radiology 135:601, 1980
32. Sniderman KW, Sos TA, Sprayregen S, et al: Percutaneous transluminal angioplasty in renal transplant arterial stenosis for relief of hypertension. Radiology 135:23, 1980
33. Sprayregen S, Sniderman KW, Sos TA, et al: Percutaneous transluminal

angioplasty of the popliteal artery branches. Am J Roentgenol 135:945, 1980
34. Szilagyi DE, Elliott JP, Hageman SH, et al: Biologic fate of autogenous vein grafts implanted as arterial substitutes. Ann Surg 78:232, 1973
35. Tegtmeyer C: Reported in Medical News of JAMA 243:99, 1980
36. Tegtmeyer CJ, Moore TS, Chandler JG, Wellons HA, Rudolf LE: Percutaneous transluminal dilatation of a complete block in the right iliac artery. Am J Roentgenol 133:532, 1979
37. Van Andel GJ: In Van Andel GJ: Percutaneous Transluminal Angioplasty. Amsterdam, Excerpta Medica, 1976
38. Velasquez G, Castaneda-Zuniga W, Formanek A, et al: Nonsurgical aortoplasty in Leriche Syndrome. Radiology 134:359, 1980
39. Weinberger MH, Yune HY, Grim CE, et al: Percutaneous transluminal angioplasty for renal artery stenosis in a solitary functioning kidney. Ann Intern Med 91:684, 1979
40. Whelton PK, Russell P, Harrington DP, William GM, Walker WG: Hypertension following renal transplantation. JAMA 241:1128, 1979
41. Wholey M: Experience with coronary and saphenous vein graft angioplasty. Lecture at Society of Cardiovascular Radiology Meeting, Phoenix, Arizona, February 4–7, 1980
42. Wierny L, Plass R, Porstmann R: Long-term results in 100 consecutive patients treated by transluminal angioplasty. Radiology 112:543, 1974
43. Zeitler E: Die perkutane rekanalisation arterielle obliterationen mit katheter nach Dotter. Dtsch Med Wochenschs 97:1392, 1972
44. Zeitler E: Transluminale verschlussrekanalisation mit angiographiekatheter. Herz/Kreisl 4:13, 1972
45. Zeitler E: Die perkutane behandlung von arteriellen durchblutungsstorungen der extremitaten mit katheter. Radiologe 13:319, 1973
46. Zeitler E: Die perkutane behandlung arterieller obliterationen mit katheter. In Heber P, Row P, Schoop W (eds): Angiologie. Grundlagen Klinik und Praxis, 2nd ed. Stuttgart, George Thieme Verlag, 1974
47. Zeitler E: In Van Andel GJ: Percutaneous Transluminal Angioplasty. Amsterdam, Excerpta Medica, 1976, p 81
48. Zeitler E: Complications in and after percutaneous transluminal recanalization. In Zeitler E, Grüntzig A, Schoop W (eds): Transluminal Vascular Recanalization. New York, Springer-Verlag, 1978, pp 120–125
49. Zeitler E: Dilatation technique of iliac artery stenoses with balloon catheters. In Zeitler E, Grüntzig A, Schoop W (eds): Percutaneous Vascular Recanalization. New York, Springer-Verlag, 1978, p 24
50. Zeitler E: Drug treatment before and after percutaneous transluminal recanalization. In Zeitler E, Grüntzig A, Schoop W (eds): Percutaneous Vascular Recanalization. New York, Springer-Verlag, 1978, pp 73–77
51. Zeitler E, Muller R: Erste ergebnisse mit der katheter-rekanalisation nach Dotter bei arterieller verschlusskrankheit. Fortscher Roentgenstr 111:345, 1969

SIX
Update on Polytetrafluoroethylene Vascular Grafts I

John J. Bergan, John P. Harris, Neil D. Rudo, and James S. T. Yao

After 5 years of use, it is appropriate to examine the role of expanded polytetrafluoroethylene (PTFE) as an arterial substitute and to summarize some of the observations made in evaluating this material in the experimental laboratory and in man. Gradually, since the 1960s, new graft materials available to clinical vascular surgeons have consisted of variations on the polyester theme. These modifications of Dacron reflected improvements in textile technology and included the introduction of woven and knitted as well as velour and double velour grafts. Graft development seemed to be based on the premise that porosity was desirable and crimping was essential to long-term success of arterial prostheses placed below the inguinal ligament. Observations indicated that loosely knitted grafts and velours allowed ingrowth of the patient's fibrous tissue into the graft itself, thus making it integral to the patient. This impression persisted even though it became known that the inner surface of vascular grafts in man consists of compacted fibrin rather than endothelium, and this was not derived from tissue ingrowth. An exception was the partial endothelialization seen to extend into the grafts for 2 to 3 mm from the anastomoses.

With these observations in mind, it was amazing to vascular surgeons to have presented to them a nonfabric expanded PTFE prosthesis, which

---

This work was supported in part by a grant in aid from the Conrad Jobst Foundation and the Northwestern University Vascular Research Fund.

was neither porous to blood nor crimped to prevent kinking at joint creases. That this graft functioned at all and that it seemed to function in the short-term in a fashion similar to saphenous vein was remarkable. This prompted a review of the status of this material at this time.

EXPERIMENTAL EVALUATION

Reports that began to appear in 1972 suggested that small arterial segments in the experimental animal could be replaced by various configurations of expanded Teflon material.[5,15,24] These experimental observations were made using grafts of 3- and 4-mm internal diameters. The pathologic studies were especially encouraging because a well-developed neointima with little surrounding inflammation was seen. In addition, the host-to-graft anastomoses were firmly bonded with continuity established by dense connective tissue. An apparent true neointima was present that contained many myointimal cells. These findings suggested that the intimal layer might function like a native arterial lining. Also, elastic fibers were observed in the connective tissue.

Later observations by Campbell and his colleagues[6] showed pore size to be the primary determinant of tissue ingrowth, neointimization, and patency. Paradoxically, a pore size of 22 μ or less in grafts was associated with 88 percent patency rates, while those with an average pore size of 34 μ or greater had a 53 percent patency rate. This indicated that in this configuration with this particular material the smaller pore size grafts, which had less tissue ingrowth, remained patent while larger pore size grafts did not. This observation clearly challenged previous graft dogma.

Since the early experiments indicated that the patency rate fell precipitously when the pore size became greater than 22 μ, it was felt that large pore size grafts allowed blood to extravasate into the interstices of the graft material where it became static and initiated the coagulation cascade.

Three different commercial configurations of PTFE grafts were evaluated by Hastings et al.[21] This study concluded that there were no differences in patency among the three materials and that each of the three types of graft showed a large amount of pannus formation. These authors concluded that the material was inferior to autologous vein grafts and specifically did not advise routine clinical use of the graft in the community hospital setting. They suggested that prospective and randomized clinical studies should be reported from centers already using the grafts. They were particularly specific in saying that PTFE grafts should not be used in preference to available autogenous saphenous vein in man.

Another word of caution was added by Roberts and Johnson[29] and by Campbell et al,[3] who reported graft aneurysms in an early PTFE configuration. In the aneurysm of expanded microporous PTFE graft reported by Roberts, the graft was manufactured by Impra Inc., and that particular graft did not have circumferentially oriented outer layers of PTFE reinforcing. No aneurysms have been reported in grafts having the external reinforcing layer.[17]

GRAFT DIFFERENCES

Because early fabrications of PTFE grafts were subject to aneurysmal degeneration and because external circumferential reinforcement of grafts was not applied to all grafts of all manufacturers, a strength study of PTFE grafts available to vascular surgeons was done.* The purpose of the study was to test the tendency for aneurysmal degeneration by measuring graft burst strength. In addition, it was considered desirable to estimate the potential for needle hole bleeding from the grafts by measuring resistance of each graft fabrication to needle tearing.

Twenty-two commercially available grafts were tested. Eleven were manufactured by Impra, Inc., and were supplied to hospitals as 8-mm tapered tubes (five grafts), 8-mm straight tubes (three grafts), 6-mm straight tubes (two grafts), and a 7-mm straight tube (one graft). All were manufactured between October, 1978 and August, 1980. Eleven grafts were manufactured by W. L. Gore & Associates, Inc. There were 6-mm tapered tubes (three grafts), 10-mm straight tubes (two grafts), 8-mm straight tubes (two grafts), 6-mm straight tubes (two grafts), and 5-mm straight tubes (two grafts). All were manufactured between June 1979 and March 1980.

Graft strength was assessed in two 15-mm sections of each graft using a destructive water entry pressure burst tester. In this test, water completely replaces air in the graft and continues to be forced into the graft until the maximum pressure/volume ratio is obtained. Tests were terminated at 256 psi.

Suture retention was tested in a longitudinal direction and transverse direction in each of two 2-cm sections of each graft using an AMTEK/Hunter Tensile Strength Tester. An 0.014-inch curved surgical needle was inserted 1 mm from the end of each graft sample, suturing through both walls. Maximum force, recorded in grams, needed for the suture

---

* Bio-Technics Laboratories, Inc., 1133 Crenshaw Boulevard, Los Angeles, California 90019.

to tear through the graft in a longitudinal and transverse direction was noted for each graft sample.

Bursting strength of each of the grafts tested is noted in Table 1. In this table, the various graft sizes of each manufacturer are displayed. The Gore-Tex grafts failed the burst test suddenly, with an aneurysm developing in a single location, while the Impra grafts gradually increased in size until a maximum pressure/volume ratio was reached. The strength of each end of tapered grafts is noted. One sees that the externally reinforced Gore grafts are three to four times as resistant to bursting as the nonreinforced Impra grafts. The coefficient of variation is 5 to 11 percent for Gore grafts and 15 to 25 percent for Impra grafts.

The longitudinal suture retention strength of the various grafts is displayed in Table 2. It can be seen that the force required to pull a single suture through 1 mm of graft wall is three to four times as great in the externally reinforced graft as compared to the nonreinforced graft. In both types of grafts, the mode of failure was by the suture tearing directly through the graft or by the suture pulling a 1-mm section from the edge of the graft. The coefficient of variation is 11 to 34 percent for Gore grafts and 11 to 37 percent for Impra grafts.

The transverse suture retention strength of the various grafts is displayed in Table 3. The nonreinforced Impra grafts exhibited a transverse suture retention force averaging 413 gm while the Gore grafts showed an average suture retention force of 1214.

It can be concluded from this testing that the externally reinforced Gore-Tex grafts withstand about three times the pressure of the nonreinforced Impra grafts before failure occurs. Similarly, suture retention strength of the Gore-Tex grafts is approximately three times that of Impra grafts in both longitudinal and transverse directions.

DESCRIPTION OF GRAFT MATERIAL

Figure 1 illustrates the standard PTFE 30-μ structure as viewed by the scanning electron microscope. Solid PTFE nodes are connected by thin PTFE fibrils and it is apparent that the graft wall is approximately 85 percent open space. Figure 2 shows the outer wall of the same commercially available product. The scanning electron photomicrograph illustrates the circumferentially oriented outer layer, or skin, of PTFE that reinforces the inner, longitudinally oriented fibrils of the same material. It is the high hoop strength of this material that prevents aneurysm formation in the clinical situation.

Figure 3 shows a scanning electron microphotograph of flattened, confluent monolayers of endothelial-like cells on a PTFE graft luminal

Table 1. Bursting Strength of PTFE Grafts (psi)

Manu-facturer	Tapered Grafts (large end/small end)				Straight Grafts			
	6 mm				10 mm	8 mm	6 mm	5 mm
Gore	153/182	163/202	156/169		176.5 160.5	132 144	163.5 153	170.5 165
	8 mm				8 mm	7 mm	6 mm	
Impra	45/56	23/50	48/48 35/41	41/43	41 43.5	42.5	43.5	48 46

Table 2. Longitudinal Suture Retention Strength of Grafts (gm)

Manu-facturer	Tapered Grafts (large end/small end)				Straight Grafts			
	6 mm				10 mm	8 mm	6 mm	5 mm
Gore	1095/1025	1090/1000	1040/1040		1137.5 1117.5	1287.5 1367.5	905 1067.5	940 882.5
	8 mm					8 mm	7 mm	6 mm
Impra	240/205	335/215	170/210 205/165	265/245		370 347.5	320 257.5	275 270

Table 3. Transverse Suture Retention Strength of Grafts (gm)

Manu-facturer	Tapered Grafts (large end/small end)				Straight Grafts			
	6 mm				10 mm	8 mm	6 mm	5 mm
Gore	925/1165	735/810	1030/1200		1202.5 1397.5	1640 1342.5	1010 1125	1087.5 1332.5
	8 mm					8 mm	7 mm	6 mm
Impra	450/385	400/355	305/345 245/250	505/360		510 467.5	487.5 377.5	437.5 445

110   Critical Problems in Vascular Surgery

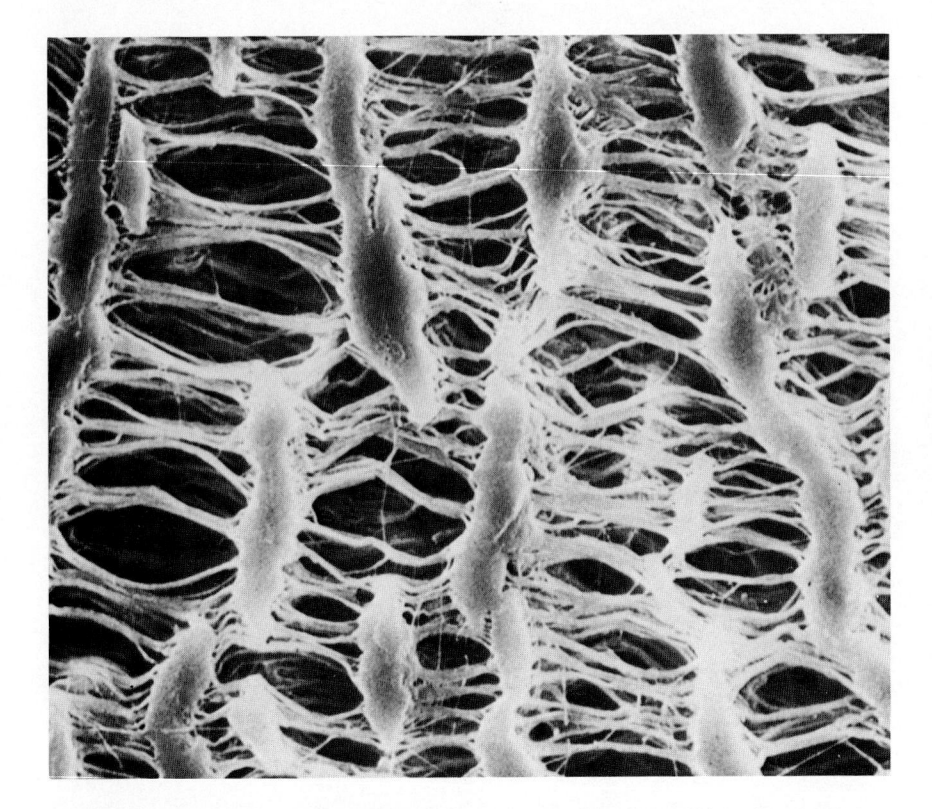

FIGURE 1. In this scanning electron photomicrograph, solid Teflon nodes are connected by thick fibrils to adjacent nodes. Note the large amount of empty air space in the expanded Teflon structure.

surface. This pavement-type orientation appears to be endothelium but precise identification of Weibel-Plade bodies has not been achieved, nor has immunofluorescent staining study for factor VIII-related antigen been done on this material.

Figure 4 shows a unique view, looking into the graft wall and onto the graft luminal surface. In this view, the continuity of nodal structures can be seen, and the interlacing fibrilar nature of graft wall is visualized. Once again, the low density of the graft material can be appreciated as one estimates that the open spaces comprise more than 80 percent of wall structure.

Figure 5 is a light photomicrograph showing endothelial-like cells on the PTFE graft luminal surface, the structure of the PTFE itself, and adventitial coverings. The entire graft is infiltrated with host tissue.

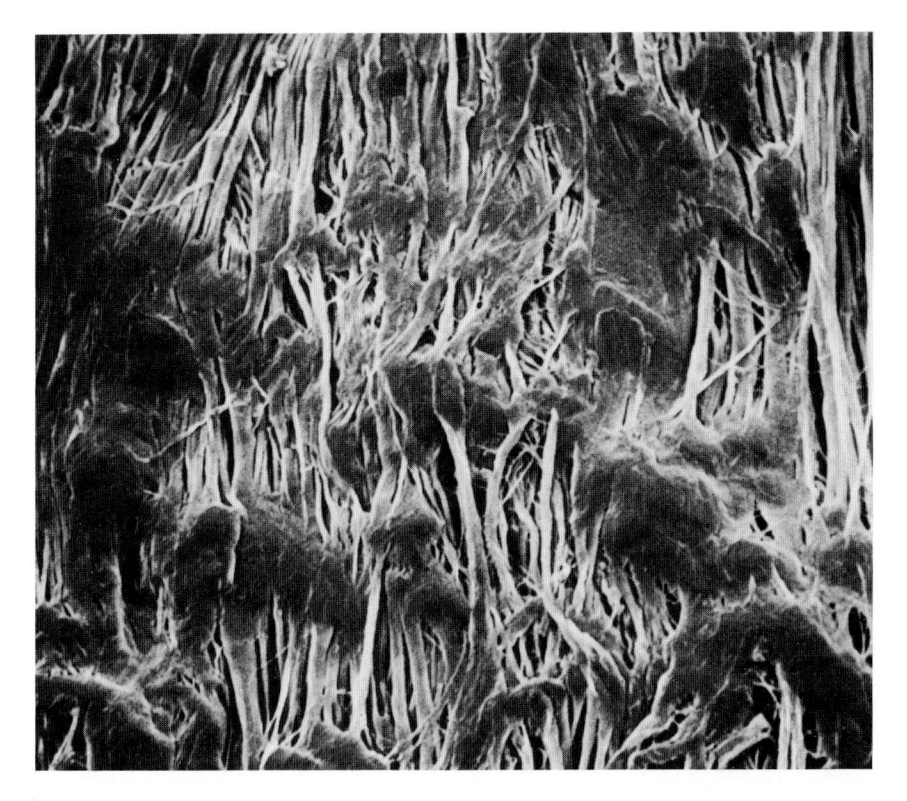

FIGURE 2. Expanded polytetrafluoroethylene that is used as an arterial substitute must have an external, circumferentially reinforced outer wall. This scanning photomicrograph illustrates the outer skin of the Gore-Tex graft.

This specimen was removed from a canine implantation of 6 months duration and clearly shows the absence of host inflammation or foreign body cells.

POLYTETRAFLUOROETHYLENE AS A FEMOROPOPLITEAL SUBSTITUTE

Except for the earliest days of arterial reconstructive surgery, vascular surgeons have had a conservative point of view with regard to reconstruction of the femoropopliteal segment. The well done, early studies of Boyd showed that 50 percent of patients with femoropopliteal occlusion and intermittent claudication would not have progression of symptom-

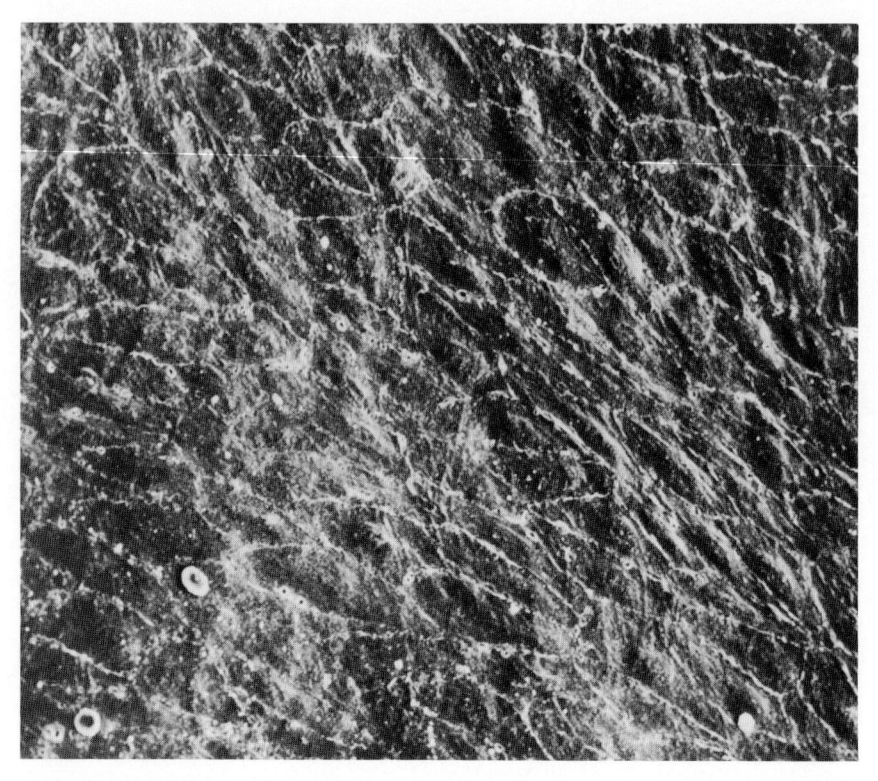

FIGURE 3. Following implantation, the inner surface of the PTFE graft achieves a pavement-like appearance. Precise endothelial markers have not been identified but the overall appearance is that of endothelium.

atology, and that approximately one-third would become asymptomatic without surgical treatment after the initial diagnosis. Accordingly, appropriate conservative care for such patients usually consists of advice regarding cessation of smoking, prescription of exercise programs, treatment of hyperlipidemia and heart disease, and advice regarding weight loss.

After 1976, a number of reports indicated that PTFE might be used as a substitute for unavailable saphenous vein in attempts to salvage limbs threatened by severe ischemia. Among these was Campbell et al.'s[3] report of 13 of 15 patients with viable extremities and a limb salvage rate of 87 percent. In this report, however, the longest observation period was 8 months. Later, Veith et al.[34,35] described a concurrent series of observations with 56 PTFE replacements compared to a similar

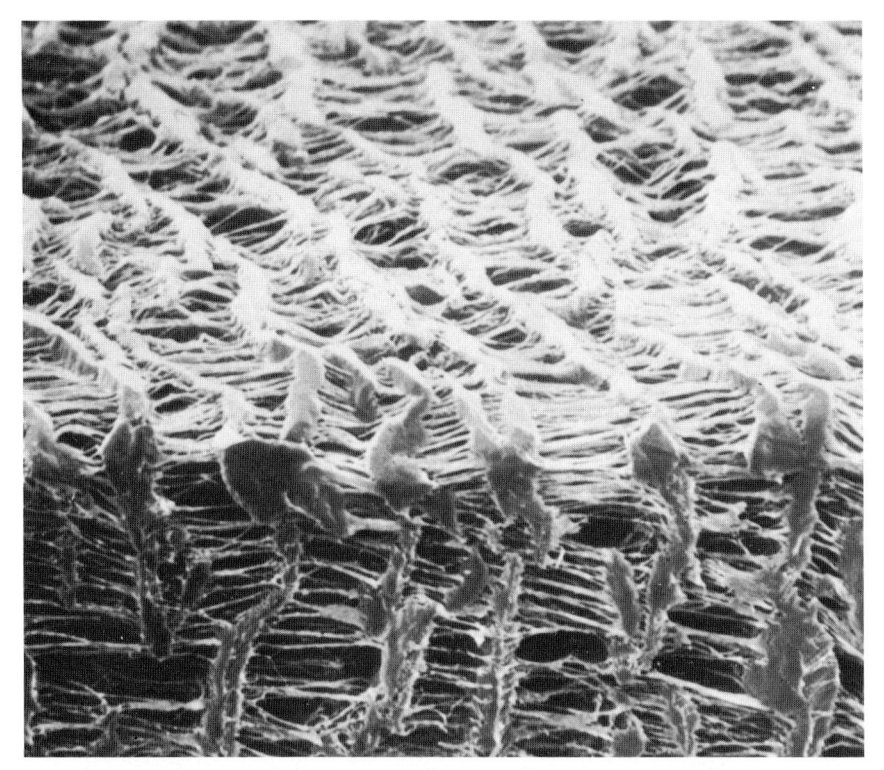

FIGURE 4. In this unique scanning electron photomicrograph, the inner graft surface and adjacent graft wall can be seen. The nodal structures and interlacing fibrils and their relationship to one another are well illustrated in this three-dimensional view.

number of autogenous saphenous vein grafts, suggesting that after 4 to 14 months follow-up, the limb salvage rate and patency rates for the two materials were comparable. Campbell et al.[4] provided a 2-year followup on 131 femoropopliteal, distal popliteal, and tibial bypasses, indicating an 82 percent overall patency rate and 75.7 percent cumulative patency rate at 28 months. Other reports[2,22] confirmed the early patency rates of expanded PTFE.

Of particular importance to long-term follow-up is the enormous experience of Raithel and Groitl,[28] who have described 743 arterial reconstructions using expanded PTFE, 601 of which involved the lower extremity. Their observations include 150 femoropopliteal grafts with an average follow-up of 19 months with an 81 percent patency rate. They cite a cumulative patency rate for 294 PTFE grafts as 76.4 percent

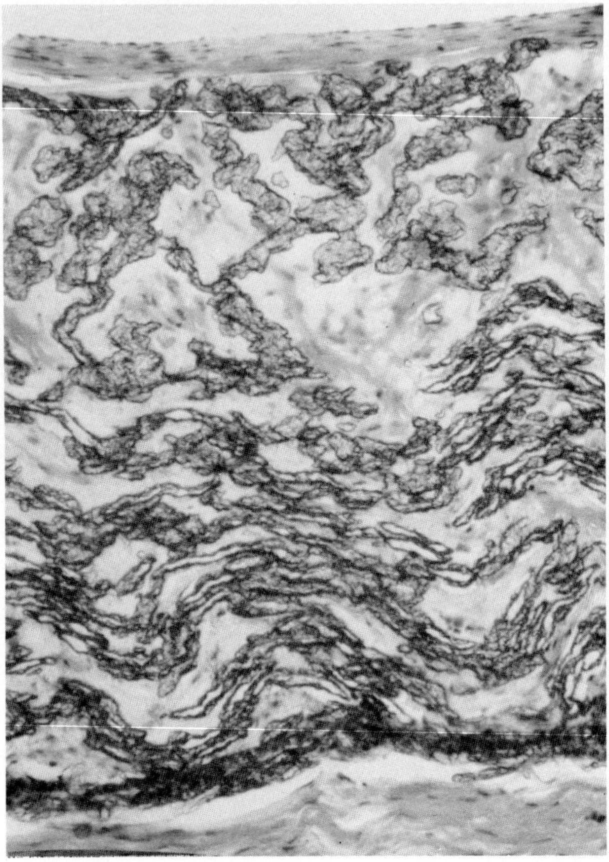

FIGURE 5. In this standard light photomicrograph of a cross-section of an implanted PTFE graft the endothelial surface (bottom) PTFE structure and adventitial coverings (top) are well seen. Host tissue infiltration is clear and absence of host inflammation and foreign body giant cells is noted. This graft had been implanted in a dog for 6 months before this biopsy.

for 36 months. In commenting on this experience, Campbell referred to the 1972 work of Darling and Linton,[8] pointing out that current results with PTFE were quite similar. Darling[20] has now reported a personal experience with 100 femoropopliteal PTFE grafts implanted primarily for limb salvage and in most instances placed to a compromised outflow tract. At 30 months, his cumulative patency rate in such grafts was 81 percent with grafts placed above the knee (28); 47 percent with femoropopliteal grafts placed below the knee (54); and 23 percent in tibial grafts (8).

It has been pointed out that an aggressive approach to occlusion of the PTFE graft can increase the number of late patencies.[32] In a later report on this same subject, Veith et al[32] described 175 PTFE femoropopliteal grafts performed for limb salvage and followed up to 3 years. Nine of these closed within 1 month and 22 closed from 1 to 23 months after operation. With reoperation, all nine early closures remained patent for long periods. Only 18 of the 22 late closures were deemed suitable for reoperation but of these, six grafts remained patent for more than 1 year after the reoperation. Life table patency rates at 3 years were increased from 62 percent to 77 percent by these reoperations on the 175 PTFE femoropopliteal bypasses. These findings, in Veith's opinion,[33] justify an aggressive approach with appropriate reoperation when expanded PTFE grafts occlude early or late in the postoperative period.

In further exploration of the use of PTFE, a survey was done by the New England Society for Vascular Surgery. Questionnaires were distributed to members of the Society, and 32 answers were received. These indicated that 186 PTFE graft insertions could be evaluated, 112 of which were in the lower limb and 106 of which were done for limb salvage. Calculated cumulative patency rates were 91 percent for above-knee and 52 percent for below-knee implantations at 6 to 9 months. A less optimistic review of PTFE grafting in the femorotibial system was presented by Edwards and Mulherin,[10] who compared PTFE with saphenous vein and glutaraldehyde-tanned human umbilical cord vein grafts. In the autogenous saphenous vein grafts, the immediate and 1-year patency rates for 57 bypasses were 92 and 82 percent, respectively. A high incidence of failure occurred in the PTFE grafts, so that 1-year patency was 24 percent of 29 grafts. The 1-year patency rate for the umbilical cord grafts was 10 percent. This experience caused Edwards to conclude that cephalic and basilic veins should be used in those patients who require arterial reconstruction for relief of severe ischemic symptomatology. It should be pointed out, however, that technical features of handling the PTFE graft are of extreme importance. The earliest experience of many individual investigators or groups is frequently bad.

Among the criticisms of the PTFE graft has been the report of intimal hyperplasia developing at and just distal to the lower anastomosis. This compromises the outflow from some grafts, and this proliferation is thought to be due to a lack of compliance of the PTFE graft in comparison to the normal artery. The hypothesis is that with each pulse wave, the more flexible artery expands and exerts a significant shear force on the suture line. This chronic stress is thought to be responsible for the development of intimal hyperplasia. Keshishian[23] has observed, however, that in the experimental situation tapering the distal anastomosis so that it enters smoothly into the distal artery prevents a jet effect from the blood flowing into the artery. A large, ovoid orifice is more effective than a small-mouthed anastomosis entering the artery at an obtuse angle. By using a distal anastomosis of 1.5 cm or larger, he was able to eliminate the distal anastomotic failure problem.

GRAFT FAILURE UNRELATED TO GRAFT MATERIAL

In reviewing the results of bypass grafting to the distal popliteal artery and tibial vessels, one cannot help but be impressed by the high rate of failure of such procedures. Clearly, a number of factors enter into production of such a high rate of failure. Several of these are clearly unrelated to the graft material itself. Among these factors are the anatomic relationship of the graft to peripheral arterial arborizations, hemodynamic failure of the graft, and graft occlusion caused by arterial embolization. With particular interest in the relationship of the graft to peripheral arterial outflow, O'Mara et al.[26] did a careful anatomic study of intraoperative arteriograms. A more precise description of foot anatomic arches was made. Furthermore, an analysis was done in which patency of proximal and/or distal arterial arches was correlated with operative results of tibial bypass grafting. When both plantar arches were present, 20 of 21 anterior tibial artery grafts, 8 of 10 posterior tibial artery grafts, and 9 of 9 peroneal artery grafts succeeded. On the other hand, when both plantar arches were absent, only 1 of 5 anterior tibial artery grafts, 1 of 7 posterior tibial artery grafts, and no peroneal artery grafts were successful.

Clinical experience has shown that the artery to which the graft is attached must be in anatomic continuity with the plantar arches, and there can be no intervening arterial occlusion. If there is such a discontinuity between the proximal arterial anatomy and the distal foot arborization, the graft is doomed to early failure. In Darling's series of 10 tibial artery PTFE grafts, 5 grafts closed very quickly after surgery. Others have also noted this. Since many investigators have superior early results with PTFE, however, factors other than graft material alone must enter into the reason for such a high rate of early failure.

Hemodynamic graft failure is known to the experienced vascular surgeon who has seen patent grafts fail to relieve foot ischemia. In the study by O'Mara et al,[27] 34 patients were identified who had hemodynamic failure of patent arterial grafts. Twenty of these were femoropopliteal or femorotibial reconstructions. In the majority of instances, outflow occlusive disease limited the hemodynamic results of the grafting procedure.

Having experienced hemodynamic graft failure in some instances, Flinn et al.[14] explored the use of sequential femorotibial bypasses in 20 patients. All of these patients had grafts inserted from the common femoral artery to the popliteal or infrageniculate level with a second arterial anastomosis performed to the distal peroneal, anterior tibial, or posterior tibial artery. Thirteen of the patients retained patency of the entire reconstruction, but seven ultimately developed occlusion of the distal limb of the graft. This distal segmental occlusion was clearly identified in each instance by a decrease in ankle pressure that was not associated with a change in low thigh pressure. In every instance, subsequent arteriographic examination confirmed the Doppler findings of distal segmental occlusion. Severe ischemia recurred in only one of these seven patients. Thus, one of the solutions to hemodynamic graft failure is employment of the sequential bypass principle that allows partial graft failure to prevent amputation in a significant number of patients.

The role of arterial embolization as a cause of graft failure has been incompletely defined. Experience with single cases confirms this concept, however. The following case is illustrative.

> A 46-year-old white man was admitted for treatment of severe left foot ischemia. This patient brought an arteriogram indicating a markedly irregular aorta and left common iliac segment. A left common iliac endarterectomy had been done that had been followed by removal of a left femoral artery embolus. When reocclusion of the left iliofemoral system occurred, a left femoropopliteal autogenous saphenous vein bypass graft was done. When this failed, the patient was referred for futher care.
>
> A PTFE graft was placed from the left common femoral artery to the distal popliteal in the region of the anterior tibial bifurcation. This graft occluded in the immediate postoperative period, and a thrombectomy was done. Following the thrombectomy, a right common femoral arterial occlusion occurred that was caused by an embolus. Treatment consisted of bilateral aortofemoral grafting with right femoral embolectomy and exclusion of the aortoiliac segment. A concomitant left femoropopliteal graft thrombectomy was also done. During the placement of the aortofemoral graft, the aorta was inspected and found to be full of loosely adherent thrombus superimposed on severe atherosclerotic disease of the aortic wall.

That arterial embolization represents an important cause of graft failure is gradually becoming recognized by centers interested in tibial artery reconstruction. Clearly, such graft failure would not be dependent upon abnormalities of the coagulation mechanism, history of smoking, development of further atherosclerosis, or the graft material itself.

USE OF POLYTETRAFLUOROETHYLENE IN EXTRA-ANATOMIC BYPASS

In the report of Veith et al[36] of their first 110 consecutive cases of limb salvage operations using expanded PTFE, a number of extra-anatomic bypasses were described. These included eight axillofemoral, seven femorofemoral, four axillopopliteal, three axillary crossover grafts to the popliteal artery, and two femoral crossovers to the popliteal. In that report, it was clear that these extra-anatomic bypasses fared far better than grafts to the femoropopliteal system. The advantages of the expanded PTFE graft in such extra-anatomic sites included its low porosity and low leakage of blood from interstices of the graft.

A larger experience with PTFE grafts for extra-anatomic bypass has been presented by the group from the Royal Prince Alfred's Hospital in Sidney.[13] Although this report consists of an early experience, the 1 year cumulative patency of 95.6 percent for femorofemoral grafts and 89.5 percent for axillofemoral grafts was most encouraging. This group pointed out that thrombectomy of graft failures could be performed using local anesthesia and was worthwhile to increase significantly the overall patency rate of these grafts. It is well known that axillofemoral grafts, in particular, have a propensity for isolated episodes of thrombosis that are unrelated to progression of distal disease. It is now known that flow can be restored without revision of either anastomosis or extension of the graft to a better outflow site. It may be that the best indication for expanded PTFE as a graft material will be in the extra-anatomic location.

POLYTETRAFLUOROETHYLENE FOR VASCULAR ACCESS

During the past five years, a number of groups have been interested in using the PTFE graft for vascular access and a very large experience has been accumulated with this material.[1,11,18,19] The general conclusions of this experience are that the material shows great promise, is easy to work with, and survives multiple punctures and even localized infections. It is not superior to autogenous tissue, however.

POLYTETRAFLUOROETHYLENE AS A VENOUS SUBSTITUTE

Early reports of use of PTFE for segmental replacement of the superior and inferior vena cava, portal and external iliac veins attracted many vascular surgeons to this material.[16,25,30,31] The report by Norton and Eiseman[25] indicated that replacement of the portal vein was possible in three cases of pancreatic carcinoma in man. This was particularly encouraging. In contrast, experimental venous replacement indicated that PTFE was not reliably useful.[12] In fact, in this report, all prosthetic grafts failed within 24 to 48 hours. Nevertheless, in Europe, Vollmar has used PTFE in venous replacement and recently in the United States, a long synthetic PTFE graft has been used as an extra-anatomic bypass of an iliac vein obstruction secondary to recurrent thrombophlebitis.[7] The graft remained patent during a 12-month period of observation. Clowes' conclusion was that the concept of long-term patency of venous grafts might be improved by deliberate insertion of a temporary distal arteriovenous fistula. As direct venous reconstruction is contemplated, this report becomes important.

CONCLUSION

It is noteworthy that not one investigator using PTFE as a femoropopliteal prosthesis advocates that this be the graft material of choice. All acknowledge that autogenous saphenous vein is superior, and none imply that in the usual circumstance, a prosthetic graft should be placed instead of an available autogenous saphenous vein. On the other hand, it is clear that a number of factors that are not related to graft material enter into failure of femoropopliteal grafting. In the modern experience, concomitant series of patients operated upon using autogenous saphenous vein in the femoropopliteal and tibial position and expanded PTFE grafts in the same location indicate that results up to 2 and 3 years are quite similar. The overall results of vein grafting in such situations are far inferior to the results obtained and reported by Darling and Linton in 1972.[8] The reasons for this are clear to surgeons performing vascular operations today. Indications for femoropopliteal arterial reconstruction at the present time are limited to limb salvage situations or relief of severe intermittent claudication. This was not true during the late 1960s, when the series of Darling and Linton was accumulated.

An important report by Donaldson and Mannick[9] suggests that indications for femoropopliteal bypass may be broadened in the future. In their report of 43 consecutive patients undergoing 51 femoropopliteal arterial reconstructions for claudication alone, all patients experienced relief of symptoms, there was no operative mortality, and there was only one case of immediate graft failure. Cumulative graft patency was 93 percent at 2 years and 88 percent at 5 years, despite the fact that 11 prostheses and one composite prosthesis and vein graft were used in these 51 procedures.

In the past, indications for femoropopliteal reconstruction have become restricted to some extent because of the acknowledged short life expectancy of patients with arteriosclerotic disease causing femoropopliteal occlusion. Yet, Bloor in the Hunterian Lecture of 1960 indicated that patients with femoropopliteal occlusive disease who were 35 to 44 years of age had a 91.8 percent 5-year life expectancy, and those who were 10 years older had a 79 percent 5-year life expectancy. In contrast, those patients over 65 had approximately a 50 percent 5-year life expectancy. These facts suggest that, in the future, indications for femoropopliteal bypass may very well be broadened, especially in situations in which an autogenous saphenous vein is available.

Since the final long-term results of grafting to the femoropopliteal segment with expanded PTFE grafts are not available, it is wise to withhold judgment on the ultimate place of this material. On the other hand, its admirable results in extra-anatomic locations and its unique characteristics that allow easy thrombectomy make it appear to be the ideal graft for extra-anatomic bypassing.

REFERENCES

1. Butler HG III, Baker LD Jr, Johnson JM: Vascular access for chronic hemodialysis: Polytetrafluoroethylene (PTFE) versus bovine heterograft. Am J Surg 134:791, 1977
2. Burnham SJ, Flanigan DP, Goodreau JJ, Yao JST, Bergan JJ: Non-vein bypass in below-knee reoperation for lower limb ischemia. Surgery 84:417, 1978
3. Campbell CD, Brooks DH, Webster MW, Bahnson HT: The use of expanded microporous polytetrafluoroethylene for limb salvage: A preliminary report. Surgery 79:485, 1976
4. Campbell CD, Brooks DH, Webster MW, et al.: Expanded microporous polytetrafluoroethylene as a vascular substitute: A two year follow-up. Surgery 85:177–183, 1979.
5. Campbell CD, Goldfarb D, Detton DD, et al.: Expanded polytetrafluoroethylene as a small artery substitute. Trans Am Soc Artif Int Organs 20:86, 1974
6. Campbell CD, Goldfarb D, Roe R: A small arterial substitute: Expanded microporous polytetrafluoroethylene: Patency versus porosity. Ann Surg 182:138, 1975

7. Clowes AW: Extra-anatomical bypass of iliac vein obstruction. Use of a synthetic (expanded polytetrafluoroethylene [Gore-tex]) graft. Arch Surg 115:767, 1980
8. Darling RC, Linton RR: Durability of femoropopliteal reconstructions: endarterectomy versus vein bypass grafts. Am J Surg 123:472, 1972
9. Donaldson MC, Mannick JA: Femoropopliteal bypass grafting for intermittent claudication. Is pessimism warranted? Arch Surg 115:724, 1980
10. Edwards WH, Mulherin JL Jr: The role of graft material in femorotibial bypass grafts. Ann Surg 191:721, 1980
11. Elliott MP, Gazzaniga AB, Thomas JM, Haiduc NJ, Rosen SM: Use of expanded polytetrafluoroethylene grafts for vascular access in hemodialysis: Laboratory and clinical evaluation. Am Surg 43:455, 1977
12. Faulkner RT, Cowan GSM Jr, Rothouse L: Early failure of expanded polytetrafluoroethyelene in femoral vein replacement. Arch Surg 114:939, 1979
13. Fletcher JP, Little JM, Loewenthal J, et al.: Initial experience with polytetrafluoroethylene for extra-anatomic bypass. Am J Surg 139:696, 1980
14. Flinn WR, Flanigan DP, Verta MJ Jr, Bergan JJ, Yao JST: Sequential femoral-tibial bypass for severe limb ischemia. Surgery 88:357, 1980
15. Florian A, Cohn LH, Dammin GJ, Collins JJ Jr: Small vessel replacement with Gore-Tex (expanded polytetrafluoroethylene). Arch Surg 111:267, 1976
16. Fujiwara Y, Cohn LH, Adams D, Collins JJ: Use of Gore-tex grafts for replacement of the superior and inferior vena cava. J Thorac Cardiovasc Surg 67:774, 1974
17. Gregory RT, Wheeler JR, Hurwitz RL: PTFE graft lower extremity arterial reconstruction. Presented to Michael E. DeBakey International Cardiovascular Society, Houston, Texas, Oct. 12–14, 1978
18. Haimov M: Clinical experience with the expanded polytetrafluoroethylene vascular prosthesis. Angiology 29:1, 1978
19. Haimov M, Giron F, Jacobson JH II: The expanded polytetrafluoroethylene graft. Three years' experience with 362 grafts. Arch Surg 114:673, 1979
20. Hallett JW, Brewster DC, Darling RC: Polytetrafluoroethyelene femoropopliteal and tibial arterial reconstruction: A three year experience. Personal communication.
21. Hastings OM, Jain KM, Hobson RW II, Swan KG: A prospective randomized study of three expanded polytetrafluoroethyelene (PTFE) grafts as small arterial substitutes. Ann Surg 188:743, 1978
22. Hobson RW II, O'Donnell JA, Jamil Z, Mehta K: Below-knee bypass for limb salvage. Comparison of autogenous saphenous vein, polytetrafluoroethylene and composite Dacron-autogenous vein grafts. Arch Surg 115:833, 1980
23. Keshishian JM: Intimal hyperplasia and the PTFE graft. Surgery 87:475, 1980
24. Matsumoto H, Fuse K, Yamamoto M, Hasegawa T, Saigusa M: Studies on the porous polytetrafluoroethylene as the vascular prosthesis. Jinkosoki (Japan) 1:44, 1972. A new vascular prosthesis for a small caliber artery. Surgery 74:519, 1973

25. Norton L, Eiseman B: Replacement of portal vein during pancreatectomy for carcinoma. Surgery 77:280, 1975
26. O'Mara CS, Flinn WR, Neiman HL, Bergan JJ, Yao JST: Correlation of foot arterial anatomy with early tibial bypass patency. Accepted for presentation, Midwestern Vascular Surgical Society Annual Meeting, Cincinnati, Sept. 26–27, 1980
27. O'Mara CS, Flinn WR, Johnson ND, Bergan JJ, Yao JST: Recognition and surgical management of patent but hemodynamically failed arterial grafts. Submitted for publication.
28. Raithel D, Groitl H: Small artery reconstruction with a new vascular prosthesis. World J Surg 4:223, 1980
29. Roberts AK, Johnson N: Aneurysm formation in an expanded microporous polytetrafluoroethylene graft. Arch Surg 113:211, 1978
30. Smith DE, Hammon J, Anane-Sefah J, Richardson RS, Trimble C: Segmental venous replacement. J Thorac Cardiovasc Surg 69:589, 1975
31. Soyer T, Lempinen M, Cooper P, Norton L, Eiseman B: A new venous prosthesis. Surgery 72:864, 1972
32. Veith FJ, Gupta S, Daly V: Management of early and late thrombosis of expanded polytetrafluorethylene (PTFE) femoropopliteal bypass grafts: Favorable prognosis with appropriate reoperation. Surgery 87:581, 1980
33. Veith FJ, Gupta S, Daly V, et al.: Three-year experience with expanded polytetrafluoroethylene (PTFE) grafts in arterial reconstructions for limb salvage. Presented to XIV World Congress International Cardiovascular Society, San Francisco, Ca., Sept., 1979, Am J Surg 140:214, 1980
34. Veith FJ, Moss CM, Fell SC, et al.: Comparison of expanded polytetrafluoroethylene and autologous saphenous vein grafts in high risk arterial reconstructions for limb salvage. Surg Gynecol Obstet 147:749, 1978
35. Veith FJ, Moss CM, Fell SC, Rhodes BA, Haimovici H: Comparison of expanded PTFE and vein grafts in lower extremity arterial reconstructions. J Cardiovasc Surg 19:341, 1978
36. Veith FJ, Moss CM, Fell SC, et al.: Expanded polytetrafluoroethylene grafts in reconstructive arterial surgery. Preliminary report of the first 110 consecutive cases for limb salvage. JAMA 240:1867, 1978

SEVEN

Update on Polytetrafluoroethylene Vascular Grafts II

Horace C. Stansel, Jr.

Polytetrafluoroethylene (PTFE) was first used as vascular grafts in 1972 by Soyer and his associates[9] for experimental venous replacement. In 1973, Matsumoto[6] reported on the use of PTFE grafts for replacement of small caliber arteries, and since that time, there has been an ever increasing number of reports on the use of this material for both venous and arterial substitutes as well as for a variety of other applications. Early enthusiastic reports on the success of the material is a vascular replacement have prompted what has probably been excessive clinical usage of PTFE grafts without adequate experimental data as justification.

A typical enthusiastic early report was that of Haimov[2] who reported the use of PTFE grafts in 13 patients who had femoropopliteal or femorotibial bypasses. In his study, 71 percent of femoropopliteal bypasses and 1 of 3 femorotibial bypasses remained open for 6 to 18 months. Later the same author[3] reported 184 PTFE grafts used as femoropopliteal reconstructions with 74 percent patency at the end of the first year and 58 percent patency at the end of the second and third year of observation. Seventeen grafts used for femorotibial bypasses had a patency rate of 40 percent at the end of 1 year. A similar report by Burnham and his associates in 1978,[1] describes 47 PTFE reconstructions to the below-knee popliteal artery with a patency rate of 65 percent at 26 months. Similar results have now been reported by many authors,[5,11,12] and it is apparent that there is general agreement that the immediate and short-term results with PTFE grafts to the popliteal artery below the knee closely approach those of autogenous saphenous vein femoropopliteal reconstructions.

CORONARY BYPASS GRAFTING

Use of PTFE in coronary bypass grafting has been reported with short-term follow-ups in a small group of humans. In 1978, Moline and his colleagues[7] reported on the use of PTFE to revascularize the right coronary artery, and the graft was shown to be patent by arteriography 3 months postoperatively. Yokoyama and his associates[14] reported five patients in which PTFE was used as coronary artery bypass grafts. All patients were alive approximately 1 year postoperatively, and 3 to 6 months postoperatively showed that four of the grafts were open.

Hancock and associates[4] at the Mayo Clinic have reported on the experimental results with PTFE grafts in dogs. In an interesting experiment, they bypassed segments of coronary arteries with 7-cm lengths of 4-mm PTFE (Gore-Tex) grafts in 42 animals. They divided these into two groups, one of which was given antiplatelet drugs, dipyridamole and aspirin in a dose of 30 mg per kg per day. Every graft closed in the group of animals that were treated without antiplatelet drugs. Of the animals treated with antiplatelet drugs, however, 64 percent had patent grafts at 1 month.

Szilagyi and associates[10] reported the use of Gore-Tex grafts between the aorta and circumflex coronary artery in two dogs. One animal was given Dicumarol and aspirin for 7 days, preoperatively and postoperatively, as well as warfarin, the latter being continued for 2 months. The nonanticoagulated dog died 3 days postoperatively with an occluded graft while the treated animal had a patent graft for 9 days by arteriography, but the graft had become occluded at the time of subsequent arteriography 54 days after operation.

VENOUS GRAFTS

The hallmark of success of any vascular graft is, of course, the capability of serving effectively for the replacement of segments of the venous system. Although the initial reports on the use of PTFE were those of Soyer and his colleagues[4] who described the replacement of segments of the venous system, there are now a number of reports that detail the use of this material as a venous graft to replace segments of the superior and inferior vena cava, the portal vein and other segments of the venous bed. A report by Smith and his associates[8] describes an 83 percent short-term patency rate for replacement of the inferior vena cava in dogs. No anticoagulants were used in the study, and, although the follow-up was relatively short, these results are highly encouraging in view of the previous high failure rate with other materials in this position. Despite these encouraging findings and a few favorable case reports, the value of PTFE grafts as venous replacements remains uncertain. More work must be done before the role of this type of graft in the venous system becomes clear.

DIALYSIS ACCESS

PTFE is being widely used to construct arteriovenous fistulae for dialysis access. Early trials have been encouraging, and many institutions are using the material almost exclusively when a graft is required. For this application, PTFE grafts have the advantage of ready availability. This probably outweighs the risk of increased infectibility, and PTFE grafts will probably continue to be used widely for this purpose in appropriate patients in whom a primary fistula cannot be constructed.

ARTERIAL REPLACEMENTS

It is obvious that the PTFE graft has many characteristics that approach the ideal arterial replacement. It is a heat-stable material that can be sterilized by a variety of techniques. It can obviously be stored at room temperature indefinitely. It comes in a variety of sizes that closely match almost any artery that the surgeon desires to reconstruct. It is easy to handle and is easier to sew than most of the fabric gafts. It is also easy to tear the material if one is rough in passing the needle through the graft wall, but with a little caution, this is not a problem. Preclotting is not required because the material is impervious to blood even in a totally heparinized patient. With all of these attractive features, one wonders why PTFE grafts have not completely replaced the autogenous saphenous vein as the best graft material.

The answer to this question can be found in the continued follow-up of patients in whom PTFE grafts have been used. We have made certain observations at the Yale-New Haven Medical Center where we have been enthusiastic users of the material as an arterial graft. At the present time, we have used PTFE grafts in reconstructive procedures for congenital heart disease (Blalock-Taussig shunts, interrupted aortic arch, or reconstructions of coarctations and a variety of other cardiac defects). In this experience which now extends over 5 years with 165 patients, we have only had one graft failure and this was almost certainly related to a technical problem.

We have also had considerable experience in the use of PTFE grafts in peripheral arterial reconstructions. Here too the initial results were quite encouraging. As these grafts have been followed for extended periods of time, however, the attrition rate becomes apparent. Indeed, of the more than 100 grafts that were used for femoropopliteal or femorotibial reconstruction, the failure rate at 3 years is approximately 80 percent:

Patency (%)	Duration (months)
85	12
60	18
50	24
40	30
20	36

Therefore, at least in our hands, while the initial patency rate during the first few months approach those of the saphenous vein there is an extremely high closure rate with continued follow-up. It should be recognized that the majority of the femoropopliteal PTFE grafts in our early experiences were reoperations and generally in patients with more advanced disease. It is also of interest that this extremely high closure rate only occurred in those long PTFE grafts that were anastomosed to small run-off vessels. When PTFE grafts were used in the chest, as in a Blalock-Taussig procedure or as a replacement for a portion of the aorta, we have not seen any failures. The difference between these two situations is, first, the length of the graft and, second, the size of the distal run-off vessel. If the run-off vessel is small and the graft is long, stasis within the graft is more likely. This may be a factor in producing graft failure.

Watanabe[13] has recently reported an interesting experiment in which grafts of PTFE with an inside diameter of 1.5 mm were used to replace the femoral artery in rabbits. He tested different anastomotic techniques including a telescoping technique in which the artery was placed inside the PTFE avoiding exposure of the cut end of the graft. He concluded that the important characteristics of the PTFE graft were its fibril length, the relative diameters of the host artery and prosthesis, and the method of anastomosis. He postulated that to minimize thrombosis it was important to avoid exposure of the PTFE material at the cut end of the graft as opposed to the surface of the graft. Whether this is true or not and whether PTFE at the cut end of the graft differs in thrombogenicity from PTFE surface material remains to be proven.

CLOSURE INDEX

It is now obvious to all that under certain conditions PTFE grafts work exceedingly well with high patency rates approaching or equal to those of the autogenous saphenous vein. In an effort to better understand why some authors have reported exceedingly high patency rates with PTFE and other authors have reported much less favorable results, we have studied in detail a large group of patients in our institution. This study has attempted to determine the factors that play an important role in long-term graft patency. The study has involved the measurement and evaluation on arteriograms of the run-off bed and the length of the graft necessary to bypass the occluded arterial segment.

Standard 40-inch arteriograms were evaluated in all patients. The popliteal run-off has been identified as "good" when the popliteal artery appeared relatively normal with at least one normal run-off artery coursing the entire length of the calf. In the case of femorotibial bypass, only those bypasses into what appeared to be "normal" tibial arteries were evaluated. The length of the graft, whether it be PTFE or autogenous saphenous vein, was determined from the operative note or from postoperative arteriograms that were available on at least 75 percent of our patients. It was then possible to derive a simple formula that appears to have a very high reliability in predicting the failure rate of most bypass grafts.

This equation, which includes the diameter of the graft, the length of the graft, and the diameter of the run-off vessel at the distal anastomosis, yields what we have termed the *closure index*. This value is obtained for PTFE grafts by multiplying the diameter of the graft in millimeters times the length of the graft in centimeters and dividing the result by the diameter of the run-off artery in millimeters as measured on a 40-inch arteriogram:

$$\frac{\text{Graft diameter (mm)} \times \text{graft length (cm)}}{\text{Run-off diameter (mm)}} = \text{Closure index}$$

If autogenous saphenous vein is used, the diameter of the run-off artery is multiplied by 2:

$$\frac{\text{Graft diameter (mm)} \times \text{graft length (cm)}}{\text{Run-off diameter (mm)} \times 2} = \text{Closure index}$$

It has been our observation that when the closure index exceeds 100, one can expect at least 90 percent of the grafts to be closed within 2 years. On the other hand, when the index is less than 50, it is likely that no graft will close over a 2-year period.

We find this index to be a very useful tool by which one can decide preoperatively whether to use PTFE grafts or whether the autogenous saphenous vein should be the graft material. When the length of the graft is short and the diameter of the run-off vessel is large as in intracavitary grafts, the closure index will always be below 100. This correlates with our experience that intracavitary PTFE grafts can be expected to stay patent indefinitely. On the other hand, when it is necessary to use a long PTFE graft and anastomose it to a 1 to 2 mm diameter run-off vessel, stasis due to the single run-off vessel and an extremely long graft will, in the vast majority of our patients, lead to early closure. In these circumstances, the closure index will be higher than 100 if PTFE is the graft material. If saphenous vein is used, however, the closure index will often be less than 100, and many such grafts will remain patent.

We therefore believe that the closure index will provide the surgeon with a preoperative guide that may be helpful in selecting those patients in whom PTFE grafts are likely to give good long-term results. However, the validity and exact role of this index have yet to be determined.

Editor's Note: Several questions regarding PTFE grafts remain to be answered. Long-term (i.e., 5-year) results with this graft are not available in significant numbers of patients. The reasons for discrepancies in reported results from different groups are unclear. Differences in case selection and surgical techniques may be important but other factors may play a role as well. The relative role of PTFE grafts in arterial surgery and the efficacy of this material in comparison to autologous saphenous vein and other prosthetic grafts will only be known when prospective randomized, controlled, and refereed studies are available to settle these issues.

REFERENCES

1. Burnham SJ, Flanigan DP, Goodreau JJ, et al: Non-vein bypass in below-knee reoperation for lower limb ischemia. Surgery 84:417, 1978
2. Haimov M: Clinical experience with the expanded polytetrafluoroethylene vascular prosthesis. Angiology 29:6, 1978
3. Haimov H, Giron F, Jacobson JH II: The expanded polytetrafluoroethylene graft. Arch Surg 114:673, 1970
4. Hancock JB, Forshaw PL, Kaye MP: Gore-Tex (polytetrafluoroethylene) in canine coronary artery bypass. J Thorac Cardiovasc Surg 80:94, 1980
5. Hearn AR, Charlesworth D: The early results of reconstruction of the femoral artery with a GORE-TEX prosthesis. Surgery 85:607, 1979
6. Matsumoto H, Hasegawa T, Fuse K, et al: A new vascular prosthesis for a small caliber artery. Surgery 74:519, 1973
7. Moline JE, Carr M, Yarnoz MD: Coronary bypass with Gore-Tex graft. J Thorac Cardiovasc Surg 75:769, 1978
8. Smith DE, Hammon A, Anane-Sefah J, et al: Segmental venous replacement:

a comparison of biological and synthetic substitutes. J Thorac Cardiovasc Surg 69:589, 1975
9. Soyer T, Lempinen M, Cooper P, et al: A new venous prosthesis. Surgery 72:864, 1972
10. Szilagyi DE, Hageman JH, Smith RF, et al: Autogenous vein grafting in femoropopliteal atherosclerosis; the limits of its effectiveness. Surgery 86:836, 1979
11. Veith FJ, Moss CM, Daly V, et al: New approaches to limb salvage by extended extra-anatomic bypasses and prosthetic reconstructions to foot arteries. Surgery 84:764, 1978
12. Veith FJ, Moss CM, Fell SC, et al: Comparison of expanded polytetralfuoroethylene autologous saphenous vein grafts in high risk arterial reconstructions for limb salvage. Surg Gynecol Obstet 147:205, 1978
13. Watanabe K: Microarterial prostheses of expanded polytetrafluoroethylene. J Microsurg 2:11, 1980
14. Yokoyama T, Gharavi MA, Lee YC, et al: Aorta-coronary revascularization with an expanded polytetrafluoroethylene vascular graft. J Thorac Cardiovasc Surg 76:552, 1978

Part Two
Graft Failures

EIGHT

Pathogenesis and Prevention of Intimal Hyperplasia

Anthony M. Imparato and F. Gregory Baumann

Intimal and neointimal fibroplasia that occur in arterial reconstructions are frequently ascribed to technical factors in the handling of vein grafts, to reaction to the performance of endarterectomy, or to suture line reaction usually at distal anastomoses.[1,4,6,8,23] Thrombus deposition may occur at suture lines, subsequently become organized, and thereafter progress to sufficient fibrous proliferation to result in occlusion of arterial reconstructions. This reaction, however, in many instances can probably be prevented by careful surgical technique to produce smooth, non-flow-obstructing suture lines and perhaps by the use of anticoagulants in the postoperative period. The similarity of these proliferative lesions, however, to spontaneously occurring fibromuscular intimal plaques, which are probably precursors to frank atherosclerosis, demand consideration of evidence supporting the idea that alterations in blood flow are related to the initiation of intimal fibromuscular lesions.[18] The following clinical and experimental considerations tend to support this concept.

Since 1962 approximately 75 early and more than 80 of the late failures in a series of approximately 5000 human arterial reconstructions including both endarterectomy and bypass operations at various sites have been systematically explored. The mechanism of failure was established by searching for the characteristic gray thrombus that forms while blood still flows, as opposed to the red or dark stasis clot that forms after blood flow has ceased. Flow thrombus was usually encountered at sites of stenosis. It was concluded that approximately 50 percent of the late

Supported by grants #NIH-HL-16290, HL22783, HL22766, HL-27784.

failures of arterial reconstructions were due to inappropriately exuberant intimal or neointimal fibroplasia in some segment of the reconstruction, while the remainder were due to progression of the atherosclerotic disease proximal or distal to the reconstruction.[18]

Analysis of early postoperative angiograms of the distribution of the hyperplastic lesions found at surgical exploration, of the microscopic appearance of hyperplastic lesions, and of the configurations of bypass grafts led to the conclusion that hemodynamic factors played a major role in the development of intimal and neointimal hyperplasia leading to failure. The distribution of obstructing lesions in venous grafts were often similar to the localization of spontaneously occurring atherosclerotic plaques; namely, at ostia, at accentuated curvatures, and at sites of taper. A few failures could be ascribed to proliferation of venous valve leaflets. A puzzling aspect was that successful arterial reconstructions with low volume flow and decreased flow velocity because of occlusions distal to the reconstructions were also subject to failure from intimal or neointimal hyperplasia. This was especially apparent in long open endarterectomy segments of the femoral and popliteal arteries with long vein roof patches in which flow was angiographically determined to be extremely slow. In these patients, lesions were found at two sites: at the terminal taper where the velocity was postulated to be greatest, and at the midportions of the endarterectomized vessels where slow flow was angiographically apparent. Failure, however, was never encountered at the common femoral artery roof patch site while it was at the origin of the profunda femoris artery. A single patient with an in situ saphenous vein bypass graft extending from the common femoral artery to the posterior tibial artery at the level of the malleolus, in whom a number of venous tributaries were permitted to remain patent to act as arteriovenous fistulae to improve flow through the graft, died 3 months after operation. The graft was recovered and found to have thickening in its most proximal portion where flow was greatest and no thickening in the most distal portion where flow appeared to be least.

The role of disordered flow patterns in this process was further emphasized by the observations upon patients with end stage kidney failure with arteriovenous fistulae created in the forearms for dialysis access. Late closures occurred in some while others remained patent for years. Intimal fibroplasia was found in those late failures that could be examined. On the other hand, the combinations of stenosis and aneurysm formation sometimes found in arteriovenous fistulae suggest that highly specific hemodynamic conditions are required for the occurrence of each and that either condition may occur with excessive flow.[27]

The lesion has been found in aortocoronary reversed bypass grafts with no clear-cut correlation with recorded intraoperative flows in the grafts, which indicates the complex nature of intimal fibroplasia.[23] Our laboratory has noted that intimal fibroplasia can occur in some internal mammary arteries implanted directly into the ventricular myocardium by the technique of Vineberg.[34] Furthermore, the long-term patency of arterial reconstructions is not related to the integrity of the outflow tract at the time of the arterial reconstruction.[21] Persons with totally unimpaired outflow tracts appear to have no greater likelihood of maintaining long-term patency than those with markedly impaired outflow tracts. Although this is not universally accepted, it has been confirmed by Szilagyi and many others for the extremities and for coronary bypass grafts as well.[6,31]

That intimal hyperplasia can occur in the body of one of paired bypass grafts to either both kidneys or both lower extremities is confusing. This attests to the probable role of local hemodynamic factors rather than to metabolic systemic disorders in the complex pathogenesis of this lesion.

On the other hand, comparisons of the morphology of intimal and neointimal hyperplasia with spontaneously occurring atherosclerosis in the same patients show definite similarities.[18] These in turn are remarkably similar to the atherosclerotic plaques removed surgically from the carotid bifurcations of patients with cerebrovascular insufficiency syndromes.[22] Autologous saphenous vein grafts removed years after operation may show frank atherosclerosis with compound plaques.[8] Because of these considerations, the metabolic disorders that show some correlation with spontaneously occurring atherosclerosis require consideration in the pathogenesis of neointimal hyperplasia. Attempts to relate lipid profiles of patients undergoing arterial reconstructions with long-term outcome do not show a close correlation. Furthermore in spite of the recognized relationship between atherosclerosis and diabetes mellitus, it is not entirely clear that the late failure of arterial reconstruction due to intimal hyperplasia occurs more frequently in the diabetic than in the nondiabetic.[21] On the other hand, psoriasis in our group of patients appears to have an adverse effect on long-term patency. Eight such carefully studied patients, who had successful arterial reconstructions for occlusive disease of the lower extremities, failed to maintain patency for more than 1 year. Moreover, lesions closely resembling the intimal fibroplasia occurring in arterial reconstructions have been found in patients who have been on long-term corticosteroid therapy.[28] It is not entirely clear, however, whether the lesions represent the natural consequence of the underlying disease or are related to therapy. Last, the progress of atherosclerosis and the failure rate of arterial reconstructions have both had a positive correlation with continued cigarette smoking.

Although the basic question of whether the earliest spontaneously occurring arterial lesion that progresses to the universally recognized compound atherosclerotic plaque begins as a fatty streak or as a fibrous plaque has not been answered definitively, the circumstantial evidence pointing to the fibromuscular intimal plaque as the primary precursor is strong.[13,16,22,26] The relationship of surgically occurring fibromuscular intimal or neointimal hyperplasia to the probable mode of evolution of atherosclerosis is also strongly supported. Brodie and his colleagues[6] have concluded that the electron microscopic appearance of late intimal thickening of vein grafts resembles atherosclerosis. Harden and his associates[16] also showed that intimal hyperplasia produced experimentally by immunologic stress in primates becomes fat laden on alteration of diet.

EXPERIMENTAL DATA

Although structural changes related to techniques of handling vein grafts can be demonstrated, these have not been correlated with the intimal proliferative changes noted in late graft failures. In the light of the self-limiting and spontaneously regressing nature of the proliferative lesions produced by forceful experimental balloon catheter trauma to the normal arterial wall,[30] it seems unlikely that such technical factors can be incriminated in the occlusions that occur months to years after operation and are a result of progressive segmental intimal thickening. It is more likely that such technical trauma results in early thrombotic failures. Late failures probably require the continued and repeated action of specific hemodynamic trauma.

Intimal hyperplasia has been experimentally produced by a variety of techniques, mainly in connection with investigations into the pathogenesis of atherosclerotic plaques. The similarity of the experimental intimal hyperplasia lesion and the lesions appearing in surgical vascular reconstructions warrants consideration of such data. Manipulations of blood vessels devised to alter vascular hemodynamics have been reported to result in intimal hyperplasia. These range from production of accentuated curvatures to production of sites of stenosis and external attachments of blood vessels to create points of fixation.[15,32] Double ligation of arteries as well as production of intimal injuries by either installation of chemical substances of an irritating nature or by stripping of intima from rabbit aortas with balloon catheters have resulted in this reaction.[16,30,33] Fry[12] has stated that intimal hyperplasia tends to occur at the sites of shear. Caro,[7] however, incriminates lack of shear. Fry has further attempted to refine the concept of shear stress leading to intimal hyperplasia by pointing out that different degrees of shear evoke different reactions, so that accentuated shear may lead to disruption of the arterial wall while lesser shear leads to endothelial stripping and fibromuscular intimal thickening. He also suggests that repeated loss of endothelial cells sets up a chronic tissue reaction resulting in marked intimal thickening.[12]

Other phenomena have been indicated, often by inference based upon hydraulic engineering principles, as occurring at sites of subsequent spontaneous intimal hyperplastic lesions and atherosclerosis. Wesolowski[36] has indicated turbulence. Texon[32] has implicated diminished lateral pressure. Gutstein[14] and LoGerfo[24] suggest boundary layer separation. Duguid[8] postulated that platelet adherence and subsequent formation of thrombus lead to fibrous organization that set the entire process in motion. Benditt[5] proposed a monoclonal theory to explain the proliferative lesion.

Metabolic alterations in experimental animals such as those that result in hypercholesterolemic states are followed by the appearance of subintimal fibrous plaques at sites of predilection for spontaneously occurring atherosclerosis. Numerous studies have attempted to relate the transport of material between the blood and the blood vessel wall and the intramural deposition of these materials to the inciting events in arterial lesion formation.[29] Ross and Glomset,[26] partly on the basis of studies of the response of arteries to balloon-catheter-induced injuries, conclude that the entire reaction of intimal fibrous proliferation results from endothelial desquamation. This is followed by platelet aggregation at the sites of desquamation.[26] The release of platelet factors and their permeation into the arterial wall along with plasma, lipoprotein, and other plasma constituents are thought to call forth the migration of smooth muscle cells from the media into the intima and their subsequent proliferation. These authors believe that this process produces a reversible lesion that might progress if trauma were repetitive. A compound atherosclerotic plaque then appears when secondary events such as hemorrhage into the plaques and calcification occur.

Our own experimental results employing hemodynamic models are not in complete agreement with Ross's formulation.[2,3,17,19,20] Although smooth muscle cell migration to the intimal site appears to be the critical factor in the formation of lesions, such migration occurs even before endothelial desquamation begins. If flow is unimpeded, platelet adherence to the specific sites of lesion formation is of short duration when it occurs at all. Smooth muscle cell mitoses have not been seen in any of the lesions examined in our hemodynamic models even after the administration of high doses of mitostatic drugs such as colchicine and vinblastine during the periods when large lesions are forming (Figs. 1–7). Figures 2 through 6 are a series of photomicrographs and electron

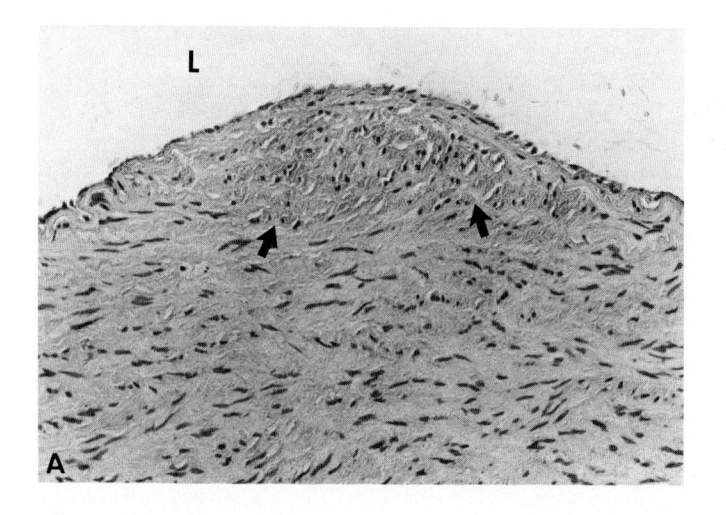

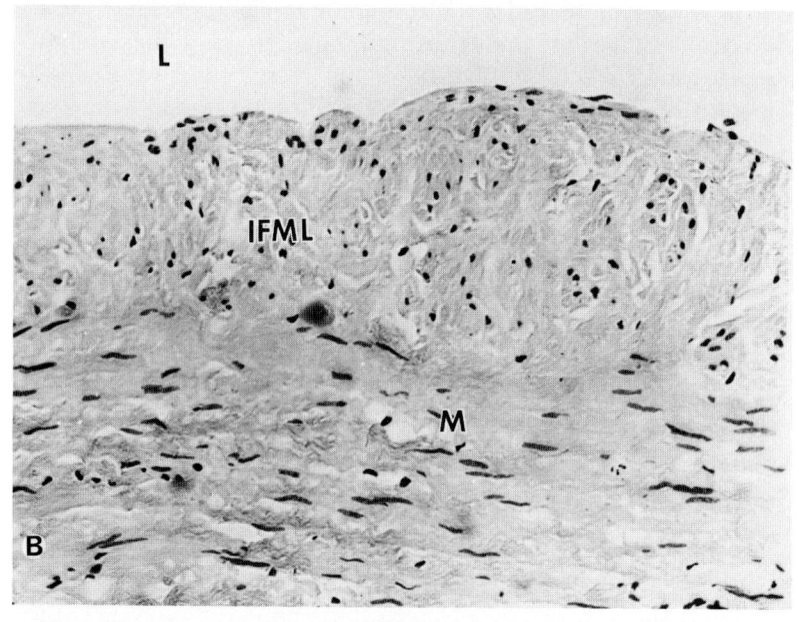

FIGURE 1. **A.** Photomicrograph of paraffin section showing discrete intimal fibromuscular lesion that has formed in a dog renal artery wall after 2 days of increased flow rate because of anastomosis of the distal renal artery to the inferior vena cava. Arrows indicate the line of demarcation between the normal arterial wall which contains circumferentially oriented smooth muscle cells and the lesion which contains longitudinally oriented smooth muscle cells. L, lumen. H&E stain ×138. **B.** Higher magnification photomicrograph of a similarly induced intimal fibromuscular lesion (IFML) in a dog renal artery after 1 week of increased flow rate. L, lumen; M, tunica media. H&E stain.

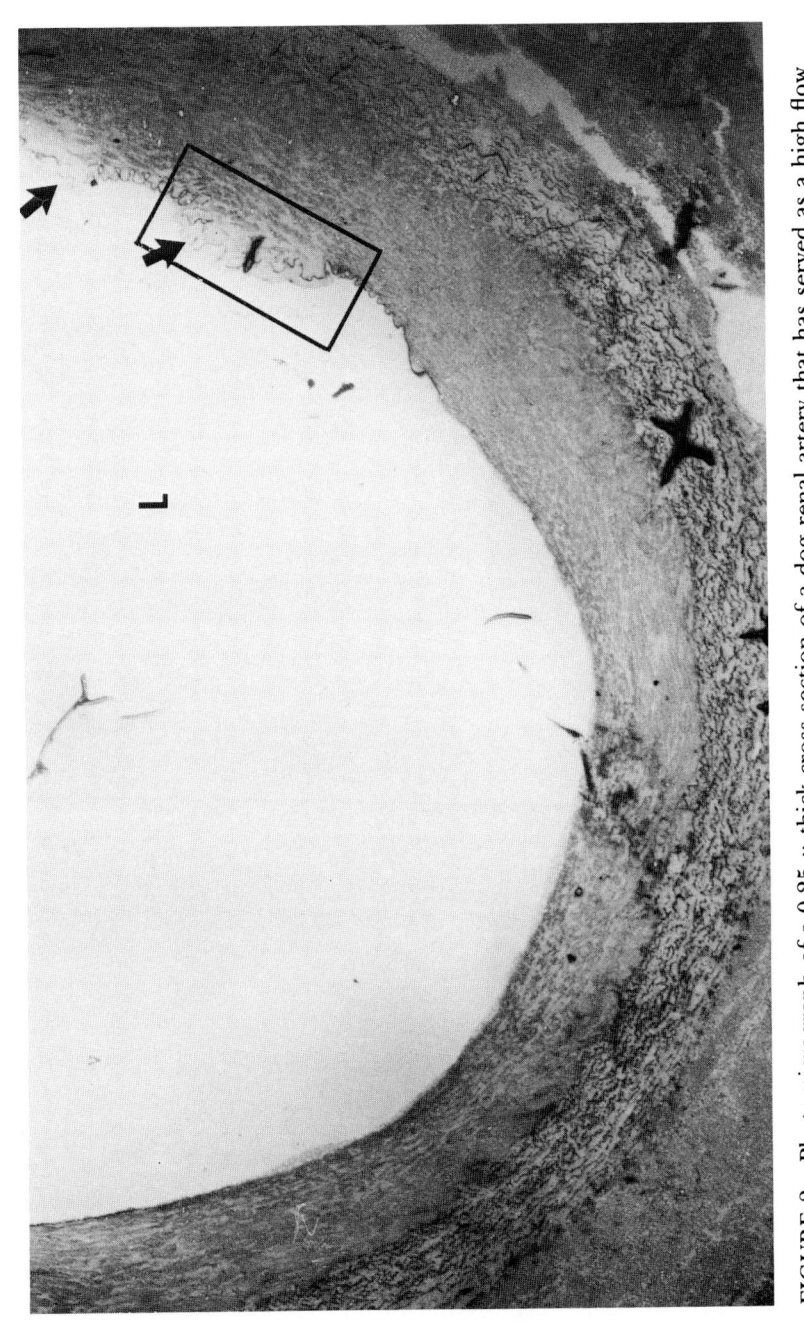

FIGURE 2. Photomicrograph of a 0.25-μ thick cross-section of a dog renal artery that has served as a high flow shunt for 2 hours. Intimal fibromuscular lesions are seen forming on the right (arrows). The lesion within the rectangle is shown at a higher magnification in the next figure. L, lumen. Polychrome stain ×90.

FIGURE 3. Higher magnification photomicrograph of lesion. Various stages in the development of a hemodynamically induced intimal fibromuscular lesion are demonstrated. The endothelium is mostly missing, the intima and inner media appear edematous, the darkly staining internal elastic lamina is broken, and reoriented modified smooth muscle cells are migrating into the intima (arrows). The area within the rectangle is shown at a higher magnification in the next figure. L, lumen. Polychrome stain ×390.

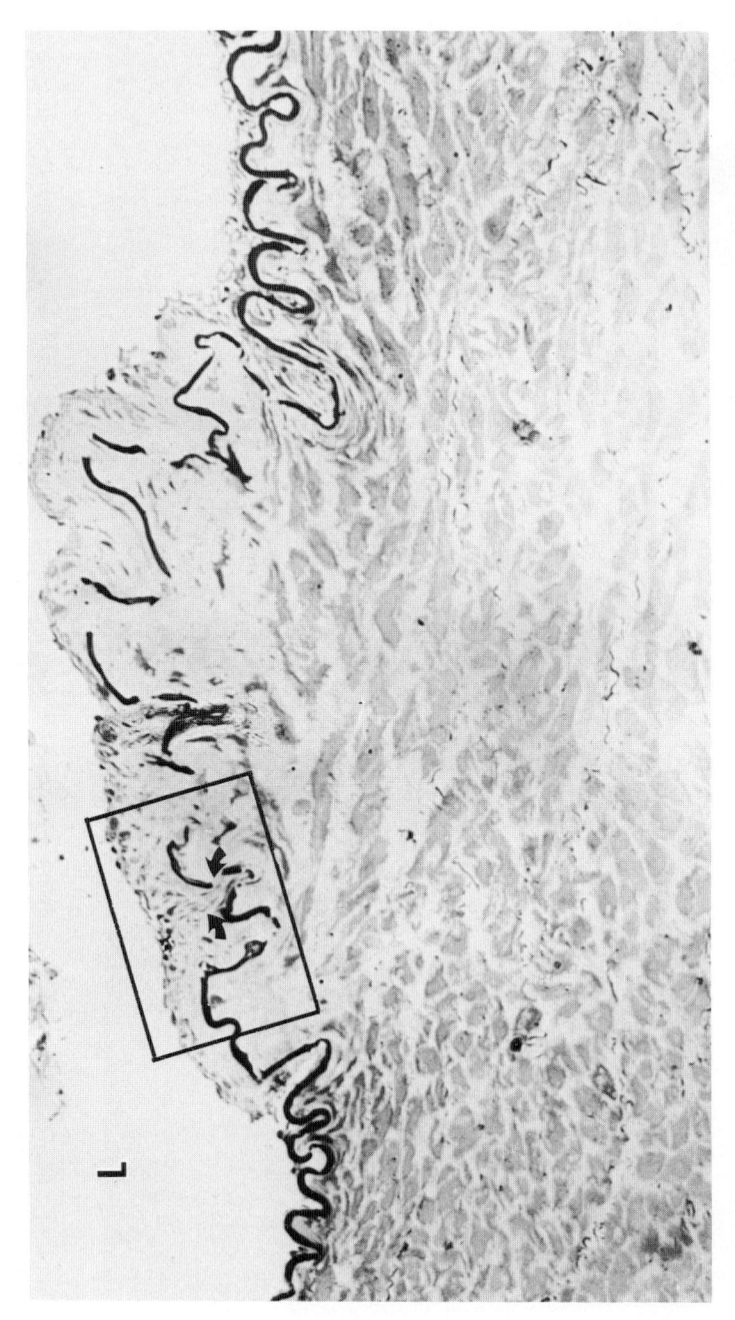

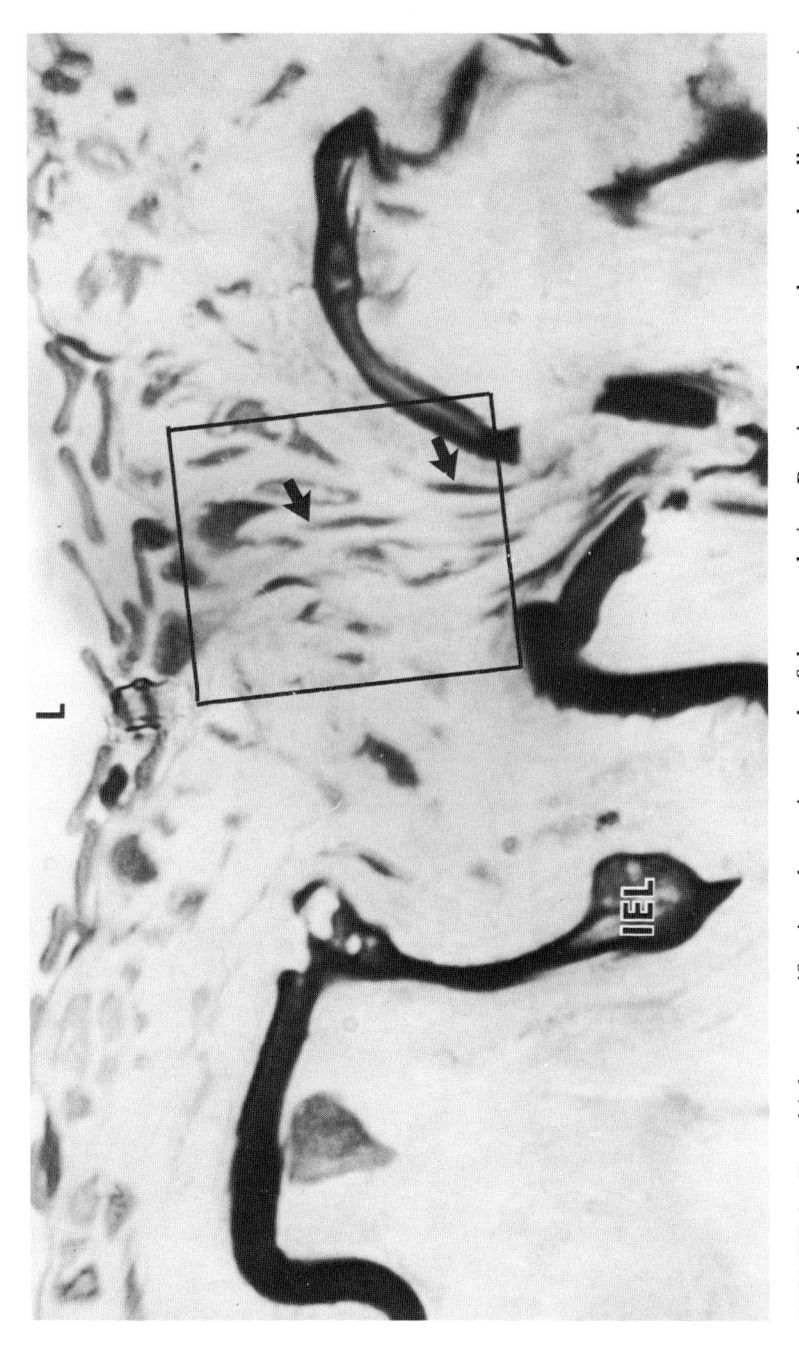

FIGURE 4. Even higher magnification photomicrograph of the same lesion. Reoriented smooth muscle cells (arrows) are passing through gaps in the degenerating internal elastic lamina (IEL) into the intima. The area within the rectangle is shown at a higher magnification in the next figure. L, lumen. Polychrome stain.

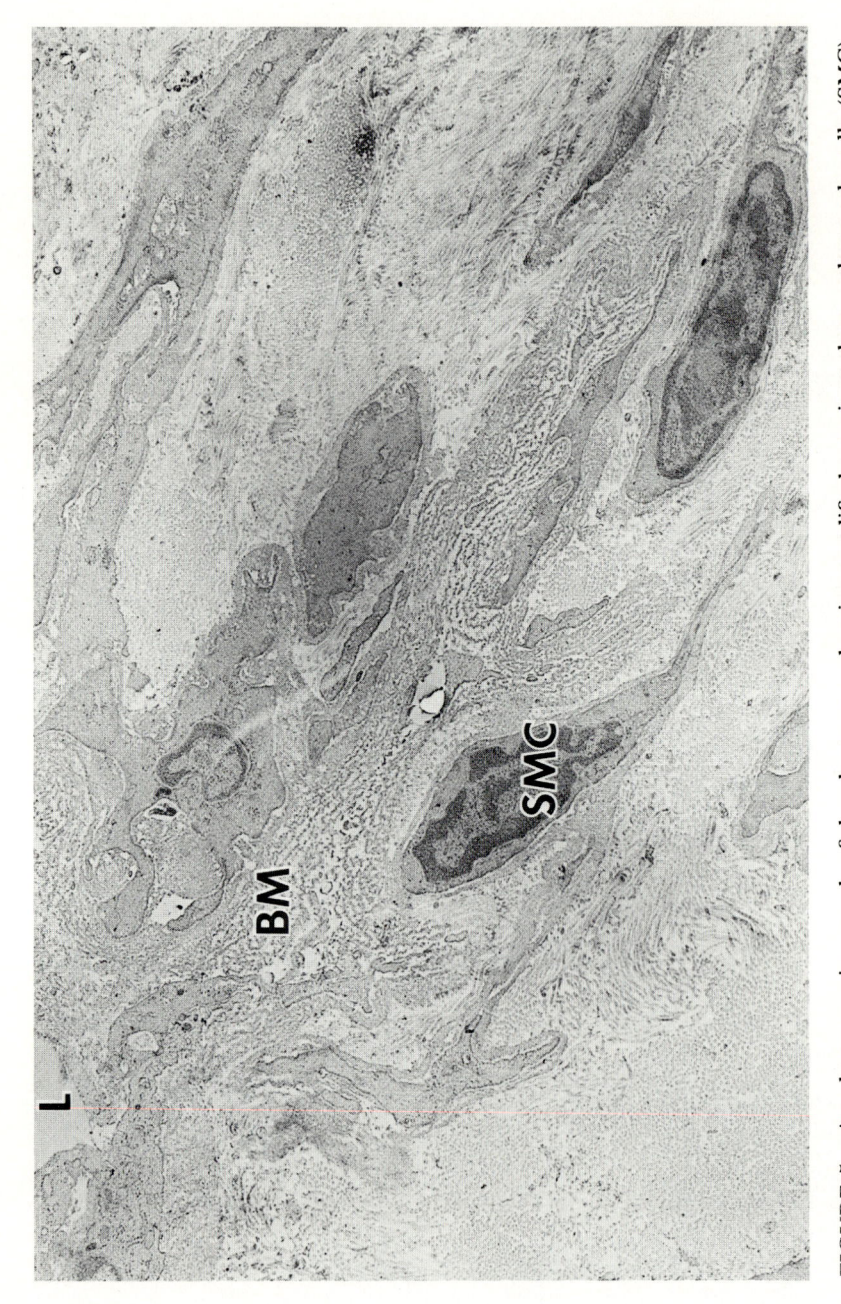

FIGURE 5. An electron micrograph of the above area showing modified, reoriented smooth muscle cells (SMC) passing into the intima. The subendothelial basement membrane (BM) is multilaminar and thickened. L, lumen. Uranyl acetate and lead citrate stain.

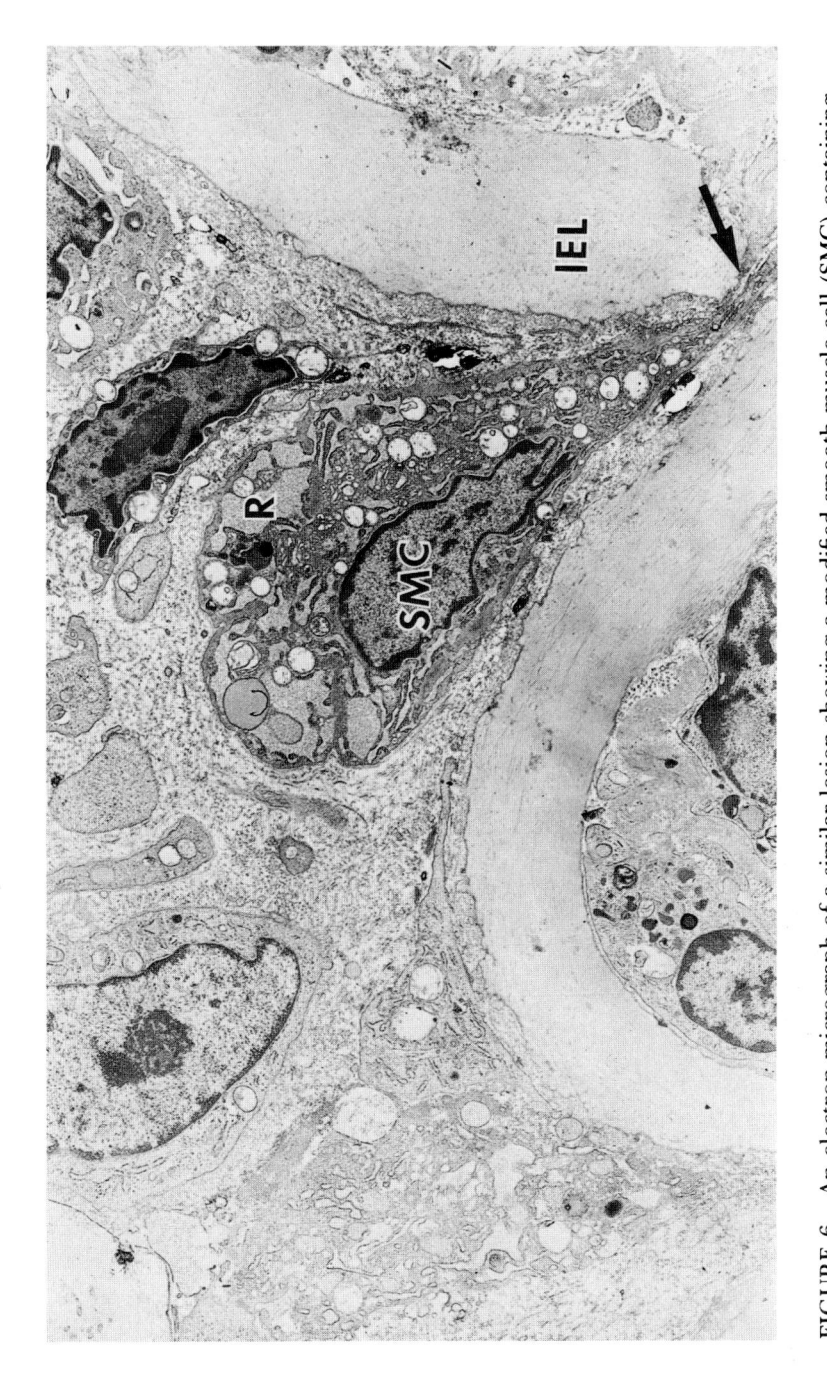

FIGURE 6. An electron micrograph of a similar lesion showing a modified smooth muscle cell (SMC) containing large amounts of rough endoplasmic reticulum (R) filled with granular electron-dense material. The smooth muscle cell is passing through a fenestration (arrow) in the internal elastic lamina (IEL). Uranyl acetate and lead citrate section.

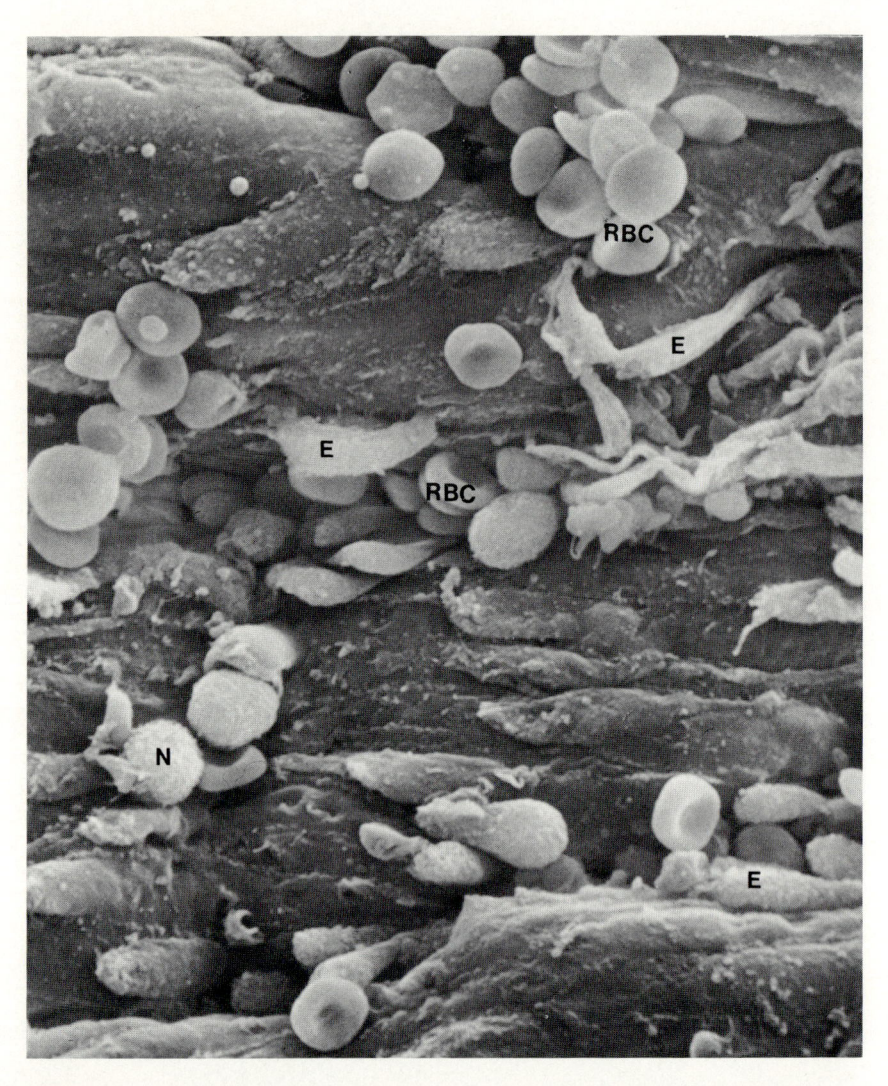

FIGURE 7. Scanning electron micrograph showing the luminal surface of a dog renal artery that has been exposed to high flow rates for 6 hours. The endothelial cells (E) are sloughing off the luminal surface. Some red blood cells (RBC) and neutrophils (N) are seen on the luminal surface, but few platelets are apparent.

micrographs of the same forming intimal fibromuscular lesion at successively higher magnifications.

Indeed, endarterectomy with removal of intima along with from one-half to the entire thickness of the media without alterations of flow usually fails to result in reorientation of residual smooth muscle cells or marked platelet adherence when studied sequentially from 2 hours to 3 weeks postoperatively. If flow is unimpeded, healing is initiated by the deposition of a thin layer of white blood cells often appearing as a monolayer. These eventually assume a flattened appearance when they are seen within the wall. As the arterial wall thickens, mitotic figures appear in the underlying smooth muscle cells. The long-term appearance of these vessels is still under observation. If, on the other hand, thrombus forms on the surface due to impaired flow, then the healing process is more complex and also involves the organization of the thrombus material with early marked thickening of the arterial wall. We still suspect from our experimental and clinical observations that when marked intimal hyperplasia occurs it does so in response to hemodynamic conditions (Fig. 8).

In accordance with the clinical observation that marked intimal or neointimal proliferation may occur in states of diminished flow, the experimental results of arterial ligations are also of interest. Weiss[35] shows that after 24 hours of arterial ligation the same progression of events was noted in other types of arterial wall injury. We noted the same progression in our accelerated flow models. The reaction is similar to that which occurs when intraluminal thrombi become organized. Our own observations on experimentally ligated arteries confirm this sequence of events and emphasize the probable role of hemodynamic factors in the distribution of the lesions proximal to ligatures. Locations and shapes of the lesions are quite characteristic for particular arteries ligated, being concentric in small vessels such as the carotid and eccentric in large ones such as the aorta and iliac arteries.

It is not unreasonable to postulate a final common pathway to explain initiation and progression of intimal fibromuscular lesions occurring under a variety of clinical and experimental situations. Our own observations, however, based upon hemodynamic experimental models that more closely simulate chronic conditions encountered in humans subjected to either surgical bypass procedures or spontaneously developing atherosclerosis, suggest that desquamation of endothelial cells as the prime initiating factor for intimal fibromuscular lesion formation has yet to be proven conclusively.

The available information regarding the response of the intima to trauma or stress suggests a similarity in the reaction of the blood vessel wall to a variety of seemingly different conditions that encompass too rapid or too slow flow, no flow, and mechanical trauma. This information does not shed any light on the reaction of an endarterectomized vessel to disordered flow states that may result in neointimal hyperplasia closely resembling the intimal hypertrophy in bypass grafts. Stripping of the intima and part or all of the media does not result in uniform and progressive hyperplasia, but rather in a relatively thin neointima that does not obstruct flow except at certain sites apparently specified by hemodynamic conditions. Full regeneration of a true intima with endothelium in humans in instances in which endarterectomy is performed from the level of the renal arteries to and including the proximal halves of the profoundafemoris artery seems unlikely. Yet, in spite of the altered permeability of the endarterectomized blood vessels resulting from the absence of a true endothelial cell lining, exuberant proliferation does not occur uniformly but rather only at particular sites. We have also recently noted that the similarity of the morphologic events leading to the normal closure of the ductus arteriosus and the development of fibromuscular intima hyperplasia are quite striking.[36] In the ductus arteriosus, the reorientation of the smooth muscle cells towards the lumen, their eventual migration in the presence of an apparently intact endothelium, and the apparent absence of mitoses are almost identical to the reaction of the adult arterial wall to alterations in flow.

Among the numerous observations made on the evolution of intimal proliferative plaques under varying experimental conditions, there seems to be uniform agreement that endothelial sloughing, fragmentation of the internal elastic membrane, and migration of smooth muscle cells to an intimal site occur. In spite of the proliferative appearance of the lesions, mitoses are rarely seen. It is not clear from any of the descriptions whether the first event in the pathogenesis of the lesions is endothelial sloughing and fragmentation of the internal elastic membrane or migration of smooth muscle cells with subsequent fragmentation of the internal elastic membrane and endothelial sloughing. The role of platelets appears to be in question. Scanning electron micrographs (Fig. 7) illustrate that, in our hemodynamic models for producing the lesion, endothelial sloughing can occur without the marked adherence of platelets if flow rates are adequate.

PREVENTION OF CLINICAL FIBROMUSCULAR INTIMAL HYPERPLASIA

It is small consolation to the operating surgeon that as yet uncontrollable hemodynamic factors may be responsible for the late failure of arterial reconstructions in a large percentage of patients and that indeed this

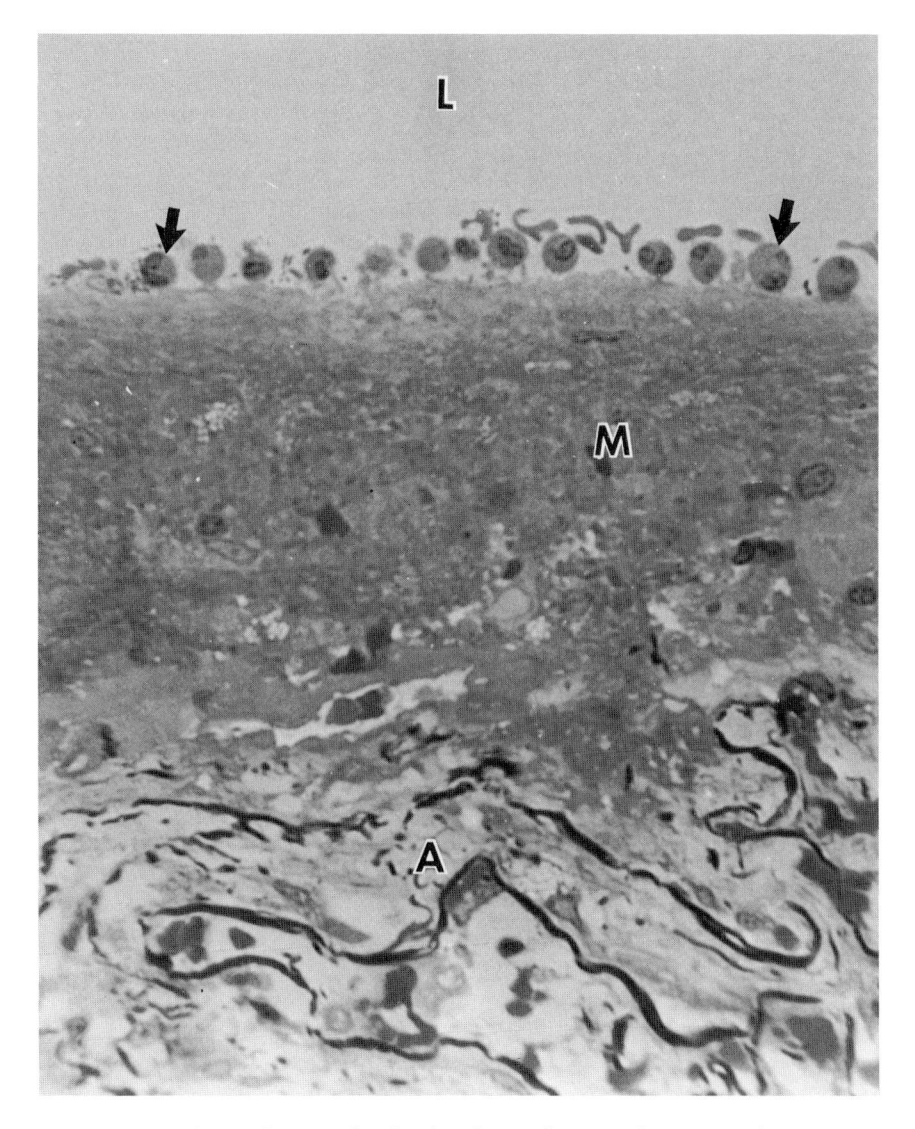

FIGURE 8. Photomicrograph of a dog femoral artery that was endarterectomized through the middle of the media 24 hours earlier after which blood flow through the artery was restored. A single layer of neutrophils (arrows) lines the endarterectomized segment. L, lumen; M, remnant of tunica media; A, tunica adventitia. Polychrome stain.

represents the result of the same disease process which initially led to the performance of the original operative procedure. Our own experimental work has failed to show that the process can be controlled with corticosteroids, mitotic inhibitors such as colchicine and vinblastine, by antimetabolites such as 5-fluorouracil, or by chronic heparin administration. In humans, neither chronic heparin therapy, coumarin therapy or aspirin and dipyridamole have prevented the late reaction from occurring in the midportions of reconstructed segments.

What is the surgeon to do? It is apparent that the arterial wall can respond in a limited number of ways to injury, stress, flow, environment, and possibly to combinations of these including metabolic factors. It can either thicken, balloon out, or develop clots that may either occlude the vessel at once or lead to later closure by organization of thrombus.

Precise surgical technique is essential to create absolutely smooth suture lines. The liberal use of vein roof patches sutured to atherosclerotic arteries to which either plastic prosthetic grafts or even vein grafts are sutured has resulted in smooth suture lines. The avoidance in bypass grafts of geometric configurations produced by accentuated curvatures would appear to be desirable. The passage of saphenous vein grafts from the subcutaneous location to the low popliteal artery around the tendon of the sartorius muscle just before its insertion on the tibial plateau has been a site of late neointimal fibrous proliferation. Perhaps surgeons should avoid placing vein grafts in the subcutaneous location where concentric rings of fibrous tissue can develop and lead to focal intimal thickening.

We feel it is beneficial to change the geometric configuration of arteries with advanced atherosclerosis if they have been subjected to endarterectomy procedures. We have elected to use vein roof patches in the carotid bifurcation, the most common site for performance of endarterectomy procedures, hoping thereby to change the hemodynamic conditions that possibly led to the initial development of lesions. Our own low incidence of recurrent stenosis perhaps attests to the efficacy of this technique. Because the occlusive process in endarterectomized arteries appears to be due to smooth muscle cell migration and transformation, we now attempt to remove all of the smooth muscle fibers at the carotid bulb during endarterectomy. Whether this could lead to subsequent aneurysm formation is unknown at this time.

Because the deposition of thrombus in injured arteries, as exemplified in our endarterectomy experiments, does lead to fibrous organization of thrombus, it may be advisable to employ not only careful surgical technique but perhaps also anticoagulant substances or antiplatelet substances during the early postoperative period.

REFERENCES

1. Abbot WM, Willand BS, Austen GW: Structural changes during the preparation of autogenous venous grafts. Surgery 76:1931, 1974
2. Baumann FG, Imparato AM, Kim GE et al: A study of the early evolution of fibromuscular lesions hemodynamically induced in the dog renal artery (15 min–2 hrs). II. Scanning and correlative transmission of electron microscopy. Artery 4:67, 1978
3. Baumann FG, Imparato AM, Kim G: A study of the evolution of early fibromuscular intimal lesions hemodynamically induced in the dog (10 mins–2 hrs). Light and transmission electron microscopy. Circ Res 39:6, 1976
4. Blaisdell FM, Lim R, Hall AD: Technical results of carotid endarterectomy. Am J Surg 114:239, 1967
5. Benditt EP, Benditt JM: Evidence for monoclonal origin of human atherosclerotic plaques. Proc Natl Acad Sci (USA) 70:1753, 1973
6. Brody WR, Angell WW, Kosek JC: Histologic fate of the venous coronary artery bypass graft in dogs. Am J Pathol 66:111, 1972.
7. Caro CG: Arterial wall shear and early atheroma in man. Nature: 223:1159, 1969
8. DeWeese JA, Rob GG: Autogenous venous bypass grafts five years later. Am Surg 174:346, 1971
9. Duguid JB: Thrombosis as a factor in the pathogenesis of aortic atherosclerosis. J Pathol Bact 60:57, 1948
10. Ferguson FC: Colchicine: general pharmacology. Arch Intern Pharm Ther 111:261, 1957
11. Fry DL: Responses of the arterial wall to certain physical factors. Ciba Found Symp 12:93, 1973
12. Fry L, McMinn RM: Action of methotrexate on skin and intestinal epithelium in psoriasis. Arch Dermatol 93:726, 1966
13. Greer JC: Fine structures of human aortic intimal thickening. Lab Invest 14:1764, 1965
14. Gutstein WH, Schneck DG: In vitro boundary layer studies of blood flow in branched tubes. Atherosclerosis 7:295, 1967
15. Gyurko G, Szabo M: Experimental investigations of the role of hemodynamic factors in formation of intimal changes. Surgery 66:871, 1969
16. Hardin NJ, Minick CR, Murphy GE: Experimental induction of atheroarteriosclerosis by the synergy of allergic injury to arterial and lipid rich diet. Am J Pathol 73:301, 1973
17. Imparato AM, Baumann FG, Pearson J et al. Electron microscopic studies of experimentally produced fibromuscular arterial lesions. Surg Gynecol Obstet 139:497, 1974
18. Imparato AM, Bracco A, Kim GE, Zeff RZ: Intimal and neointimal fibrous proliferation causing failure of arterial reconstruction. Surgery 72:1007, 1972
19. Imparato AM, Lord JW, Texon M, Halpern OM: Experimental production

of atherosclerosis by alteration of blood vessel configuration. Surg Forum 12:245, 1961
20. Imparato AM, Baumann FG, Riles TR: An electron microscopic study of healing of the endarterectomized arterial wall. In press.
21. Imparato AM, Bracco A, Kim GE: Comparisons of three techniques for femoral-popliteal arterial reconstruction. Ann Surg 177:375, 1973.
22. Imparato AM, Riles TS, Gorstein F: The carotid plaque. Stroke 10:238, 1979
23. Johnson WD, Auer JE, Tector AJ: Late changes in coronary vein grafts. Am J Cardiol 26:640, 1970
24. LoGerfo SW, Soncrant T, Teel T, Dewey CF Jr: Boundary layer separation in models of side-to-end arterial anastomoses. Arch Surg 114:1369, 1979
25. Poole JCF, Gronwell SB, Benditt EP: Behavior of smooth muscle cells and formation of extracellular structures in the reaction of arterial walls to injury. Am J Pathol 62:391, 1971
26. Ross R, Glomset JA: The pathogenesis of atherosclerosis. New Engl J Med 295:369, 420, 1976
27. Stephens WE: Blood vessel changes in chronic experimental arteriovenous fistulas. Surg Gynecol Obstet 127:327, 1968
28. Schmid FR, Cooper NS, Ziff M, McEwen C: Arteritis in rheumatoid arthritis. Am J Med 30:56, 1961
29. Steiner A, Kendall FE Bevas M: Production of arteriosclerosis in dogs by cholesterol and thiouracil feeding. Am Heart J 38:34, 1949
30. Stemerman MB, Ross R: Experimental arteriosclerosis. I. Fibrous plaque formation in primates, an electronmicroscopic study. J Exp Med 136:769, 1972
31. Szilagy ED, Smith RF, Whitney DG: The durability of aortic-iliac endarterectomy. Arch Surg 89:827, 1964
32. Texon M, Imparato AM, Lord JW, Helpern M: Experimental production of arterial lesions. Arch Intern Med 110:50, 1962
33. Williams G: Experimental studies of arterial ligation. J Pathol Bact 71:569, 1956
34. Vineberg A, Afridi S, Sahi S: Direct revascularization of acute myocardial infarction by implantation of left internal mammary artery into infarcted left ventricular myocardium. Surg Gynecol Obstet 140:44, 1975
35. Weiss P, Kranz D, Marx I, Fuhrman I: Electron microscopic observations in doubly ligated abdominal aortas of rabbits and cats. Exp Pathol 5:70, 1971
36. Wesolowski S: Significance of turbulence. Surgery 57:155, 1965
37. Yoder MJ, Baumann FG, Grover-Johnson NM, et al: A morphological study of early cellular changes with closure of the rabbit ductus arteriosus. Anat Rec 192:19, 1978

NINE

Anastomotic Neointimal Fibrous Hyperplasia: Pathogenesis and Prevention

James A. DeWeese

The healing of small arterial prostheses is initiated by the formation of a thin layer of thrombus that becomes compressed by the blood flow through the graft to become a neointima. The thrombus is rapidly replaced by fibrin. Nonthrombogenic endothelial linings are deposited on the fibrin either from bloodstream sources or, more commonly, as a panus ingrowth from the adjacent vessel. Although the endothelial lining completely coats the lining of the grafts of some species, it rarely, if ever, completely coats grafts in humans.[21]

The late thrombosis of graft materials has frequently been observed to be associated with a diffuse thickening of the neointima because of fibrous hyperplasia. It has been observed in endarterectomized arteries, in radial arteries used as aortocoronary bypass grafts, and in autogenous veins in the femoropopliteal or aortocoronary position. In many instances, however, late failure of grafts was associated with a significant hyperplasia at the anastomosis without excessive thickening of the remainder of the neointima. This anastomotic neointimal fibrous hyperplasia or ANFH was recognized by us in short plastic grafts of 4 to 6 mm in diameter that were used to bypass ligated canine femoral arteries in 1961.[19] The ANFH was most prominent in the Dacron and Teflon grafts, which thrombosed, but appeared insignificant in vein grafts whether they remained patent or occluded.

Subsequent to our early laboratory experience, ANFH has been observed by ourselves as well as others as a frequent cause of the late failures of grafts in humans. It has been observed in failed Dacron grafts, bovine heterografts, and, most recently, in Gore-Tex grafts.[6,24] It is still occasionally observed in autogenous venous grafts. As long as the cause and prevention of neointimal fibrous hyperplasia at anastomoses as well as along the entire graft surface remains undetermined, the search for the ideal vascular graft will continue.

CAUSES OF ANFH

Potential factors that might contribute to ANFH include 1) operative trauma, 2) thrombogenicity of the grafts, 3) delayed endothelialization of the thrombogenic graft, 4) hemodynamic factors associated with the anastomosis, and 5) mechanical mismatch between that grafting material and host artery. Each of these factors will be discussed in turn.

Operative Trauma

During Carrel's early experiences with vascular grafts,[4] he recognized that operative trauma could result in thrombus formation at anastomotic suture lines. He was the first to recognize that this thrombus formation could be avoided by careful approximation of the intima of one vessel to the intima of the other vessel by the gentle handling of the vessels without crushing or dessication and by the use of fine suture materials. Although anastomotic intimal thrombus may cause acute graft thrombosis, no direct evidence is available that nonoccluding thrombus in the early postoperative period progresses to the later intimal hyperplasia causing late occlusion of grafts. We have observed, in fact, the late appearance of ANFH in grafts with normal arteriograms in the early postoperative period.

Thrombogenicity of Grafts

Thrombogenicity of grafts is well recognized and, in fact, it is a necessity that plastic grafts, with their multiple small holes that are porous to blood, be thrombogenic. That different materials have different thrombogenicity has also been demonstrated. In Sauvage's experimental model,[22] umbilical vein grafts were found to be the most thrombogenic with crimped Dacron, Gore-Tex, uncrimped Dacron, and autologous artery demonstrating progressively less thrombus formation.

An experimental model consisting of the bypass of ligated canine femoral arteries with short grafts has been used in our laboratory for comparing the patency rates of different materials for the past several years. In these experiments, performed by several different surgeons, the overall comparative patency rates are as follows: autogenous veins

92 percent, homograft veins 68 percent, internal velour grafts 65 percent, Gore-Tex grafts 56 percent, knitted Dacron grafts 53 percent, bovine heterografts 39 percent, and umbilical veins 37 percent.[2,3,7,8,11,16,17,25] In these experiments, the graft materials with the lower patency rates demonstrated the most severe ANFH. Only minimal hyperplasia was observed, on the other hand, in anastomoses between autogenous veins and femoral arteries. These observations suggest that thrombogenicity or some other characteristic of the graft material used may have something to do with the development of ANFH.

Delayed Endothelialization

Because endothelialization of the entire inner surface of nonautogenous grafts does not occur in humans, it has been suggested that the thrombogenicity of the nonendothelialized neointima is responsible for a generalized neointimal fibrous hyperplasia and thrombosis.[21] This concept has led to some interesting evaluations of the seeding of endothelium on the inner surfaces of grafts to promote instant endothelialization.[10] Delayed endothelialization could explain neointimal fibrous hyperplasia, but it cannot explain progressive ANFH because the growth of endothelium from the adjacent normal artery across the anastomoses occurs during the first few weeks of graft healing and ANFH is a later occurrence.

Hemodynamic Factor

Several interesting studies have been done suggesting that hemodynamic factors are the cause of the atherosclerotic plaque and also possibly ANFH. Imparato et al[12] described neointimal fibrous hyperplasia in endarterectomized arteries and other arterial reconstructions. They were able to produce intimal hyperplasia in end-to-side anastomoses between the renal artery and vena cava.[13] They suggested that the end-to-side anastomosis and the high flow of the arteriovenous fistula resulted in the repeated stripping of endothelial cells with subendothelial injury that explained the progressive proliferation. LoGerfo et al[14] studied models of end-to-side anastomoses and found that the boundary layer separated from the wall of the vessel at bifurcations, at anastomoses, or with sudden changes in vessel diameter. A low wall shear stress was in the separation zone, and they felt that this low wall shear might result in a decreased endothelial cell stimulation, platelet adhesion to exposed subendothelium, and the consequent stimulation of fibroblasts and smooth muscle cells. Although LoGerfo could not demonstrate turbulence in his models, others have implicated the turbulence that might occur in these separation zones as being responsible for the endothelial cell damage. Whether the endothelial cell damage occurs as a result of high flow, low flow, or turbulence, considerable agreement exists that damage to endothelium and adherence of platelets to the subendothelial layer are responsible for the stimulation of fibroblasts and smooth muscle cells resulting in intimal hyperplasia.

Although the hemodynamic factors remain a very attractive theory, we have made some observations that suggest they cannot completely explain the process. In studying short bypass grafts of canine femoral arteries by cineangiograms, Phillips et al[19] noted that with cobra mouth anastomoses, marked turbulence was demonstrated in both venous and plastic grafts. Despite turbulence in both types of graft, significant ANFH was observed only when plastic graft materials were used. These observations suggest that some characteristics of the materials used as well as hemodynamic factors may be responsible for the more significant examples of ANFH.

Mechanical Mismatch

Mechanical mismatch has been postulated by Clark et al.[5] to explain why different graft materials might produce different degrees of endothelial trauma, platelet adherence to subendothelium, stimulation of fibrous tissue and smooth muscle cells, and subsequently ANFH. Clark indicates that materials with different mechanical properties that are joined together and placed in a cyclic stress system, such as is seen with arterial pulsations, can result in bending or buckling at the site of the coaption or at the anastomosis and may result in a chronic recurring injury to the vessel wall. Since the elastic modules of normal arteries are slightly different in the longitudinal than in the circumferential direction, they evaluated grafts with such elastic modules in canine arteries and found a higher incidence of patency at one year in those grafts that were more like normal arteries.

Abbott et al.[1] have also presented evidence that elasticity of grafts as measured by their compliance can influence patency. In their animal model, arterial and venous autografts, double velour Dacron grafts, and Gore-Tex grafts were compared. Patency rates ranged from 100 percent in the most compliant arterial autografts to 14 percent in the Gore-Tex grafts, which had the lowest compliances. Siefert et al.[23] also constructed prostheses made of elastic urethane copolymers and found the prostheses in which the elasticity best matched those of the normal artery had the best patency rates.

It would appear that the mismatch of mechanical properties is an important reason for the occurrence of ANFH. It most quickly explains why lesions are more frequently found with the prosthetic grafts than with autologous grafts, why the most severe lesions we have observed occurred in rigid, glutaraldehyde-treated heterografts, and why intimal hyperplasia might be observed in anastomoses where normal thin-walled elastic veins have been implanted into a rigid atherosclerotic artery.

Both hemodynamic alterations and the mismatch of mechanical properties may result in trauma to the endothelium, and it is now generally agreed that it is the subsequent platelet reaction with their aggregation to the subendothelium and subsequent "release reaction" that stimulates the growth and migration of fibroblasts and smooth muscle cells and the progressive nature of ANFH.[9]

PREVENTION OF ANFH

If platelets are indeed responsible for ANFH, then it is logical to assume that antiplatelet drugs might be effective in preventing ANFH. Aspirin inhibits secondary platelet aggregation by blocking the production of the prostaglandin endoperoxides, PGG_2, PGH_3, and thrombaxane A_2. This effect is achieved only by low concentrations of aspirin. Higher doses of aspirin inhibit synthesis of the prostaglandin antithrombotic factor, prostacycline, and may therefore actually promote intravascular thrombosis. Aspirin may produce inhibition of platelet aggregation and prostaglandin synthesis for as long as 4 to 7 days after ingestion of as little as 300 mg of the drug. Dipyridamole, conversely, inhibits primary platelet adherence as well as secondary platelet aggregation. In addition, a synergistic effect occurs if both aspirin and dipyridamole are administered.[20]

An experimental evaluation of the effects of aspirin and dipyridamole on graft healing has been undertaken. Internal velour Dacron grafts and Gore-Tex grafts were used to bypass ligated canine femoral arteries. Nine animals received aspirin and dipyridamole and were followed for 4 months; all grafts remained patent. In animals without medication, on the other hand, only 10 of the 15 grafts remained patent. In a separate study, aspirin and dipyridamole were shown to increase the patency rate of umbilical vein grafts from 10 to 60 percent.[7] ANFH was demonstrated in the control animals and was not observed in the treated animals. Clinical studies of the use of the drugs in patients undergoing aortocoronary bypass grafts have been reported with conflicting results. Pantley et al.,[18] in a small group of patients in a controlled randomized study, found that 27 of 33 grafts (82 percent) were patent in patients treated with aspirin and dipyridamole and 50 of 61 grafts (82 percent) were patent at 6 months in the control patients. Mayer et al.[15] observed a larger number of patients: 86 of 92 grafts (93.5 percent) were patent in patients treated with aspirin and dipyridamole, whereas only 98 of 120 (81.6 percent) were patent in the control group.

We have initiated a clinical study in patients requiring lower extremity bypass grafts. The study will be performed on patients who have unsuitable veins and, therefore, will receive a Gore-Tex graft. Treated patients will receive 325 mg of aspirin each day and dipyridamole, 75 mg t.i.d., preoperatively, and as soon as oral intake is resumed postoperatively. Thirty patients have been entered into the study but thus far the results are not known, and we do not expect to break the code until at least 50 patients have been included.

In conclusion, 1) ANFH is frequently associated with late graft failures; 2) possible causes of the lesion are operative reaction, thrombogenicity of grafts, delayed endothelialization, hemodynamic factors, and mismatches of mechanical properties; 3) aspirin and dipyridamole have decreased the severity of the lesions experimentally; and 4) controlled trials are indicated to determine the clinical usefulness of these drugs.

REFERENCES

1. Abbott WM, Bouchier-Hayes DJ: The role of mechanical properties in graft design. In Dardik H (ed): Graft Materials in Vascular Surgery. Miami, Fla, Symposia Specialists, 1978
2. Barner H, DeWeese, JA, Schenk, EA: Fresh and frozen homologous venous grafts for arterial repair. Angiology 17:389, 1966
3. Benson RW, Payne DD, DeWeese JA: Evaluation of prosthetic grafts of different porosity for arterial reconstruction. Am J Surg 129:665, 1975
4. Carrel A, Guthrie CC: Anastomosis of blood vessels by the patching method and transplantation of the kidney. JAMA 47:1648, 1906
5. Clark RE, Apostolou S, Kardos JL: Mismatch of mechanical properties as a cause of arterial prostheses thrombosis. Surg Forum 27:208, 1978
6. Echave V, Koornick AR, Haimov M, Jacobson JH: Intimal hyperplasia as a complication of the use of the polytetrafluoroethylene graft for femoral-popliteal bypass. Surgery 86:791, 1979
7. Feins RH, Roedersheimer LR, Green RM, DeWeese JA: Platelet aggregation inhibition in human umbilical vein grafts and negatively charged bovine heterografts. Surgery 85:395, 1979
8. Green RM, Thomas M, Luka N, DeWeese JA: A comparison of rapid-healing prosthetic arterial grafts and autogenous veins. Arch Surg 114:944, 1979
9. Harker LA: Platelet mechanisms in the genesis and prevention of graft-related vascular injury reactions and thromboembolism. Nature of the vascular interface. Sawyer PN, Kaplitt MJ (eds): Vascular Grafts. New York, Appleton-Century-Crofts, 1978

10. Herring M, Gardner A, Glover, J: Seeding endothelium onto canine arterial prostheses. Arch Surg 114:679, 1979
11. Hoepp LM, Elbadawi A, Cohn M, Dachelet R, Peterson C, DeWeese JA: Steroids and immunosuppression. Arch Surg 114:273, 1979
12. Imparato AM, Bracco A, Kim GE, Zeff R: Intimal and neointimal fibrous proliferation causing failure of arterial reconstructions. Surgery 72:1007, 1972.
13. Imparato AM, Baumann, FG, Rearson J, et al: Electron microscopic studies of experimentally produced fibromuscular arterial lesions. Surg Gynecol Obstet, 139:497, 1974
14. LoGerfo FW, Soncrent T, Tell T, Forbes D: Boundary layer separation in models of side-to-end arterial anastomoses. Arch Surg 114:1369, 1979
15. Mayer JE Jr, Lindsay WG, Castaneda W, Nicoloff DM: Influence of aspirin and persantine on patency of coronary artery bypass. Presented to the Society of Thoracic Surgeons, January 21–23, 1980
16. Oblath RW, Buckley FO Jr, Donnelly WA, Green RM, DeWeese JA: Human umbilical veins and autogenous veins as canine arterial bypass grafts. Ann Surg 188: 158, 1978
17. Oblath RW, Buckley FO Jr, Green RM, et al: Prevention of platelet aggregation and adherence to prosthetic vascular grafts by aspirin and dipyridamole. Surgery 84:37, 1978
18. Pantley GA, Goodnight, SH Jr, Rahimtoola SH, et al: Failure of antiplatelet and anticoagulant therapy to improve patency of grafts after coronary artery bypass. N Engl J Med 301:962, 1979
19. Phillips CE Jr, DeWeese JA, Campeti FL: Comparison of peripheral arterial grafts. Arch Surg 82:38, 1961
20. Rajah SM, Penny AF, Crow MJ, et al: The interaction of varying doses of dipyridamole and acetyl salicylic acid on the inhibition of platelet functions and their effect on bleeding time. Br J Clin Pharmacol 8:483, 1979
21. Sauvage LR, Berger KE, Wood, SJ, et al: Interspecies healing of porous arterial prostheses. Arch Surg 109:698, 1974
22. Sauvage, LR, Walker MW, Berger K, et al: Current arterial prostheses. Arch Surg 114:687, 1979
23. Seifert KB, Albo D Jr, Knowlton H, Lyman DJ: Effect of elasticity of prosthetic wall on patency of small-diameter arterial prostheses. Surg Forum 30:206, 1979
24. Veith FJ: Discussion of Echave et al: Intimal hyperplasia as a complication of the use of the polytetrafluoroethylene graft for femoral popliteal bypass. Surgery 86:791, 1979
25. Weyman AK, Plume SK, DeWeese JA: Bovine heterografts and autogenous veins as canine arterial bypass grafts. Arch Surg 110:746, 1975

TEN

Thrombosis of Infrainguinal Grafts

Frank J. Veith and Sushil K. Gupta

Femoropopliteal bypasses and arterial reconstructions to vessels distal to the popliteal artery can occlude in the early postoperative period or any time thereafter. Early graft thromboses are those that occur within 30 days of operation. Although the incidence of early failures may be minimized by intraoperative angiography at the time of the original reconstruction, such failures still occur in 5 to 15 percent of cases even in the best of hands. They may be a result of technical defects, unrecognized distal or proximal disease, or a transient decrease in cardiac output.

If the original reconstruction was performed for limb salvage, detection of early graft thrombosis is usually simple. The original ischemic manifestations will again become obvious. In some instances, however, particularly in the immediate postoperative period or if the reconstruction was performed for intermittent claudication, the clinical appearance and temperature of the extremity and examination of distal pulses can be unreliable indices of graft patency. Objective criteria such as Doppler determined ankle blood pressure measurements, pulse volume recordings, isotope angiography, or contrast angiography may be required to diagnose graft thrombosis with certainty.[6] These objective criteria, especially the noninvasive ones, should be evaluated frequently during the first several postoperative days when most early graft failures occur.

This work was supported in part by a grant from the John Hilton Manning and Emma Austin Manning Foundation.

Comparison of these results with those obtained preoperatively and immediately postoperatively will almost always be an accurate index of graft patency.

Prompt detection of early graft thrombosis is important because, if the original operation was justified, immediate reoperation is also indicated. With saphenous vein graft reconstructions, such reoperations have the best chance of success if they are performed as soon after thrombosis has occurred as possible, since changes that predispose to rethrombosis probably begin to occur in the vein wall after a few hours. With thrombosis of prosthetic graft reconstructions, prompt reoperation is also indicated to minimize propagation of clot into the arterial tree distal to the graft insertion, although this does not always occur.

The method of reoperation for early failure of a saphenous vein or fabric prosthetic graft is similar to the operative technique that will be described below for early failure of expanded polytetrafluoroethylene (PTFE) grafts with the exception that simple thrombectomy usually cannot be expected to restore persisting graft patency. Unless the thrombosis was clearly due to an episode of hypotension, some form of anastomotic revision or vein or outflow tract reconstruction is invariably required to provide any hope of long-term success.[2,15] This is so because defects in these areas, unrecognized at the time of the original operation, usually account for the early failure of vein grafts. Intraoperative angiography following thrombectomy may reveal such a defect. Although these may be corrected by some form of local procedure, such as angioplasty or interposition graft, they sometimes require replacement of the entire graft or extension to a more distal arterial segment.

When late thrombosis of a femoropopliteal or more distal reconstruction occurs, reoperation is only indicated when the limb is in jeopardy. Even if the original procedure was for limb salvage, graft failure may not threaten the limb. When the original operation was for claudication, on the other hand, graft failure can occasionally place the limb in jeopardy because the thrombus in the graft extends into the outflow tract or is due to disease progression in the arteries supplied by the graft. The management and outcome of late thrombosis of PTFE grafts differ somewhat from the treatment and fate of similar failures that occur after reconstructions performed with autologous saphenous veins or Dacron fabric grafts. Because of this and because we have over the last 4 years had an extensive experience with PTFE grafts, much of the remainder of this chapter will be devoted to a detailed consideration of early and late thrombosis of PTFE femoropopliteal arterial reconstructions.

In the last 4 years, more than 200 of our patients have undergone femoropopliteal bypass with 6-mm PTFE tubular grafts for limb-threatening ischemia with gangrene, a nonhealing ulcer, or severe ischemic rest pain with pregangrenous changes. Distribution of local and systemic risk factors, techniques of initial operative and postoperative management, and methods for patient observation and determination of graft patency were similar to those previously reported.[11,12]

The first 175 patients undergoing operation have now all been observed over 1 year. In this group, there were 3 deaths within 1 month of operation and 25 late deaths from causes unrelated to the operation. Patency rates calculated by the life table method up to 3 years are shown in Figure 1.[1] Nine of these 175 femoropopliteal bypasses occluded *early* or in the first postoperative month, and 32 occluded *late* or from 1 to 40 months after operation. An additional recent patient had a graft fail within 4 hours of operation. She succumbed from a myocardial infarction following a graft thrombectomy.

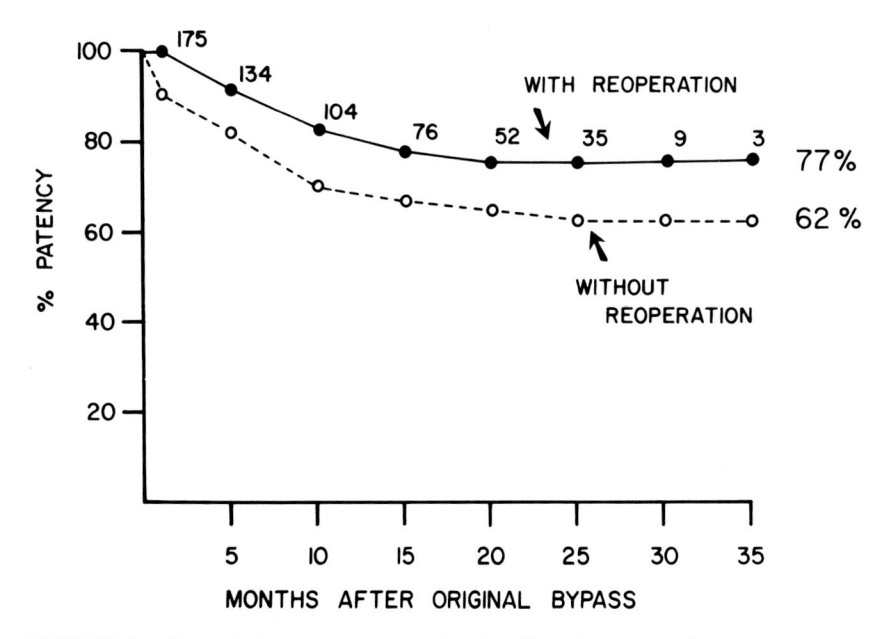

FIGURE 1. Cumulative patency rates by the life table method[1] for 175 PTFE femoropopliteal bypasses. The number above each time point indicates the cases actually observed for that time after operation. If successfully reoperated cases are considered patent, the upper line results. If all grafts that thrombose are considered nonpatent whether or not reoperation restores patency, the lower line results. (From Veith FJ, Gupta SK, Daly V: Surgery 87:581, 1980.)

PLAN OF MANAGEMENT FOR EARLY PTFE GRAFT OCCLUSION

Early PTFE graft occlusion occurred within 24 hours of operation in 7 patients, within 2 to 7 days in 2 patients, and on postoperative day 28 in 1 patient.[13] The limb was again jeopardized in all 10 patients, 7 of whom had insertion of their graft below the knee joint. Repeat angiography was not performed. Intravenous heparin, 7500 IU, was usually administered, and reoperation was undertaken within 3 hours to 30 days after graft occlusion. Under regional or general anesthesia, the distal incision was opened, and the distal anastomosis visualized. A 1.5-cm vertical incision was made in the graft to within 2 or 3 mm of the tip of its distal beveled end. Through this incision, the graft was thrombectomized proximally, and the popliteal artery was gently thrombectomized proximally and distally using balloon catheters with only partial inflation of the balloon. The distal anastomosis was completely inspected from within for intimal flaps or narrowing, the opening in the graft was closed with 6-0 polypropylene, and an arteriogram of the distal anastomosis and outflow tract obtained through a needle in the graft. In 5 patients, no anastomotic defect or distal stenosis was identified, and the reoperation was terminated. In 5 patients, a stenosis of the distal popliteal artery or impaired outflow was identified and a segment of PTFE graft, 4 mm or 6 mm in internal diameter, was used to extend the bypass from the previous opening in the graft to a more distal arterial segment. No postoperative anticoagulation was administered although patients received 0.9 g of aspirin and 100 to 375 mg of dipyridamole daily. Observation of graft patency by previously described objective methods has been complete in all 10 patients.[11,12]

PLAN OF MANAGEMENT FOR LATE PTFE GRAFT OCCLUSION

In 6 patients in whom late occlusion occurred from 2 to 10 months after operation[13] (Fig. 2), the original ischemic lesion had healed, the limb was not again threatened, and no further diagnostic or therapeutic interventions were performed. In 26 patients in whom graft occlusion occurred from 1 to 37 months after operation (Fig. 3), the limb was again in jeopardy although this took from several hours to 3 months to become apparent. Once limb survival was deemed unlikely, preoperative femoral angiography was performed with visualization of the arterial tree from the aorta to the forefoot. In this way, inflow problems proximal

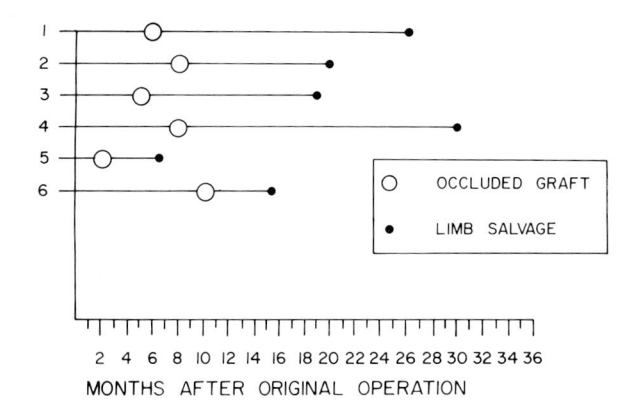

FIGURE 2. Management and outcome in each of the six patients whose PTFE femoropopliteal bypass thrombosed 30 days or more after operation and whose limbs were not placed in jeopardy by the graft occlusion.

to the graft insertion could be assessed, and the character and patency of arteries distal to the graft insertion could be determined.

Under regional or general anesthestia, the patient was given 7500 IU of heparin sodium, and the previous distal incision was opened. The graft was identified and traced distally until the anastomotic sutures could be seen. As much of the artery as possible was dissected free for 1 to 2 cm proximal and distal to the anastomosis. This dissection was often difficult because of scarring and adjacent veins and occasionally could not be accomplished completely. A vertical incision, as already described, was then made in the graft to permit thrombectomy of the graft and popliteal artery, and to provide visualization of the interior of the distal anastomosis and the arterial lumen. In 22 of 26 cases, it was possible to restore unimpeded proximal flow from this approach, while in the remaining 4 it was necessary to open the proximal incision to thrombectomize the proximal graft with or without revision of the proximal anastomosis or correction of a stenosis proximal to the anastomosis.* In no instance was it necessary to replace the occluded graft.

After proximal flow was re-established and all clot removed, attention was directed to the distal anastomosis to determine the cause of graft occlusion so that appropriate corrective maneuvers could be performed (Table 1). If intimal hyperplasia narrowed the recipient artery at or near the distal graft insertion (Fig. 4), the graft incision was extended

* Two patients required a proximal procedure during the first reoperation while 2 others required it during the second reoperation.

164 Critical Problems in Vascular Surgery

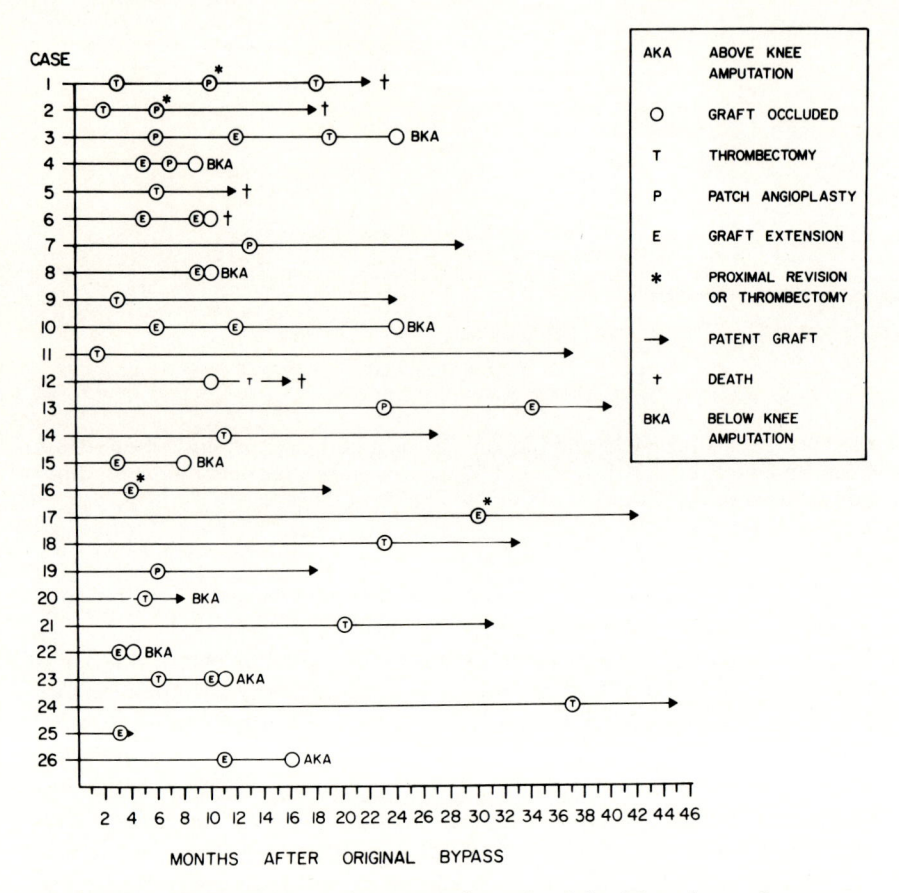

FIGURE 3. Management and outcome in each of the 26 patients whose femoropopliteal bypass thrombosed 30 days or more after operation and whose limbs were placed in jeopardy by the graft occlusion. All patients had one or more reoperation.

Table 1. Appropriate Operative Treatment and Incidence in 26 Primary and 8 Secondary Reoperations of Late PTFE Femoropopliteal Bypass Occlusions

Cause	Treatment	Number	Incidence (%)
Intimal hyperplasia	Incision and patch graft	7	21
Progression of distal disease	Graft extension	15	44
None found	Thrombectomy alone	12	35

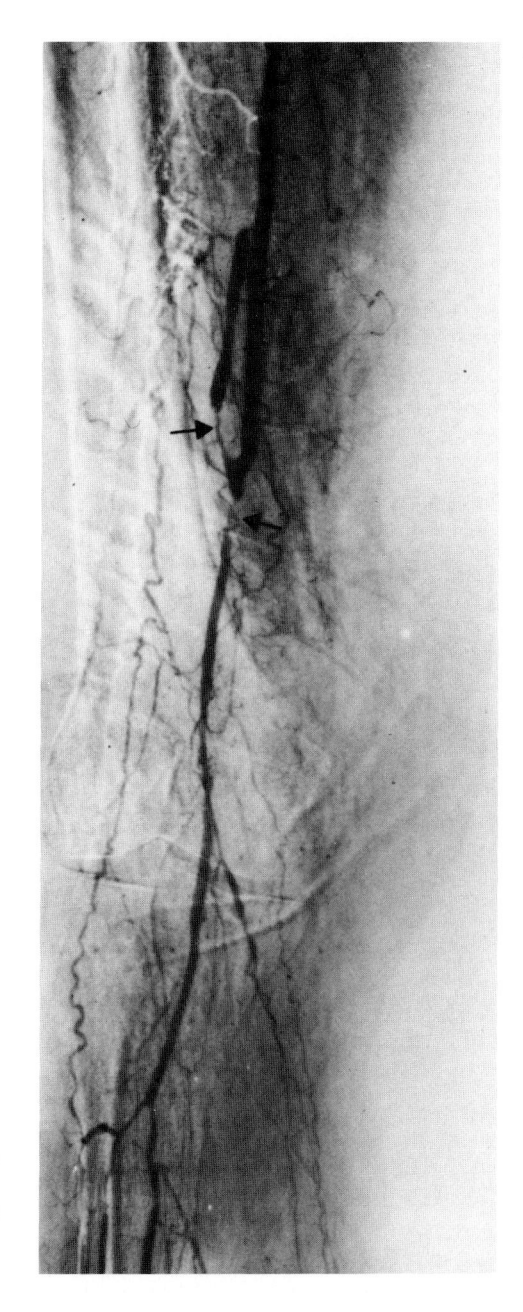

FIGURE 4. Femoral arteriogram demonstrating intimal hyperplasia producing narrowing of the popliteal artery proximal and distal (arrows) to the site of bypass insertion. This graft thrombosed 4 days after this arteriogram.

distally across its apex and down the recipient artery until its lumen was no longer narrowed. A PTFE patch was inserted in the graft and artery incision to widen the lumen, and an arteriogram was obtained to assure adequacy of the repair and outflow. If no intimal hyperplasia was present at or beyond the distal anastomosis, the graft incision was closed and an operative arteriogram was obtained. If this revealed any stenotic lesion because of disease progression distal to the anastomosis, a segment of PTFE graft, 4 mm or 6 mm in internal diameter, was inserted side-to-end into the old graft to extend the bypass to a patent artery below the stenotic lesion. Often the preoperative arteriogram was helpful in identifying such a lesion (Fig. 5). If no cause of late graft closure could be identified by direct inspection of the distal anastomosis and preoperative and operative angiography, the operation consisted of thrombectomy alone. Postoperative management and patency evaluation were as described for early graft occlusion.

The fate of 10 patient whose grafts failed during the first postoperative month and were treated by reoperation is shown in Figure 6. There were one early death and two late deaths with patent grafts, 3 and 14 months after operation, respectively. Six of the seven other grafts were patent for 5 to 37 months or a mean of 30 months, and the seventh patient had a viable limb 12 months following the original reoperation, although the graft closed after 8 months. The outlook for the patients treated by simple thrombectomy was as good as for those in whom graft extension was required.

The results of our policy of management for the late PTFE graft closures is shown in Figures 2 and 3. A conservative approach to a graft that did not place the limb in jeopardy was justified by the continued survival for 5 to 22 months of all six limbs in this category (Fig. 2). Figure 3 shows the results of our reoperations for late PTFE graft occlusion, which places the limb in jeopardy. In 24 of 26 cases, graft patency was reestablished for at least 2 months. In 16 of the 26 patients (62 percent) this patency has persisted until death or the present. The range of patency following reoperation in this group of 16 patients is 2 to 36 months with a mean of over 13 months, although four patients have requried a secondary reoperation to maintain graft patency and limb viability (Fig. 3). Twelve grafts have remained patent more than 1 year after reoperation. Sustained graft patency for more than 1 year was achieved in some patients treated initially with simple thrombectomy (five patients) as well as those requiring an initial patch graft (four patients) or graft extension (three patients). Ultimate graft failure and amputation within 1 year, however, appeared more likely in those patients requiring an extension at the primary reoperation (7 of 11) than those having thrombectomy alone (1 of 11) or patch grafting (0 of 4).

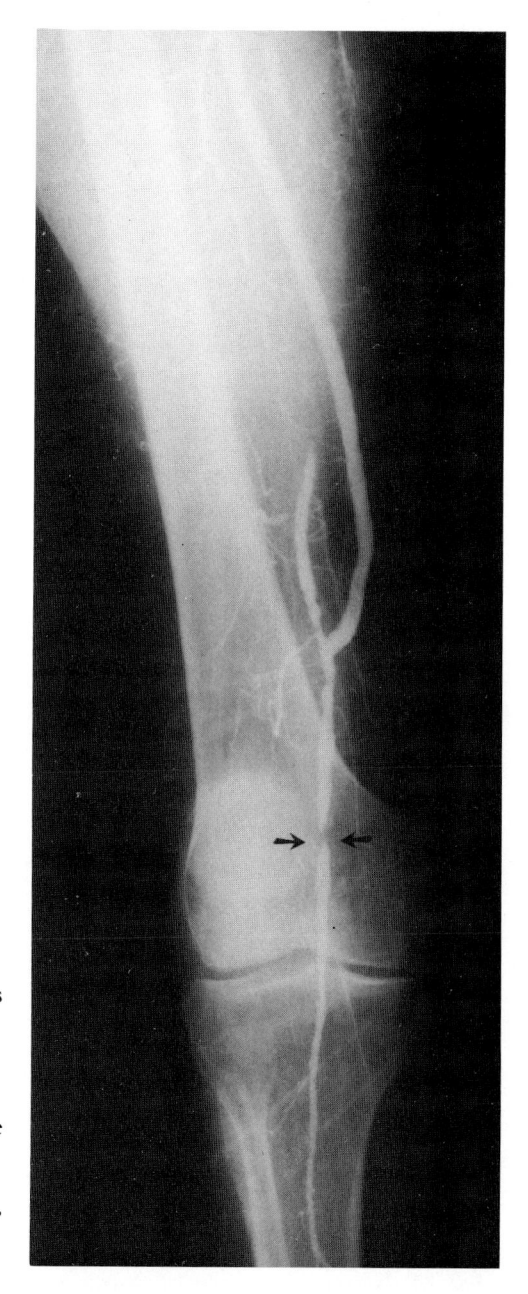

FIGURE 5. Femoral arteriogram obtained 18 months after a PTFE femoropopliteal bypass. A stenotic lesion (arrows) that was not originally present has developed in the popliteal artery distal to the site of the original operation. The graft thrombosed 4 weeks after this arteriogram. (From Veith FJ, Gupta SK, Daly V: Surgery 87:581, 1980.)

168 Critical Problems in Vascular Surgery

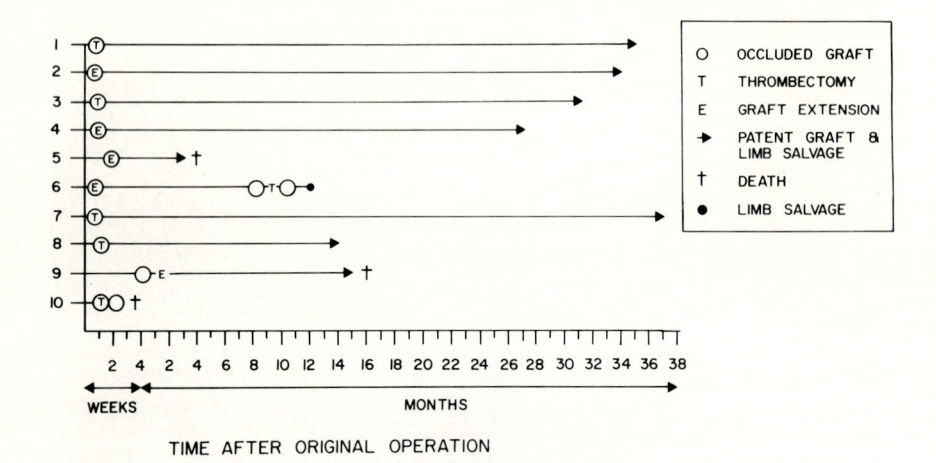

FIGURE 6. Treatment and outcome in each of the 10 patients whose PTFE femoropopliteal bypass thrombosed within 1 month of operation.

Only 8 of 32 patients in whom late graft occlusion occurred ultimately required major amputation, and in all but two instances this could be successfully performed below the knee. There was one postoperative death that occurred from a myocardial infarction 1 week after a secondary reoperation, yielding an operative mortality of 3 percent for all 34 primary and secondary reoperations. Four patients with functioning grafts died from unrelated causes, and one patient with a functioning graft required below-knee amputation.

These results show that PTFE femoropopliteal bypasses that occlude within the first month after operation or any time thereafter can often be treated effectively by aggressive reoperation. If the reoperation is appropriately performed and monitored by intraoperative angiography, long-term graft patency can result.

EARLY THROMBOSIS OF SAPHENOUS VEIN FEMOROPOPLITEAL BYPASSES

The results of reoperation for early failure of PTFE femoropopliteal grafts contrast sharply with the results of autologous saphenous vein and Dacron femoropopliteal bypasses that require early reoperation for thrombosis. Craver and his associates[2] reported on the results in patients whose femoropopliteal bypass grafts failed within 30 days of operation. Most of their grafts were of autologous saphenous vein. Failure was usually due to technical defects at an anastomosis, defects in the graft, judgmental errors regarding the adequacy of inflow or outflow from the graft, or low cardiac output. Of 66 patients subjected to reoperation for thrombosis, only 28 percent had a patent graft after 1 year. Furthermore, simple thrombectomy of a graft when no cause of early failure could be identified and corrected was always followed by rethrombosis.[2] These findings contrast sharply with the present observation that reoperation for PTFE femoropopliteal bypasses that thrombose within 30 days can restore graft patency that usually persists whether or not a cause of the thrombosis is identified. Thus, PTFE femoropopliteal bypasses appear to be unique in that thrombectomy alone, even when delayed up to 30 days after closure, can sometimes restore long-term patency after early thrombosis.

INTIMAL HYPERPLASIA AND PTFE GRAFTS

We have previously noted that intimal hyperplasia at or just beyond the distal anastomosis is a major cause of PTFE graft closures that occur several months or more after operations.[12] This process, which has been reported in almost all types of small- and medium-sized vessel reconstructions in all locations, may or may not be more common with PTFE grafts than other vascular substitutes.[3,5,9] Echave and his associates[4] have also noted that intimal hyperplasia causes failure of tapered femoropopliteal PTFE grafts, and this group has recommended treatment by graft thrombectomy and extension to a distal artery. Our findings and management concepts concerning this lesion differ in some regards from those of this group. We have observed intimal hyperplasia as a cause of PTFE graft failure even when uniform tubes 6 mm in diameter are employed. In addition, we have not found intimal hyperplasia to be the predominant cause of late PTFE femoropopliteal bypass failure (Table 1). Furthermore, we believe that, because incision and patch grafting leaves the maximal amount of undisturbed distal artery should subsequent operation be required and because the results seem to be superior, it is a better technique than graft extension for managing this lesion.

Although the etiology of intimal hyperplasia is not clearly defined, it may be related to anastomotic geometry and flow factors that produce local vessel injury.[5] The role of platelets has also been implicated, and the experimental observations of Oblath and his colleagues[7] have indicated that treatment with aspirin and dipyridamole may decrease the incidence of this lesion in experimental arterial grafts. Whether or not this is true in patients remains to be demonstrated conclusively, although we have observed a lower late failure rate in our recent femoropopliteal bypass patients all of whom receive preoperative and postoperative aspirin and dipyridamole. This operation in previous patients had a higher failure rate, and they did not receive these drugs. The two groups of patients were neither concurrent nor randomized, however.

LATE OCCLUSION OF SAPHENOUS VEIN AND DACRON FEMOROPOPLITEAL GRAFTS

The outlook for restoring patency to an autologous saphenous vein or Dacron fabric femoropopliteal bypass that fails after the immediate postoperative period is generally regarded as bleak. There are two main causes of late vein graft failure that occurs within 5 years in 20 to 35 percent of femoropopliteal reconstructions. Failures during the first year after operation are usually due to progressive changes in the vein graft itself. These changes have been well described by Szilagyi and his associates[9] and include intimal thickening or hyperplasia, vein valve fibrosis, and fibrotic stenoses some of which are thought to be due to clamp injury. The second cause of vein graft failure is progression of atherosclerotic occlusive disease within the vessels proximal or distal to the graft or occasionally within the vein itself.[9] These atherosclerotic changes usually result in vein graft failure after the first postoperative year.

When a return of symptoms, a timely examination, or routine noninvasive studies reveal circulatory deterioration, or when routine angiography is performed, it may be possible to detect all these lesions before they cause graft thrombosis. Operative revision consisting of a vein patch angioplasty, an interposition vein, or an extension vein bypass can result in salvage of the original vein graft.[9,15] The prognosis for long-term patency after such reoperations is good with an 86 percent 5-year cumulative patency being reported in one series of 8 patients.[15] Recently, we have been employing transluminal angioplasty to correct stenotic lesions in or distal to vein grafts before thrombosis occurs, and early results have been good.[14] The prognosis for long-term patency, however, of other secondary operations performed after vein grafts or Dacron grafts thrombose from the same causes is far worse. A completely new secondary bypass or reconstruction has been regarded as the only option for alleviating limb-threatening ischemia in such cases. Although some early success with these seconday procedures has been reported, the late results are poor with less than 50 percent 2-year patency.[8,10,15] Recently, however, Whittemore and his associates[15] have reported on a series of 72 primary reoperations and 34 secondary reoperations for failed femoropopliteal saphenous vein grafts. They recommended angiography following thrombectomy of the vein graft. They performed a vein patch angioplasty in 18 patients with short stenosis in the thrombectomized vein. Cumulative patency in these 18 patients was 39 percent at 2 years and 19 percent at 5 years. In 18 other cases, they were able to use an additional segment of autologous vein as an extension of the original graft to bypass a long stenosis or a defect at/or distal to the anastomosis. This restored patency to 50 percent of their patients at 2 years and 36 percent at 5 years by life table analysis.

Apart from this experience, which would be applicable to only a minority of vein graft failures, an entirely new secondary bypass is usually the only option for reversing ischemia when a saphenous vein or Dacron femoropopliteal bypass occludes after 1 month. Adequate autologous saphenous vein may be obtained from the ipsilateral or contralateral leg for such a secondary bypass. Because of the symmetrical nature of peripheral arteriosclerosis, we have felt it unwise to use vein from the opposite extremity. Frequently, it is difficult to find a suitable and adequate length of ipsilateral greater saphenous vein, and lesser saphenous vein, arm veins, composite grafts of arm and leg veins, and prosthetic grafts of Dacron, modified umbilical vein, or PTFE may be used. Our present preference is for the latter. Thus, although the results of reoperation for late thrombosis of a saphenous vein or Dacron femoropopliteal graft are only fair at best, reoperation is indicated if the limb is in jeopardy; and a substantial number of limbs may be salvaged by an aggressive approach with appropriate reoperation.[8,10,15]

MANAGEMENT OF THROMBOSIS OF BYPASSES TO ARTERIES BELOW THE POPLITEAL

The results with reoperation for femoropopliteal bypasses differ from those with reoperation for thrombosis of grafts inserted into arteries below the popliteal. Simple thrombectomy of saphenous vein or PTFE grafts, however, that thrombose immediately after operation due to hypotension, decreased cardiac output, or other unknown factors may occasionally (15–30 percent) result in prolonged patency. Intraoperative angiography should be performed after thrombectomy, and occasionally a correctable defect will be found. If such a defect can be corrected, long-term patency may result, but secondary reoperations on small vessel bypasses are frequently unrewarding.

If graft failure occurs after the first postoperative week, the same principles of management outlined for femoropopliteal grafts should be followed. The success rate will be lower with reoperation, however, resulting in protracted graft patency in less than 30 percent of cases.

CONCLUSION

Problems associated with early and late thrombosis of infrainguinal graft are among the more difficult in vascular surgery. By following appropriate principles of management and employing careful and correct reoperative techniques, many limbs can be salvaged for important additional periods of time.

Reoperation for early or late occlusions of PTFE femoropopliteal bypasses is particularly important. If appropriately conducted and combined with preoperative and intraoperative angiography, such reoperations usually restore graft patency for important periods of time. Graft replacement is almost never required even when reoperation is delayed up to 3 months after graft thrombosis. Moreover, patency can be maintained more than 1 year in many reoperated patients. The sustained effectiveness of appropriate reoperation when PTFE femoropopliteal grafts fail substantially increases the overall patency rates as indicated in Figure 1. The incidence and period of effective limb salvage and palliation is thereby augmented at a low cost in the risk of reoperation.

REFERENCES

1. Colton T: Statistics in Medicine. Boston, Little, Brown, 1974, p. 237
2. Craver JM, Ottinger LW, Darling C, et al: Hemorrhage and thrombosis as early complications of femoropopliteal bypass grafts: Causes, treatment, and prognostic implications. Surgery 74:839, 1973
3. Deweese JA: Anastomotic intimal hyperplasia. In Sawyer PN, Kaplitt MJ (eds): *Vascular Grafts.* New York, Appleton-Century-Crofts, 1978, pp 147–152
4. Echave V, Koornick A, Haimov M, Jacobsen JH: Intimal hyperplasia as a complication of the use of the polytetrafluoroethylene graft for femoralpopliteal bypass. Surgery 86:791, 1979
5. Imparato AM, Bracco A, Kim GE, Zeff R: Intimal and neointimal fibrous proliferation causing failure of arterial reconstructions. Surgery 72:1007, 1972
6. Moss CM, Rudavsky A, Veith FJ: The value of scintiangiography in arterial disease. Arch Surg 111:1235, 1976
7. Oblath RW, Bucklet FO, Green RM, et al: Prevention of platelet aggregation and adherence to prosthetic vascular grafts by aspirin and dipyridamole. Surgery 84:37, 1978
8. Painton JF, Avellone JC, Plecha FR: Effectiveness of reoperation after late failure of femoropopliteal reconstruction. Am J Surg 135:235, 1978
9. Szilagyi DE, Elliott JP, Hageman JH, et al: Biologic fate of autogenous vein implants as arterial substitutes: Clinical, angiographic and histopatho-

logic observations in femoropopliteal operations for atherosclerosis. Ann Surg 178:232, 1973
10. Szilagyi DE, Elliott JP, Smith RF, et al: Secondary arterial repair: The management of late failures in reconstructive arterial surgery. Arch Surg 110:485, 1975
11. Veith FJ, Moss CM, Fell SC, et al: Comparison of expanded polytetrafluoroethylene and autologous saphenous vein grafts in high risk arterial reconstructions for limb salvage. Surg Gynecol Obstet 147:749, 1978
12. Veith FJ, Moss CM, Daly V, et al: New approaches to limb salvage by extended extra-anatomic bypasses and prosthetic reconstructions to foot arteries. Surgery 84:764, 1978
13. Veith FJ, Gupta SK, Daly V: Management of early and late thrombosis of expanded polytetrafluoroethylene (PTFE) femoropopliteal bypass grafts: Favorable prognosis with appropriate reoperation. Surgery 87:581, 1980
14. Veith FJ, Sprayregen S, Gupta SK: Unpublished observations
15. Whittemore AD, Clowes AW, Couch NP, Mannick JA: Complications of vascular repair below the inguinal ligament. In Bernhard VM, Towne JB, (eds): Complications in Vascular Surgery. New York, Grune & Stratton, 1980, pp 97–105

ELEVEN

Indications for Use of Alternative Vascular Prostheses in Infrainguinal Arterial Reconstruction

Robert W. Hobson II, Zafar Jamil, and Thomas G. Lynch

It is generally believed that with the aid of modern chemistry the perfect prosthesis will be developed which will replace natural vascular grafts. The advantage of having available all lengths and sizes of such replacements is almost a utopian dream, inconceivable today to the vascular surgeon.

Robert R. Linton, M.D.
Presidential Address (1955)
Society for Vascular Surgery

Although 25 years have passed since Linton[16] predicted future availability of an ideal vascular prosthesis, the goal of developing a prosthesis as a substitute for the autogenous saphenous vein for bypass or replacement of small- to medium-sized arteries such as the femoropopliteal system has not yet been achieved. Characteristics of an ideal vascular prosthesis should include immediate availability in variable sizes and shapes, biocompatibility allowing rapid endothelialization, and adequate durability to insure long-term patency without aneurysmal degeneration. The material must be flexible, easily sutured, and cross joint spaces without undue kinking. One of its most important characteristics may be a compliance comparable to autogenous arteries and veins, particularly at the anastomosis between the prosthesis and the artery.[3,10,27] Until such a prosthesis is available for clinical use, surgeons must continue to be cautious in recommending preferred use of any material other than autogenous saphenous vein for small- or medium-sized arterial reconstruction.

During recent years, however, as an aggressive approach toward arterial revascularization of the ischemic lower extremity has evolved, availability of alternative vascular prostheses has become a necessity under a variety of clinical circumstances. These include absence or unsuitability of an autogenous saphenous vein, elective utilization of an alternative vascular prosthesis in the higher-risk patient undergoing complex revascularization to shorten operative time or to preserve a satisfactory vein for future use, and unwillingness to use arm veins for lower extremity revascularization in the absence of a suitable saphenous vein. The purpose of this chapter will be to review these various factors and evaluate their importance in selecting an alternative vascular prosthesis.

ABSENT OR UNSUITABLE SAPHENOUS VEIN

The overall incidence of absent or unsuitable autogenous saphenous vein ranges from 30 to 70 percent depending on the author and clinical report. The higher percentages of unsuitability may be related to lack of diligence in the search for a suitable saphenous vein. Causes of unsuitability or absence include prior operation, varicosities, duplications, sclerosis secondary to previous phlebitis or trauma, as well as inadequate diameter and length. Dale,[7] Darling,[9] and Kakkar[14] have noted that approximately one-third of their patients may require use of an alternative prosthesis. In our own clinical series,[13] we utilized autogenous saphenous vein in 50 percent of cases because of a high incidence of reoperation after previously failed saphenous vein reconstructions. Ferris and Cranley[11] reported that 70 percent of saphenous veins were inadequate in their recent clinical series, perhaps because of selection of only the "larger and more adequate saphenous veins." Despite its imperfections and a relatively high incidence of unsuitability, the autogenous saphenous vein remains the graft of choice when available. Although most surgeons would agree with this statement, a controversy develops when one is faced with the decision to use a marginally acceptable autogenous vein. Precise prospective data on the recommended minimal size for autogenous saphenous vein are not available; however, approximations from retrospective analyses have shown that grafts should exceed 4 to 5 mm in least diameter for their successful use in vascular reconstructions.[15,21] Saphenous veins that are less than 4 mm in diameter or are segmentally sclerotic due to phlebitis, intravenous infusions, or other causes may be less desirable than other currently available arterial prostheses. A recent case report from our clinical experience illustrates this point:

> The patient was a 62-year-old man admitted for rest pain involving the right forefoot. At operation, the ipsilateral autogenous saphenous vein was utilized to revascularize the lower extremity by femoral to below-knee popliteal arterial bypass. The vein was moderately thickened in places but measured 3 to 4 mm in diameter throughout its length following hydrostatic dilation. As demonstrated by operative arteriography (Fig. 1), the saphenous vein graft in the thigh was small; however, arterial run-off was excellent and the anastomosis was technically satisfactory. Nevertheless, peripheral pulses were not palpable postoperatively and ankle systolic pressure increased from a preoperative value of 40 mm Hg to only 50 mm Hg. During the immediate postoperative period, the graft occluded and thrombectomy was performed on two occasions. At the second thrombectomy, a decision was made to replace the autogenous saphenous vein graft with a 6-mm polytetrafluoroethylene prosthesis. Return of palpable peripheral pulses and increase in ankle systolic pressure to 120 mm Hg were observed immediately after operation. A segment of the autogenous saphenous vein was removed for pathologic examination (Fig. 2). Chronic inflammatory changes were noted within the wall of the vein and intimal disruption was apparent perhaps from use of overly high distension pressures during preparation of the graft.

This case report is reflective of the opinion expressed by many surgeons that use of a marginal saphenous vein is inferior to an alternative vascular prosthesis.

The ill-advised traumatic surgical excision and preparation of the saphenous vein may convert a suitable saphenous vein into a marginal performer. Acinapura and co-workers[2] demonstrated reductions in fibrinolytic activity of the endothelium of vein grafts subjected to clamping, stretching, or inadvertent suturing. Since loss of fibrinolytic activity may affect patency adversely, care must be exercised to avoid direct trauma to the vein. This can be best accomplished by use of a long medial thigh incision for full exposure of the saphenous vein coupled with precise and careful ligation and division of tributaries. Once the vein has been excised, use of a chilled (4 C) heparinized balanced salt solution[1] or blood[20] is recommended for irrigation and hydrostatic dilitation to minimize endothelial damage. Traditional forceful hydrostatic dilatation of the vein is to be avoided, however, and should be used sparingly.[20] Malone and associates[17] demonstrated substantial endothelial distortion

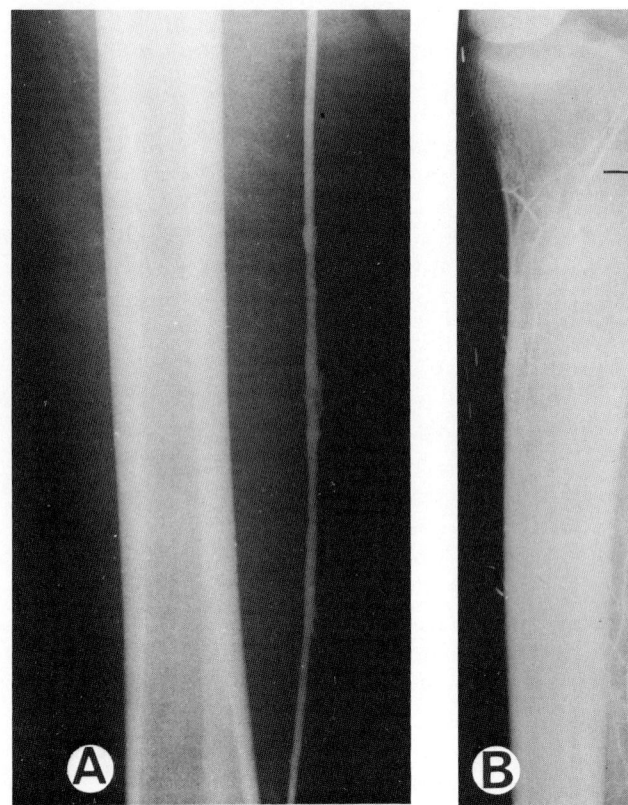

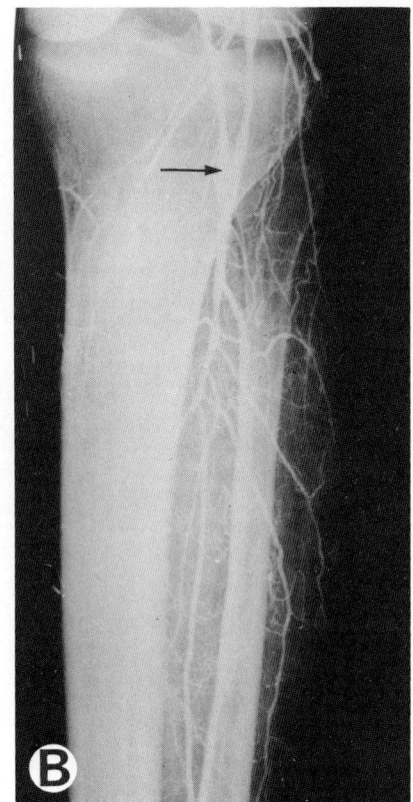

FIGURE 1. Operative arteriogram demonstrating the saphenous vein graft in the thigh (left), distal popliteal anastomosis (arrow, right), and satisfactory arterial run-off.

and damage after venous dilatation at pressures in excess of 700 mm Hg. Fibrinolytic activity was also reduced significantly at this distension pressure. These investigators recommended a distension pressure of less than 500 mm Hg. Boncheck[5] has developed a balloon device to limit maximal pressure to 300 to 400 mm Hg during venous distension to minimize endothelial damage. Use of such a device plus conscientious efforts to minimize hydrostatic dilatation of the vein graft during its preparation should be helpful in improving patency and preventing conversion of a satisfactory saphenous vein to an unsatisfactory graft.

Use of preoperative saphenous venography is an innovative technique that may assist the surgeon in determining suitability of a saphenous vein in selected patients. Veith and associates[25] have demonstrated the value of the technique to predict adequacy of the saphenous vein preoperatively. All veins measuring 2 mm or more at venography dilated to

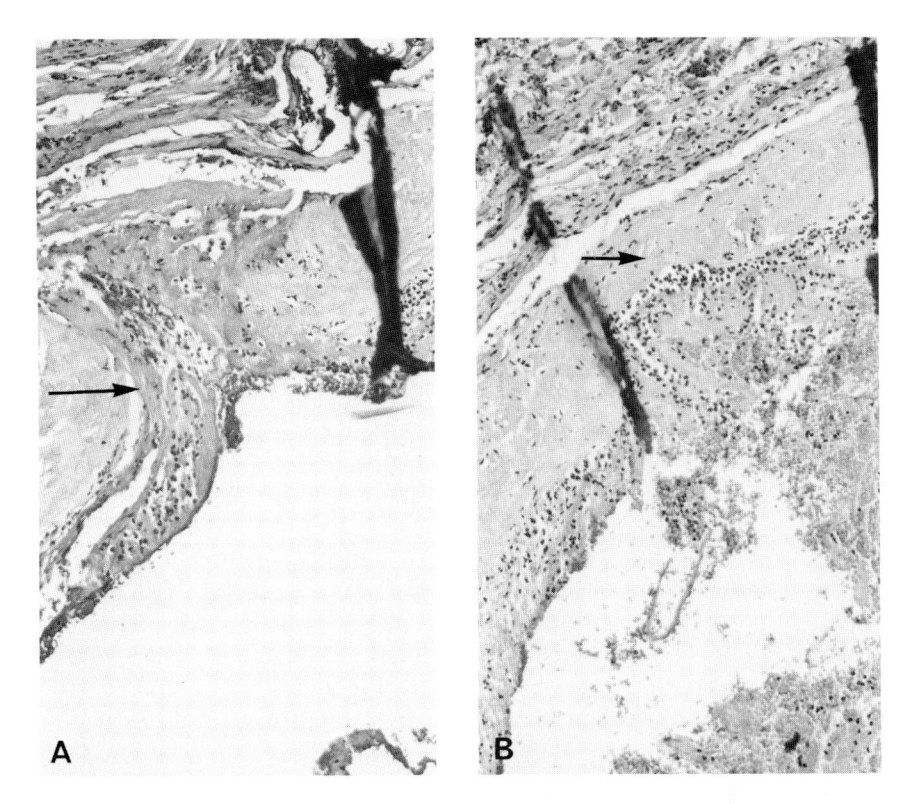

FIGURE 2. **A.** Intimal fracture (arrow) is shown with early thrombus formation. **B.** Subintimal fibrosis (arrow) is present, and thrombus has become attached to the venous wall in an area of denuded intima.

4 mm or more at operation and were suitable for femoropopliteal or distal arterial bypass. Whether or not an autogenous saphenous vein measuring less than 5 mm in transverse diameter should be used remains controversial.[18,25] With the availability of the newer prosthetic alternatives, however, it is our current recommendation that prostheses such as expanded polytetrafluoroethylene and perhaps umbilical vein should be used preferentially to saphenous vein grafts of less than 4 mm transverse diameter.[8,11,13]

REDUCTION IN OPERATIVE TIME: ELECTIVE PRESERVATION OF THE SAPHENOUS VEIN

Cardiac complications are among the most common cause of perioperative morbidity and mortality after major elective vascular reconstruction.[4] The incidence of coronary arterial occlusive disease ranges from 15 to

55 percent in patients with atheroslerotic peripheral vascular disease.[19,24] The presence of symptomatic coronary artery disease may result in a recommendation to use an alternative vascular prosthesis to reduce operative time by eliminating the need to harvest an autogenous saphenous vein or arm veins. Similarly, preoperative pulmonary insufficiency may result in an increased incidence of postoperative complications that might be reduced by decreasing operative time. Although postoperative cardiorespiratory complications will continue to occur as operative procedures are extended to higher-risk patients, it is uncertain whether a reduction in operative time by the 30 to 60 minutes required to remove and prepare the saphenous vein will be beneficial.

Ferris and Cranley[11] used 13 of 70 umbilical vein grafts (19 percent) in complex revascularizations, which included simultaneous performance of inflow and outflow procedures in many cases. These authors observed that the use of a substitute for the saphenous vein conserved approximately 1 hour of operative time that in their cases was "frequently worthwhile." In addition, Haimov and associates[12] recommended use of polytetrafluoroethylene as the prosthesis of choice in high-risk patients because of "expedience." Although some surgeons would argue that the saphenous vein can be harvested and prepared by a second operative team thereby reducing the requirement for additional operative time, the advantage of selecting an alternative vascular prosthesis to expedite the operative procedure may be compelling enough to recommend its use in highly selected individuals. Controlled data are not available on this question, however, and the decision must remain with the individual surgeon in consultation with his medical conferees.

Finally, surgeons may choose to preserve the saphenous vein for future use in coronary or tibial arterial revascularizations.[22] This position suggests acceptability of alternative vascular prostheses including Dacron and possibly polytetrafluoroethylene or umbilical vein for femoropopliteal bypass, preserving the autogenous saphenous vein for the longer distal tibial or peroneal bypasses.[8,11-13,22,26]

USE OF ARM VEINS

Cephalic and basilic veins have been recommended for use in femoropopliteal reconstruction.[6,14,23] In the most recent review, Clayson and associates[6] reported 32 operations using arm veins, 11 of which were used for arterial reconstruction in the lower extremity. Seven of these grafts were patent at 24 months of follow-up suggesting a favorable outcome. The cephalic vein is notable for its thinness, however, particularly in the proximal segment. In addition, it may be more difficult to manipulate and complete a technically satisfactory anastomosis with cephalic vein than with saphenous vein. As a result, several surgeons would suggest use of an alternative prosthesis when arm veins are the only autogenous alternative graft to an unsuitable saphenous vein. Although use of an arteriovenous fistula at the wrist has been suggested as a method to arterialize the cephalic vein and thereby improve its handling characteristics, this requires time and is frequently not an available option in patients requiring expeditious revascularization. Although we have used the cephalic vein in composite Dacron-vein grafts, we currently prefer to use polytetrafluoroethylene before considering Dacron vein composites or arm veins.[13]

While the search for ideal vascular prostheses continues, caution must be exercised in their evaluation and acceptance. Previous experience would indicate that carefully conceived clinical trials comparing newer prostheses with the autogenous saphenous vein or established synthetics such as Dacron are desirable before generalized clinical application of the material.

REFERENCES

1. Abbott WM, Wieland S, Austen WG: Structural changes during preparation of autogenous venous grafts. Surgery 76:1031, 1974
2. Ancipura AJ, Porter JM, Futrell W, Silver D: The effect of local vascular trauma on fibrinolysis. Ann Surg 32:762, 1966
3. Baird RN, Abbott WM: Vein grafts: A historical prospective. Arch Surg 134:293, 1977
4. Bonchek LI: Prevention of cardiac complications during peripheral vascular operations. In Bernhard VM, Towne JB (eds): Complications in Vascular Surgery. New York, Grune & Stratton, 1980
5. Bonchek LI: Consequences of trauma to saphenous veins during their preparation for use as arterial grafts. In Bernhard VM, Towne JB (eds): Complications in Vascular Surgery. New York, Grune & Stratton, 1980
6. Clayson KR, Edwards WH, Allen TR, Dale WA: Arm veins for peripheral arterial reconstruction. Arch Surg 111:1276, 1976
7. Dale WA: Autogenous vein grafts for femoropopliteal occlusion. JAMA 196:120, 1966
8. Dardik H, Ibrahim IM, Darkik I: Evaluation of glutaraldehyde-tanned human umbilical cord vein as a vascular prosthesis for bypass to the popliteal, tibial, and peroneal arteries. Surg 83:577, 1978
9. Darling R, Linton R, Razzuk M: Saphenous vein bypass grafts for femeropopliteal occlusive disease. A reappraisal. Surg 61:31, 1967
10. Edwards, WS: Arterial grafts: Past, present, and future. Arch Surg 113:1225, 1978

11. Ferris EB, Cranley JJ: Use of umbilical vein graft as an arterial substitute. Arch Surg 114:694, 1979
12. Haimov H, Giron F, Jacobson JH II: The expanded polytetrafluoroethylene graft. Arch Surg 114:673, 1979
13. Hobson RW, O'Donnell JA, Jamil Z, Mehta K: Below-knee bypass for limb salvage. Arch Surg 115:833, 1980
14. Kakkar V: The cephalic vein as a peripheral vascular graft. Surg Gynecol Obstet 128:551, 1969
15. Koontz TJ, Stansel HC: Factors influencing patency of the autogenous vein-femoropopliteal bypass graft: An analysis of 74 cases. Surg 71:753, 1972
16. Linton RR: Some practical considerations in the surgery of blood vessel grafts. Surg 38:817, 1955
17. Malone JM, Gervin AS, Kischer CW, et al: Venous fibrinolytic activity and histologic features with distension. Surg Forum 29:479, 1978
18. Miller VM: Femoral popliteal bypass graft patency: An analysis of 156 cases. Ann Surg 180:35, 1974
19. Minken SL, DeWeese JA, Southgate WA, et al: Aortoiliac reconstruction for atherosclerotic occlusive disease. Surg Gynecol Obstet 126:1056, 1968
20. Ramos JR, Bergen K, Mansfield PB, Sauvage LR: Histologic fate and endothelial changes of distended and nondistended vein grafts. Ann Surg 183:205, 1976
21. Ray SS, Lape CP, Lutes CA, Dillihunt RC: Femoropopliteal saphenous vein bypass grafts: Analysis of 150 cases. Am J Surg 119:385, 1970
22. Reichle FA: Criteria for evaluation of new arterial prostheses by comparing vein with Dacron femoropopliteal bypasses. Surg Gynecol Obstet 146:714, 1978
23. Stipa S: The cephalic and basilic vein in peripheral arterial reconstructive surgery. Ann Surg 175:581, 1972
24. Tomatis LA, Fierens EE, Verbrugge GP: Evaluation of surgical risk in peripheral vascular disease via coronary arteriography: A series of 100 cases. Surg 71:429, 1972
25. Veith FJ, Moss CM, Sprayregen S, Montefusco C: Preoperative saphenous venography in arterial reconstructive surgery of the lower extremity. Surg 85:253, 1979
26. Veith FJ, Moss CM, Fell SC, et al: Comparison of expanded polytetrafluoroethylene and autologous saphenous vein grafts in high risk arterial reconstructions for limb salvage. Surg Gynecol Obstet 147:749, 1978
27. Wright CB, Hiratzka LF: Introduction to the vascular symposium. Arch Surg 114:665, 1979

Part Three
Reconstructive Venous Surgery

TWELVE

Reconstructive Venous Surgery: Diagnosis and Techniques

John J. Bergan, Neil D. Rudo, John P. Harris, and James S. T. Yao

The recent awakening of interest in direct venous surgery has allowed a complete rethinking of the problems of venous stasis. Facts obtained from older investigations are now falling into place to explain the phenomena observed and pathophysiology noted in venous stasis. It is appropriate, therefore, for us to re-examine the status of testing of venous physiology and note its application to diagnosis and surgical treatment of patients with venous stasis disease.

In general terms, three conditions occur alone and in combination to produce the final product that is called venous stasis. These conditions include chronic obstruction of major veins such as is seen in the common iliac vein and in the superficial femoral vein; each of these obstructions can be treated by autogenous bypass. A second condition, which may coexist with the first, is deep vein valvular incompetence. Such valvular incompetence may be primary, as described and corrected by Kistner,[13] or secondary to recanalization of acute thrombosis, such as occurs in the natural evolution of superficial femoral thrombophlebitis. The third condition, which may exist with either or both of the other two, is valvular incompetence of communicating veins. It is this particular form of venous insufficiency that has been the target of surgical therapy in the past.

Just as bypass of chronic obstruction can be performed, so, too, can reconstruction of valves be achieved by valvuloplasty and by transposi-

---

This work was supported in part by a grant in aid from the Conrad Jobst Foundation and the Northwestern University Vascular Research Fund.

tion of veins so that the venous stream is directed through competent valves. Both methods, singly and in combination, eliminate valvular incompetency. The older techniques, which focus upon perforator incompetence, remain crucially important to treatment of venous stasis, as does removal of superficial varices when these alone produce severe venous stasis.

DIAGNOSTIC TESTING

Objectives of diagnostic testing in patients with chronic venous insufficiency are twofold. The first is to clarify the diagnosis and separate those cases of pure superficial venous insufficiency from those of deep venous insufficiency. The second is to quantitate the degree of venous stasis in order to assess the value of therapeutic maneuvers.

Although the clinical diagnosis of deep venous thrombosis has been known to be unreliable for a long time, it has only been appreciated in recent years that the diagnosis of chronic venous stasis disease caused by the postphlebitic syndrome is also subject to error. The clinical combination of edema, superficial varicose veins, cutaneous pigmentation, and skin eczema or ulceration had seemed to indicate unequivocally the postphlebitic syndrome. When such a diagnosis was made, the condition was thought to be incurable, even though it could be treated conservatively and surgically. Now, accurate noninvasive evaluation of venous pathophysiology has taught us that the hallmarks of the postphlebitic state may be caused by superficial venous insufficiency in the presence of normal deep venous anatomy. Thus, the condition becomes not only treatable but curable.

Venous Pressure Determinations

Since venous cannulation is such a simple procedure, the study of venous pressure has been available for many years and has been used by some surgeons interested in the surgery of venous insufficiency for more than 25 years. The test can be performed with the patient supine, sitting or standing, during or after exercise, and can be combined with the application of tourniquets at the leg and thigh in order to separate venous flow into its superficial and deep components.

In the normal extremity, pressures are equal in the superficial, deep, and perforating veins. In the erect position, the venous pressure at the ankle is approximately equal to the pressure exerted by a column of blood extending from the right atrium to the point on the limb in which the venous system is cannulated. Standing venous pressure at the ankle approaches that of the arterial system and is in the range of 100 to 120 mm Hg. In the normal limb, calf exercise causes emptying of the veins, with a reduction in standing venous pressure during such calf compression. The drop in pressure will be 30 to 40 percent of the resting value. The time it takes to regain normal standing venous pressure can be used as an estimate of venous insufficiency.

Patients with primary varicose veins will have a normal standing venous pressure. Walking or other calf exercise, however, does not reduce venous pressure by as great a degree as in the normal limb. Venous pressure recovery time with cessation of exercise is markedly shortened in patients with varicose veins because of reflux through the superficial venous system in a distal direction. Application of a tourniquet above or below the knee will eliminate the superficial venous incompetence. When this is done in patients with primary varicose veins, walking venous pressure will fall in response to exercise as it does in the normal limb, and the recovery time of venous pressure will be prolonged as it is in a normal person. In patients with chronic deep-vein insufficiency, on the other hand, application of tourniquets above and below the knee during exercise testing and venous pressure measurement will not produce as great a venous pressure fall as in the normal person. Recovery time to baseline levels remains quite short because blood refluxes through the deep venous system in a retrograde direction.

Photoplethysmography

The venous photoplethysmograph can provide information similar to that of venous pressure studies, especially with regard to venous refilling time, and in a less cumbersome fashion. The photoplethysmograph (PPG) consists of a transducer, amplifier, and strip-chart recorder. The PPG emits infrared light that is directed through underlying tissues. Reflected light is detected by a photodetector and is proportional to the largely venous blood content of the subpapillary plexus. The content of this vascular plexus is affected by arterial inflow, venous outflow, and venous reflux.

In clinical use, the PPG records changes of skin blood content before, during, and after exercise, just as has been done with venous pressure recordings. Abramowitz and colleagues[1] established the fact that absolute volume change of the subpapillary plexus is not determined accurately by the photoplethysmographic technique. Refill time after exercise, however, was entirely comparable to venous pressure refill time. The high degree of correlation between simultaneous measurements suggested that the PPG technique could be substituted for venous pressure determinations. Normal patients had a venous refill time of greater than

23 seconds, while abnormal patients with venous reflux had a refill time of less than 20 seconds.

In application of this technique, the patient is examined in a sitting position with the legs dependent. He is asked to contract his calf muscles by flexing and extending the foot five times. Photoplethysmographic tracings are taken before, during, and after exercise, and these tracings are done before and after application of a tourniquet above the knee and then below the knee. The tourniquet is inflated to 50 mm Hg to occlude superficial veins.

The PPG technique of assessing venous insufficiency can be used in three ways (Fig. 1). First, it can assist in differentiating between superficial and deep venous insufficiency. Second, it can quantitate the degree of venous insufficiency before surgery in patients with superficial venous

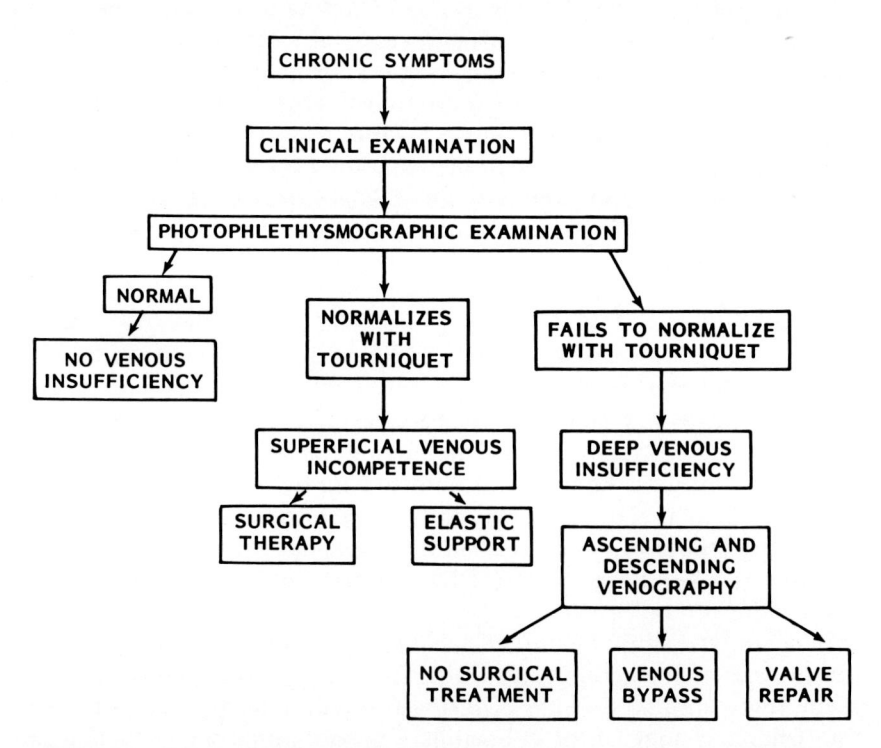

FIGURE 1. This schema shows how clinical evaluation, diagnostic testing, and ascending and descending phlebography are used in evaluation of patients with venous stasis. (From Bergan JJ, Yao JST: Noninvasive assessment of venous disease. In Greenhalgh RM (ed): Hormones and Vascular Disease. London, Pitman Medical Ltd, 1980.)

incompetence and can measure the results of simple varicose vein surgery. Third, the technique can be used to give objective evaluation of venous insufficiency in patients with the postphlebitic state. In those patients subjected to direct venous reconstruction, the method allows objective evaluation of this surgery. Thus, in a preliminary study, we examined 15 patients who had pure saphenous venous insufficiency with primary varicose veins. Photoplethysmographic refill time was measured before and after vein stripping. Thirteen of the patients had venous refill time improved preoperatively during tourniquet application while being tested. All but one of these patients were found to have normalization of venous refill time after vein stripping. This one patient clearly did not derive maximum benefit from vein stripping. Also, in this group of 15 patients, it was clear that two patients had a component of deep venous insufficiency in addition to superficial venous incompetence.

Experience in separating patients into the two groups, those with only superficial incompetence and those with only deep venous incompetence, has been valuable. For example, it has been found that some patients with severe cutaneous ulceration, with or without stasis dermatitis and with cutaneous pigmentation at the ankle, have normalization of their PPG testing by superficial tourniquet application. This is surprising but has important implications since these patients can be benefitted by extensive superficial venous stripping. Furthermore, this experience has shown that clinical evaluation of patients may be erroneous. Some patients carrying a diagnosis of incurable postphlebitic state have a condition that can be markedly improved by simple venous stripping.

Phlebography

Direct repair of venous insufficiency is dependent upon excellent ascending and descending venography. Ascending venography, done by the technique of Rabinov and Paulin,[22] allows demonstration of patency of existing veins. The technique does this but does not assess valve function. Descending venography determines whether or not a competent valve is present in the proximal saphenous vein, superficial femoral vein, or profunda femoris vein. The examination is done with the patient standing and a catheter placed in the common femoral vein. As contrast media is injected, the patient performs a strong Valsalva maneuver, and the flow of contrast media is watched during fluoroscopy on an image intensification screen. Films are taken for a permanent record. In this examination, the contrast agent is heavier than blood and tends to settle in the direction of gravity unless it is prevented from doing so by a competent valve. Experience has shown that during descending venography a spectrum of valve function is seen. This ranges from valves that are totally competent to those that are so grossly incompetent that reflux occurs down the venous system as far as the ankle. Such an assessment allows a choice of valve for subsequent valve transposition or valvuloplasty.

BYPASS GRAFTING FOR VENOUS OCCLUSION

In 1950, Jean Kunlin[16] described a venous bypass using a free transplant of saphenous vein to connect an external iliac vein with the contralateral common iliac vein. While thrombotic obstruction occurred in his case, patency was demonstrated to be present for 3 weeks. Subsequently, Creighton Hardin[8] described saphenous vein bypass grafts for the relief of venous obstruction in the extremity in 1962. Hardin's procedure was a common femoral-to-vena cava bypass with a free saphenous vein transplant with a venous patch added at the lower end to widen the origin of the venous graft. Eduardo Palma of Montevideo[19,20] receives credit for the ingenious idea of crossover femorofemoral grafting with a single venovenous anastomosis.

A large experience has accumulated from which some conclusions can be derived about femorofemoral crossover grafting. In Dale's experience,[2-4] only 6 of 42 patients failed to obtain any relief from the crossover graft and, in 22 of the cases, complete relief of symptoms was obtained. Husni's treatment of postphlebitic disease by crossover bypass grafting in 85 cases is also noteworthy as he demonstrated 83 percent patency of his reconstructions.[12]

It is apparent that in performing this operation bilateral femoral venous pressure measurements must be taken because the pelvic veins must be be grossly obstructed to ensure patency of the graft. There must be a gradient of pressure between the affected limb and the recipient venous bed. The best results are obtained when the thigh and leg veins are patent on the affected side, with the thrombosis limited mainly to the pelvic veins. It is in this ideal situation, however, that the patient may be relatively asymptomatic.

While Kunlin was the first to show experimentally that a temporary arteriovenous fistula would improve patency of the venous anastomosis, others have confirmed this work. Among these is documentation by Dost[5] in 1968, the confirmation of his work by Dumanian,[6] and the wider clinical application of this by Vollmar.[23] Vollmar's most recent modification of the technique is to use a tributary vein to create a small arteriovenous fistula that feeds the venous anastomosis.

Many feel that the temporary arteriovenous fistula represents the decisive advance in the bypass procedure of Palma. The Northwestern group, however, believes this technique to be unnecessary, and instead performs the Palma operation with careful venovenous anastomosis using magnification and 7–0 polypropylene suture without creation of an arteriovenous fistula.

Femoropopliteal Bypass

In attempting to correct the venous insufficiency of superficial femoral venous occlusion, Warren and Thayer[24] transplanted the great saphenous vein to the submuscular compartment and in one-half of these patients anastomosed the popliteal vein to the greater saphenous. Husni's experience with this operation is extensive.[9-11] He demonstrated 66 percent patency of the graft in 24 instances, and indicated that, in all cases in which the graft thrombosed, there was acute or subacute phlebitis in the popliteal vein or its tributaries at the time of the reconstruction.

A similar experience has been described by Frileux et al.[7] In their series, 23 patients were operated upon, 15 were improved and 2 were unimproved, but 6 patients were lost to follow-up. In another relatively large series, May[17,18] described 16 patients, 14 of whom were improved by the procedure, and 2 were unimproved.

Several steps in this procedure are of importance. A medial approach is made to the popliteal vessels below the knee, carefully avoiding the saphenous vein. The crural fascia is incised, and the gastrocnemius-soleus muscle complex retracted posteriorly as in exposure of the popliteal vessels for arterial anastomosis. In patients with the postphlebitic state, the dissection may be difficult because of perivenous adhesions. The saphenous vein is best identified above the knee through an anteromedial thigh incision directly over the vein. Its tributaries are ligated, and enough length is dissected free to allow the vein to lie in a tunnel parallel to and adjacent to the popliteal vein posterior to the knee. The divided saphenous vein is gently irrigated with dilute heparin solution; the patient is given systemic heparin; the vein is tunnelled through the previously prepared anatomic tunnel along the neurovascular bundle behind the knee; and an end of saphenous vein-to-side of popliteal vein anastomosis is performed using continuous 7–0 monofilament vascular suture with the aid of magnification. This modification of Husni's technique prevents acute angulation of the vein at the level of the crural fascia.

VENOUS VALVULOPLASTY

The diagnosis of valve incompetence of the proximal veins of the lower extremities is dependent upon excellent phlebography. Once such evaluation has been made and ascending phlebography has been done to rule out venous occlusion, attention can be turned toward proper correction of the venous insufficiency. Kistner[13,15] made several important observations including the fact that establishing one competent valve in the deep venous system of the lower extremity at the femoral level markedly improves abnormal venous function. This is crucial to an understanding of why a single valvuloplasty is performed.

In Kistner's technique, valve repair is done through a longitudinal incision in the femoral vein, which is exposed from above the saphenofemoral junction down to the junction of the upper and middle thirds of the superficial femoral vein near the midthigh. Usually, the highest valve in the superficial femoral system is chosen for repair. Once the venous segment is exposed, the adventitia is carefully cleaned from the vein wall and the valve cusp insertion visualized through the intact vein wall. Kistner has described that this insertion appears as a white line around the circumference of the vein and has a semilunar shape with the convexity directed downward. Great care must be taken to identify the precise line of insertion of the valve cusp. A marking suture is placed at the juncture or commissure of the two valve cusps.

The venotomy is done meticulously in order that the incision through the vein wall goes through the commissure of the cusps and does not damage the valve in any way. The venotomy is eventually 6 to 8 cm in length and allows careful inspection of the valve cusp. The abnormality of the valve is usually an elongation or stretching of the cusp. Once this is identified carefully, multiple interrupted sutures of 7–0 prolene are placed to shorten the leading edge of the cusp itself. Loop magnification is used and the number of sutures placed is sufficient to remove all of the vertical folds of the valve. Exact coaptation of the commissure is done during venotomy closure, which is effected with 7–0 monofilament suture also.

The upper half of the venotomy is closed first so that competence of the valve can be checked by releasing the proximal venous clamp. An ideal repair will produce a valve cusp that fills with blood without reflux. After full closure of the venotomy, competency of the valve is checked by milking blood through the vein and then exerting back pressure by digital compression of the proximal vein. Systemic heparinization, which is initiated before venotomy, is continued through the early postoperative phase of convalescence.

VALVE TRANSPOSITION

Because primary venous valvular incompetence is relatively rare and postphlebitic recanalization-induced valvular incompetence is so common, development of the procedure of valve transposition has been welcome. The objective of this operation is to provide a functionally competent venous valve at the femoral level. Planning for the procedure depends on excellent ascending and descending venography. This is supplemented by Doppler ultrasonic evaluation of the competence of the saphenofemoral valve.

A vareity of procedures can be done, but the important principle of the operation is to provide a competent valve through which mainsteam venous flow is directed.[15,21] The most useful procedure is transection of the superficial femoral vein and saphenous vein with anastomosis of the distal end of the transected superficial femoral vein to the proximal end of the saphenous vein. This directs flow from the superficial femoral vein into the saphenous vein with its competent saphenofemoral valve (Fig. 2). Variations of this operation can include anastomosis of the distal end of the transected saphenous vein to the superficial femoral vein, with or without anastomosis of the profunda femoris vein to the superficial femoral vein as well. When a profunda femoris vein contains a competent valve, the superficial femoral vein may be anastomosed

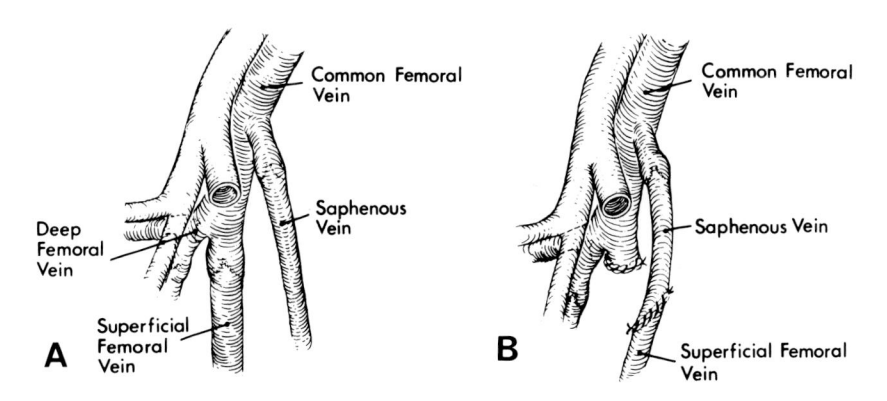

FIGURE 2. **A.** In the normal situation competent valves may be present in the three tributaries to the common femoral vein. One method of correcting superficial femoral venous incompetence is shown in **B.** This is transposition of the superficial femoral venous stream through a competent saphenofemoral valve. (From Queral LA, Whitehouse WM Jr, Flinn WR, et al: Surgical correction of chronic deep venous insufficiency by valvular transposition. Surgery 87:688, 1980; used with permission.)

end-to-end or end-to-side to the profunda femoris vein (Fig. 3A). Kistner has also suggested that any of these procedures can be combined with valvuloplasty in order that competence can be achieved in one of the several available valves.

In at least one situation, superficial femoral vein ligation may prove to be the procedure of choice. This is encountered when gross valvular incompetence of the superficial femoral vein is found, and the patient has a competent valve at the junction of the profunda system with the common femoral vein. Ligation of the superficial femoral vein in this situation causes the deep venous circulation to return to the profunda system, in which a competent valve is present (Fig. 3B).

RESULTS

Early assessment of the results of venous valve transposition, ligation of the superficial femoral vein when appropriate, and valve repair has been gratifying in several respects. Patient satisfaction with the procedure is the most prominent feature of the early postoperative recovery period. A decrease in bursting pain in the extremity with dependency, a decrease in edema, and a decrease in the sense of fullness and heaviness is noted by virtually every patient.

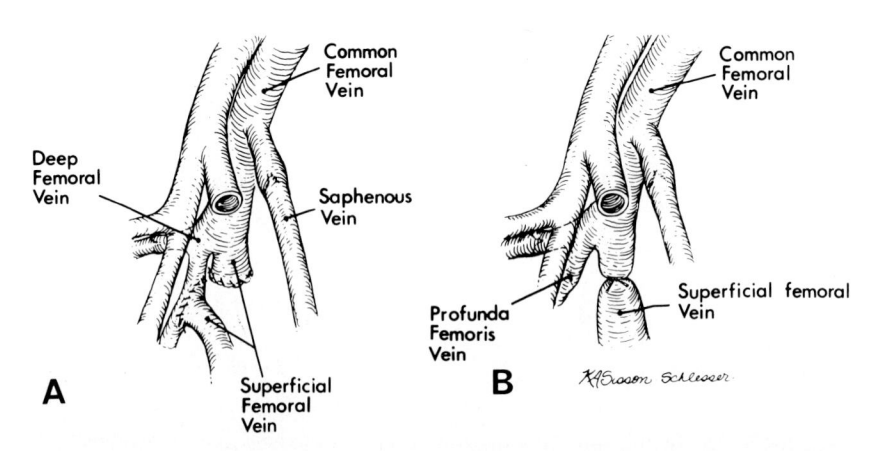

FIGURE 3. **A.** Profunda venous transposition. **B.** Superficial femoral ligation. Variations on venous transposition may be useful in solving individual patient problems. Superficial to profunda transposition is shown, as is simple ligation of the superficial femoral vein. This latter operation may be done when profunda femoris valvular competence is present. (From Queral LA, Whitehouse WM Jr, Flinn WR, et al: Surgical correction of chronic deep venous insufficiency by valvular transposition. Surgery 87:688, 1980; used with permission.)

Objective proof of benefit of the procedure is more difficult to document. Insufficient time has elapsed to determine whether years of freedom from sequelae of stasis disease will be present. On the other hand, some objective measurements of improvement have been observed. Among these is PPG recovery time and venous pressure recovery time. Table 1 shows that venous pressure recovery times were usually significatnly improved by reconstruction of the femoral valve system. The PPG recovery time along with the venous pressure recovery time was much improved. Careful measurement of venous pressures indicated, however, that after valve transposition the degree of drop of venous pressure after exercise was unchanged. That directional Doppler examination of popliteal venous valvular competence has shown that bidirectional venous flow has been corrected in 6 of 11 cases operated upon at the femoral level was of some interest. That perforator incompetence, present in each of these cases, was not corrected was additionally interesting. Valve transposition alone was the procedure done and evaluated.

It is encouraging that some dynamic parameters of deep venous function have been improved after valve repair at the femoral level. The final test of effectiveness of this procedure will be persistent relief of symptomatology. Ultimately, only absence of ulcer recurrence, return to previous employment, and/or the reversal of need to wear elastic

Table 1. Postexercise Hemodynamic Recovery in 12 Patients Undergoing Venous Valve Transposition (sec)

Case No.	Preoperative PPG	Preoperative Venous Pressure	Postoperative PPG	Postoperative Venous Pressure
1	9.5	11.0	20.0	24.0
2	7.6	8.0	20.0	21.0
3	10.3	9.4	31.3	28.0
4	6.6	7.0	18.2	19.3
5	8.8	9.0	23.4	24.8
6	8.6	7.3	22.0	24.0
7*	20.0	18.5	36.0	34.8
8*	9.0	8.3	23.0	24.0
9	14.0	15.0	21.0	22.6
10	9.0	10.0	18.0	18.0
11	12.0	14.0	7.0	7.0
12	10.0	11.0	16.0	15.0

* Superficial femoral vein-to-profunda femoris vein anastomosis thrombosed during re-exploration. The superficial femoral vein was transected after assuring that the profunda vein was patent.

support will be the final tests. On the other hand, early striking hemodynamic improvement in the small number of limbs operated upon and assessed suggests that direct venous valvular repair may be important to those surgeons who are dedicated to care of patients with venous stasis disease.

REFERENCES

1. Abramowitz HB, Queral LA, Flinn WR, et al: The use of photoplethysmography in the assessment of venous insufficiency: a comparison to venous pressure measurements. Surgery 85:434, 1979
2. Dale WA: Crossover grafts for iliofemoral venous occlusion. In Bergan JJ, Yao JST (eds): Venous Problems. Chicago, Year Book, 1978, pp. 411–420
3. Dale WA, Harris J: Cross-over vein grafts for venous occlusion. Ann Surg 168:319, 1968
4. Dale WA, Harris J: Cross-over vein grafts for iliac and femoral venous occlusion. J Cardiovasc Surg 10:458, 1969
5. Dost K: Druck-und Flussgeschwindigkeit in der Vene bei plastischem Venenersatz. Angiologica 5:271, 1968
6. Dumanian AV: Cross-over saphenous vein graft combined with a temporary femoral a.v. fistula. Vasc Surg 2:116, 1968
7. Frileux, D, Pillot-Bienayme P, Gillot C: Bypass of segmental obliterations of iliofemoral venous axis by transposition of saphenous vein. J Cardiovasc Surg 15:409, 1972
8. Hardin CA: Bypass saphenous grafts for the relief of venous obstruction of the extremity. Surg Gynecol Obstet 115:709, 1962
9. Husni EA: In situ saphenopopliteal bypass graft for incompetence of the femoral and popliteal veins. Surg Gynecol Obstet 130:279, 1970
10. Husni EA: Venous reconstruction in postphlebitic disease. Circulation 43 (Suppl 1): 147, 1971
11. Husni EA: The postphlebitic limb. Hospital Med 7:73, 1971
12. Husni EA: Clinical experience with femoropopliteal venous reconstruction. In Bergan JJ, Yao JST (eds): Venous Problems. Chicago, Year Book, 1978, pp 485–491
13. Kistner RL: Transvenous repair of the incompetent femoral vein valve. In Bergan JJ, Yao JST (eds): Venous Problems. Chicago, Year Book, 1978, pp 493–509
14. Kistner RL, Ferris EB: Technique of surgical reconstruction of femoral venous vein valves. In Bergan JJ, Yao JST (eds): Operative Techniques in Vascular Surgery. New York, Grune & Stratton, 1980
15. Kistner RL, Sparkuhl MD: Surgery in acute and chronic venous disease. Surgery 85:31, 1979
16. Kunlin J: Le retablissement de la circulation veineuse par greffe en cas d'obliterative traumatique ou thrombophlebitique: greffe de 18 cm entre

la veine saphene interne et al veine iliaque externe; thrombose apres trois semaines de permeabilite. Mem Acad Chir 79:109, 1950
17. May R: Surgical treatment of the postthrombotic state by a femoral bypass. VASA 1:267, 1972
18. May R: Femoral bypass for the postphlebitic state. Phlebologie 27:469, 1974
19. Palma CE, Esperon R: Tratamiento del sindrome posttrombo-flebitico mediante transplante de safena interna. Angiologia 11:87, 1959
20. Palma CE, Esperon R: Vein transplants and grafts in the surgical treatment of the postphlebitic syndrome. J Cardiovasc Surg 1:94, 1960
21. Queral LA, Whitehouse WM Jr, Flinn WR, et al: Surgical correction of chronic deep venous insufficiency by valvular transposition. Surgery 87:688, 1980
22. Rabinov K, Paulin S: Roentgen diagnosis of venous thrombosis in the leg. Arch Surg 104:134, 1972
23. Vollmar J: Die Rekonstruktion unilateraler Beckenvenenverschlusse. Acta Chir 5:79,1970
24. Warren R, Thayer TB: Transplantation of the saphenous vein for postphlebitic stasis. Surgery 35:867, 1954

THIRTEEN
Reconstructive Venous Surgery

W. Andrew Dale

In the 1960s, our attention was attracted to the field of reconstructive venous surgery for patients with lower extremity venous insufficiency for which little or no help was available beyond restrictive measures that often led to a life of semi-invalidism. While there had been occasional reports of successful operations dating back to 1906,[9] venous surgery was little known and poorly understood.

Experiments in the animal laboratory were therefore conducted to learn the general principles in this field of surgery and over 100 of these were summarized in 1963.[8] Our observations included certain instances of recanalization of an initially thrombosed vein graft,[4] the importance of pressure differential and internal flow to maintenance of graft patency (rather than external splinting or graft rigidity), and the long-term successes of properly placed venous grafts.

Of particular interest was the crossover graft described in 1959 by Eduardo Palma of Montevideo, Uruguay.[17] Our animal experiments with this procedure produced good results and led to the clinical cases reported in 1968.[7]

Interest in reconstructive venous surgery has continued, but experience has accumulated slowly because of caution with new procedures as well as difficulties in delineating appropriate candidates with venous obstruction from the large numbers of postphlebitic patients whose veins have partially recanalized and do not appear to be suitable for such operations.

REPAIR OF LARGE VEINS

Animal experiments as well as occasional patients show successful results in repairing injuries of the vena cava and iliac and femoral veins. Suture of lateral injuries of these veins is well known and certainly preferable to their ligation. Lateral patch grafts may be used if a portion of the wall is missing or requires debridement.

While synthetic grafts do not usually remain open when used to replace small peripheral veins, such prosthetic tubes have successfully replaced both the superior and inferior vena cava damaged by tumor or by injury. Figure 1 is a postoperative phlebogram showing a patent Dacron tube

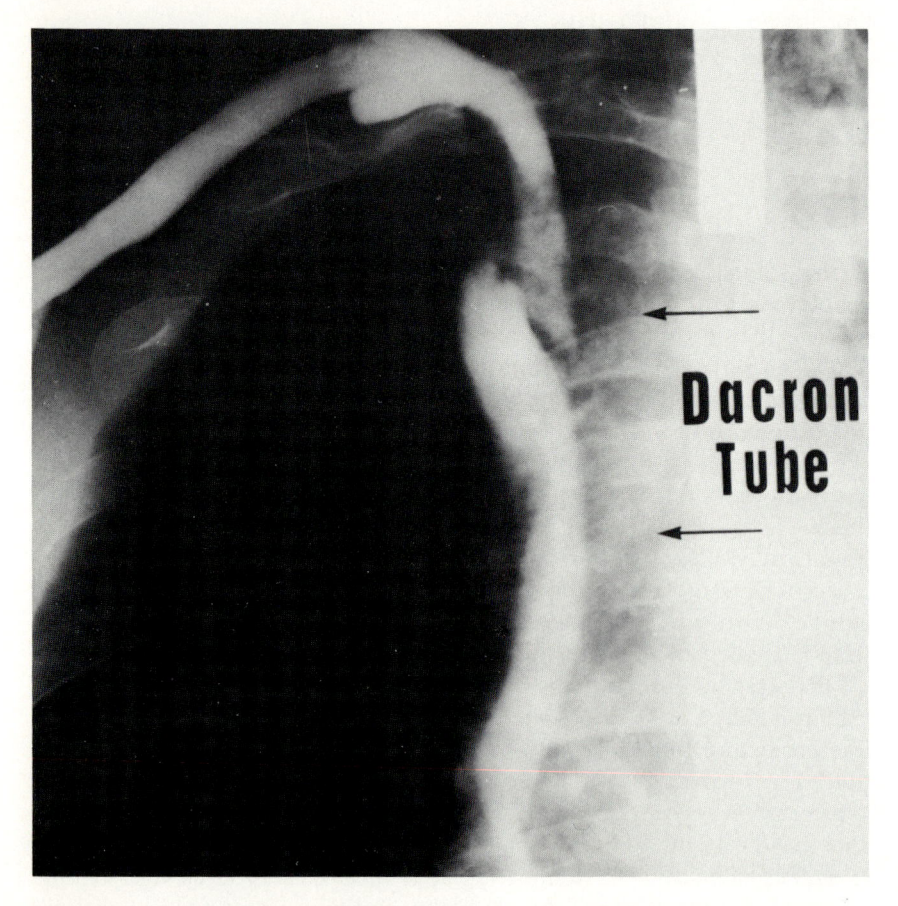

FIGURE 1. Postoperative phlebogram shows a knit Dacron tube bypassing the superior vena cava from the subclavian vein to the right atrial appendage within the pericardial sac.

bypass to relieve venous hypertension of the head and upper extremities. In this case the obstruction was caused by malignant occlusion of the superior vena cava. Such a palliative bypass is occasionally helpful.

The patent polytetrafluoroethylene graft replacing the traumatized inferior vena cava in Figure 2 illustrates that success may be achieved with this procedure. The numbers of such cases are small and the patency rate is not known since it is quite likely that successes are reported while failures are never shown. Nevertheless, the feasibility of such procedures must be recognized.

We have no personal experience with the use of a large venous graft constructed from panels of saphenous vein or with the spiral placement of the vein over a mandril to achieve a larger diameter, but these operations have been reported.[1]

Venous bypasses in the portal system whereby a large diameter Dacron tube has been used to form an H mesocaval shunt have been well-described in the literature[10] and we have found them to be useful. Less recognized are longer shunts from a high pressure vein within the abdomen to one of the low pressure veins within the chest to alleviate the portal hypertension following hepatic vein occlusion (Budd-Chiari syndrome). A number of variations of such procedures have been reviewed and reported. Our single experience with such a Dacron bypass from the umbilical vein within the abdomen to the azygos vein within the chest remained patent only 6 months, yet it allowed palliation of the patient during the crucial time needed for the development of further collaterals so that a reasonable life continued even after failure and removal of the bypass.[6]

VENOUS RECONSTRUCTION IN THE ILIAC AND FEMORAL VEINS

Most of our experience in the venous field has consisted of bypasses of the chronically occluded iliac and/or femoral veins. The etiology of all 65 cases operated upon to date is shown in Table 1; most of these were iliofemoral blocks. As shown in the table, a variety of malignant tumors can cause such venous obstruction. Tumor should be immediately suspected when sudden edema appears in a middle aged or elderly patient's lower extremity. Results of bypassing procedures for such tumorous obstructions have been even better than similar procedures for the postphlebitic state so that their use is worthwhile even if the long-term results are only palliative because of the tumor.

The plan of management of patients with chronic iliac and/or femoral occlusion is summarized in Table 2. Tumors should be carefully consid-

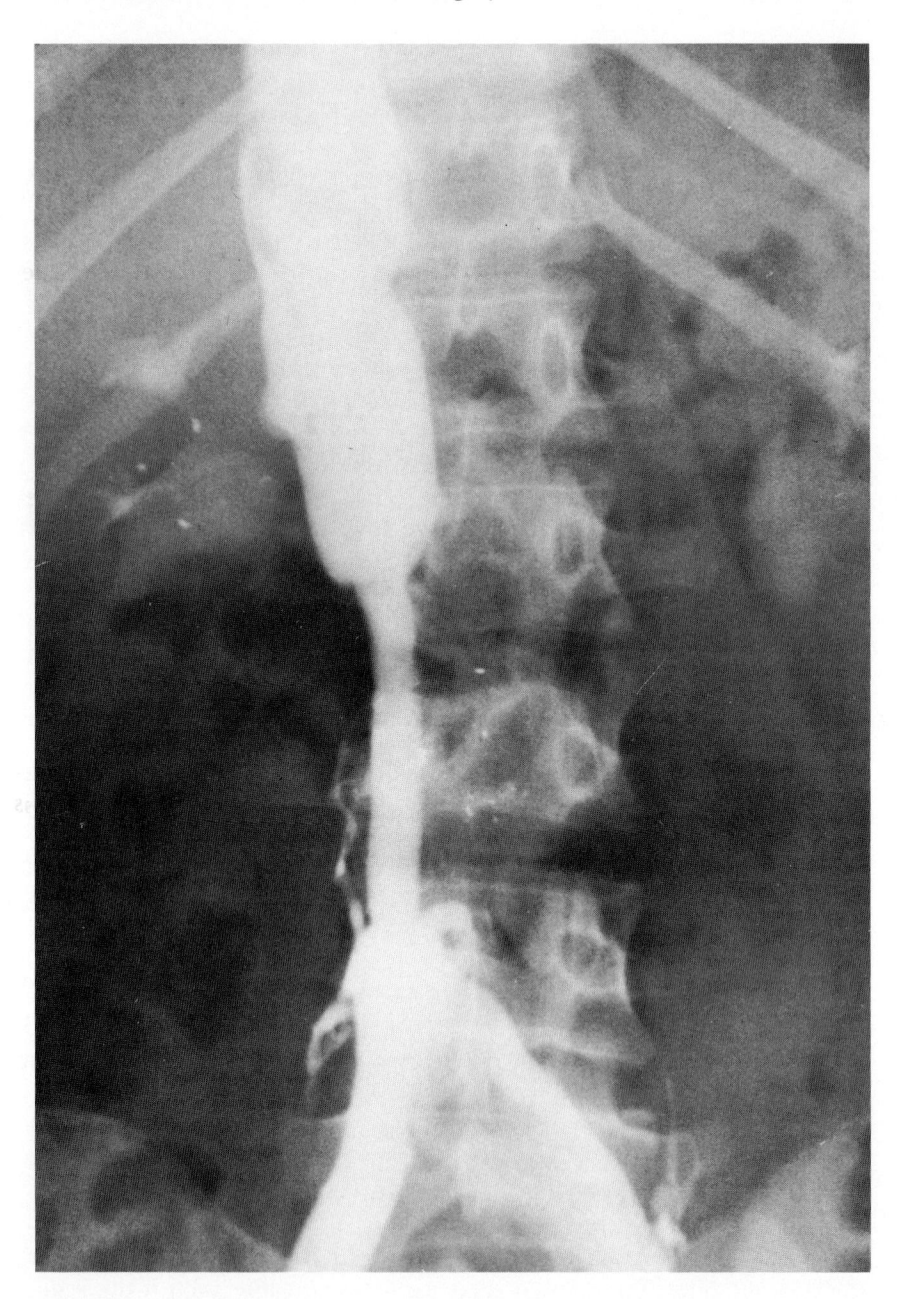

FIGURE 2. Eight-mm polytetrafluoroethylene graft replacing the inferior vena cava that was shot away by a rifle bullet. This 4-month postoperative phlebogram documents its patency. Surgery was performed by Dr. Richard Terry.

Table 1. Etiology of 64 Surgical Cases

Tumor		
Cervix	7	
Lymphoma	4	
Bladder	3	
Rectum	2	
Prostate	1	
Pancreas	1	
Total	18	(28%)
Postphlebitic	43	(66%)
Iliac vein compression	4	(6%)

Table 2. Plan of Management

Diagnosis: Tumor or phlebitis?
  Examination, includes pelvic and rectal
  Visceral x-rays, IVP, barium enema
  Cystoscopy, sigmoidoscopy
  Exploration
Delineation of venous block by phlebography
  Site and extent
  Contralateral patency
Treatment: Crossover vein graft if
  Venous thrombosis is stable and not recanalized
  The patient has a tumor with life expectancy of 6 months or longer

ered and laparotomy or extraperitoneal exploration may occasionally be necessary to find them.

The importance of complete phlebography has been noted previously, and there are several techniques by which this can be achieved.[15] Repetitive examination at 6-month or longer intervals is sometimes helpful in determining whether recanalization is improving the situation or whether there is an unchanging pattern that will require an early venous reconstructive procedure.

While ambulatory venous studies are not always critical to the management of these patients, they are not difficult to perform and may contribute to additional understanding of the overall venous problem.

TECHNIQUES AND RESULTS

The several operations available for peripheral venous reconstruction will be discussed under five categories.

Cross-over Saphenofemoral Vein Grafts

The normal contralateral saphenous vein is dissected to whatever length is needed, its tributaries ligated and it is tunneled across the suprapubic fat pad and anastomosed to the femoral vein distal to the iliac or common femoral obstruction (Fig. 3). The femoral vein is often encased in a fibrotic fascial sheath, and its walls are thickened. The lumen may contain postphlebitic webs and bands that should be trimmed away after the vein is opened. If the proximal portion of the femoral system in the groin is not patent by phlebogram, a more distal site in the midthigh should be selected. Occasionally the only patent vein in a limb distal to the occlusion is the saphenous. In such cases, it may be used for the anastomosis that is performed with a 6–0 continuous polypropylene suture. The patient is heparinized during the operation but not afterwards for fear of hematoma formation and tamponade of the graft. A special U-shaped venous clamp is of technical importance since the dissection is simplified when the entire circumference of the femoral vein does not require dissection.[7]

The procedure requires 1½ to 2 hours and is easily done under spinal

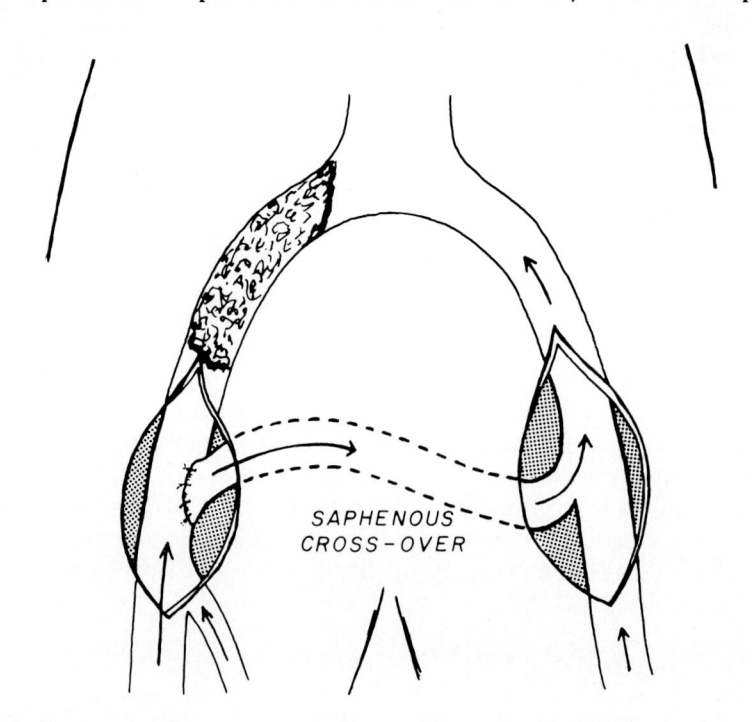

FIGURE 3. The cross-over saphenous vein graft uses a normal saphenous vein from the contralateral extremity to bypass an iliac or femoral occlusion.

anesthesia. There has been no mortality and only an occasional complication of seroma or hematoma that should be prevented by proper intraoperative hemostatis and the use of a suction drain for 24 hours if there is any evidence of continued ooze as the wound is being closed.

Our success rate in 50 cross-over vein grafts was 78 percent as indicated by either complete or partial relief of the patient's edema. Postoperative phlebograms are important in evaluating the results since clinical signs alone may be inaccurate. Our failure to obtain these universally parallels the experience of others and reflects difficulties in persuading patients to undergo an angiographic procedure that most consider to be somewhat unpleasant and to have some slight risk (see Chap. 2).

Our longest term postoperative phebogram obtained 12 years following operation shows a patent venous reconstruction (Fig. 4). The patient had been asymptomatic throughout the 12-year postoperative period. Our patency rate is similar to statistics published by others in Table 3.[12,19]

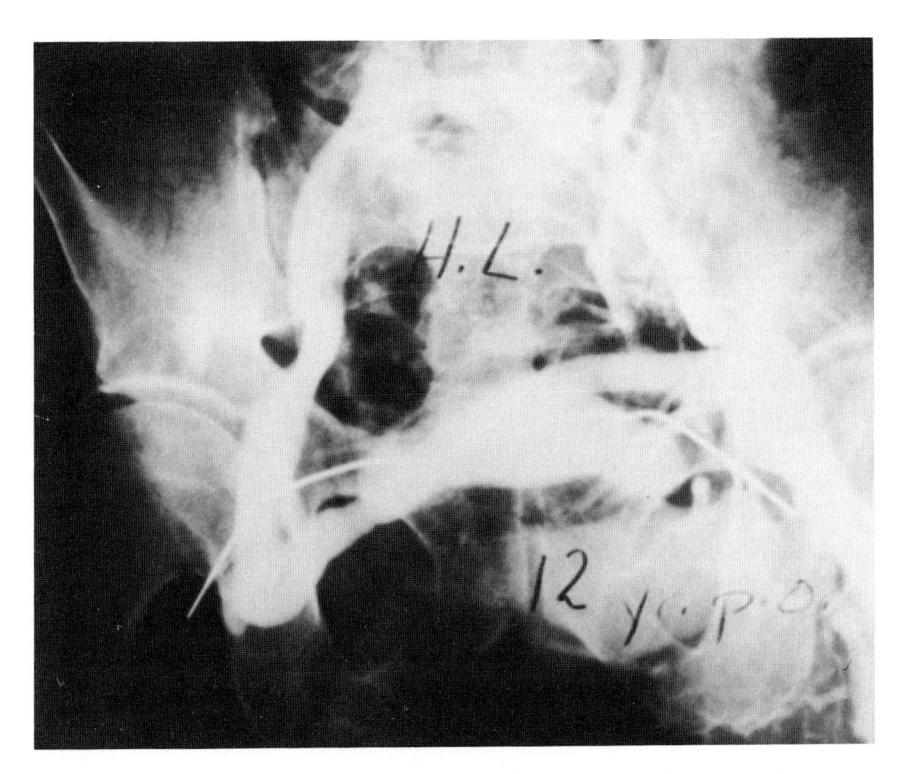

FIGURE 4. Phlebogram shows excellent patency 12 years following replacement of a cross-over vein graft to bypass postphlebitic femoral venous occlusion.

Table 3. Reported Results of Cross-Over Saphenofemoral Vein Grafts

	No.	Excellent	Good	Failure
Smith, Trimble, 1977[19]	100	59 (59%)	17 (17%)	24 (24%)
Husni, 1978[12]	39		33 (85%) patent	
Dale, 1980 (unpublished)	50	30 (60%)	9 (18%)	11 (22%)

Saphenopopliteal Anastomoses

The superficial femoral vein is a common site of continued venous occlusion after deep venous thrombosis. If this is persistent and symptomatic, a bypass may be constructed by joining the ipsilateral saphenous vein to the patent distal popliteal vein to carry blood around the obstructed superficial femoral vein.

The operation consists of dissection of the saphenous vein through a medial incision just below the knee. Saphenous tributaries are ligated and a sufficient 8 to 10 cm length is freed to allow its anastomosis to the popliteal vein through the same incision. Whether a lateral or end-to-side anastomosis is preferable is not yet known. Either is performed with continuous 6–0 polypropylene suture. The lateral anastomosis without interruption of the saphenous vein has theoretic advantages but requires more dissection and may result in tightness and angulation at the anastomosis. The operation bypassing the femoral vein may also be combined with the cross-over saphenous vein graft when that is indicated.

Our results with saphenopopliteal anastomosis are summarized in Table 4. Three of six anastomoses have been phlebographically patent in the postoperative period. Figure 5 shows a phlebogram on one of the patients after operation. Other reported results with this operation are also summarized in Table 4.[12,19]

Brachial to Jugular Bypass for Subclavian Venous Occlusion

The axillary and/or subclavian veins occasionally thrombose following indwelling arm catheterization, arm injuries, or as acute manifestations of the shoulder-girdle compression (thoracic outlet) syndrome. Most of these venous occlusions recanalize spontaneously or become asymptomatic. However, occasional ones persist and produce pain and swelling of the upper extremity that may be correctible by a venous bypass.

A reversed free saphenous vein graft is oriented properly, tunneled appropriately, and placed between a patent portion of the brachial vein in the upper arm and the external jugular vein in the neck. If there

Reconstructive Venous Surgery   207

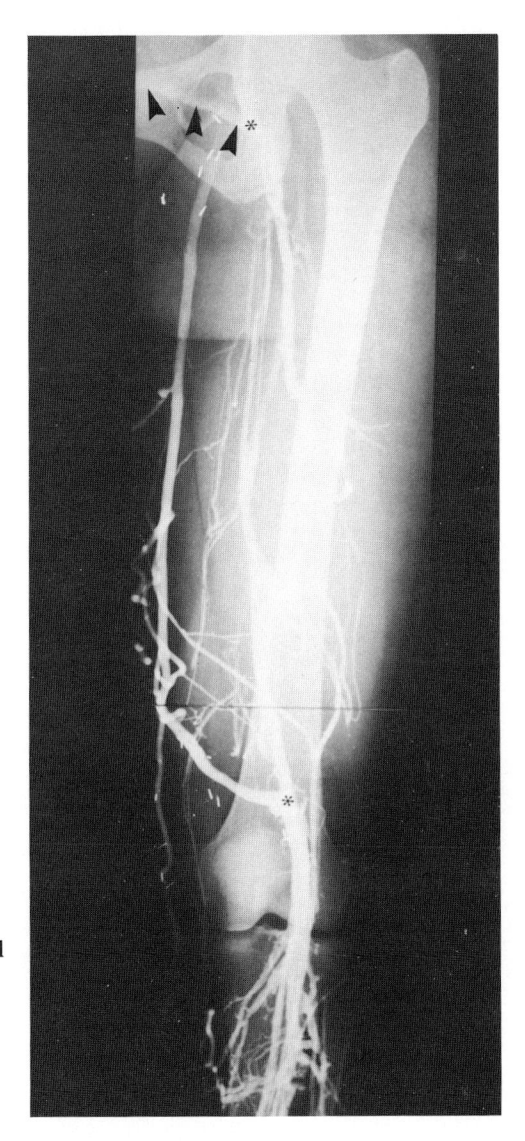

FIGURE 5. Postoperative phlebogram shows the patent anastomosis between the saphenous vein and the popliteal vein at the knee. This patient also had a cross-over graft. Attachment to the common femoral vein in the groin is demonstrated at the top of the phlebogram.

Table 4. Reported Results of Saphenopopliteal Vein Anastomoses

Report	No.	Success Rate (%)
Smith, Trimble, 1977[19]	59	76
Husni, 1978[12]	18	66
Dale, 1980 (unpublished)	6	50

are intraluminal webs and adhesions these should be trimmed out before placement of the anastomosis, which is made with continuous 6–0 polypropylene (Fig. 6).

Our experience with this procedure consists of only two cases. Both patients have been clinically improved. A phlebogram has been obtained in one patient and demonstrates that the graft has failed (despite clinical improvement). The other patient has not yet had postoperative phlebography.

Bypass of the Inferior Vena Cava by Arm Vein to the Femoral Vein.

The completely occluded inferior vena cava with ambulatory venous hypertension of the lower extremity often causes severe disability as a result of edema, pain, varicose veins, and the other sequelae of venous hypertension. Attempts to replace the inferior vena cava directly by an

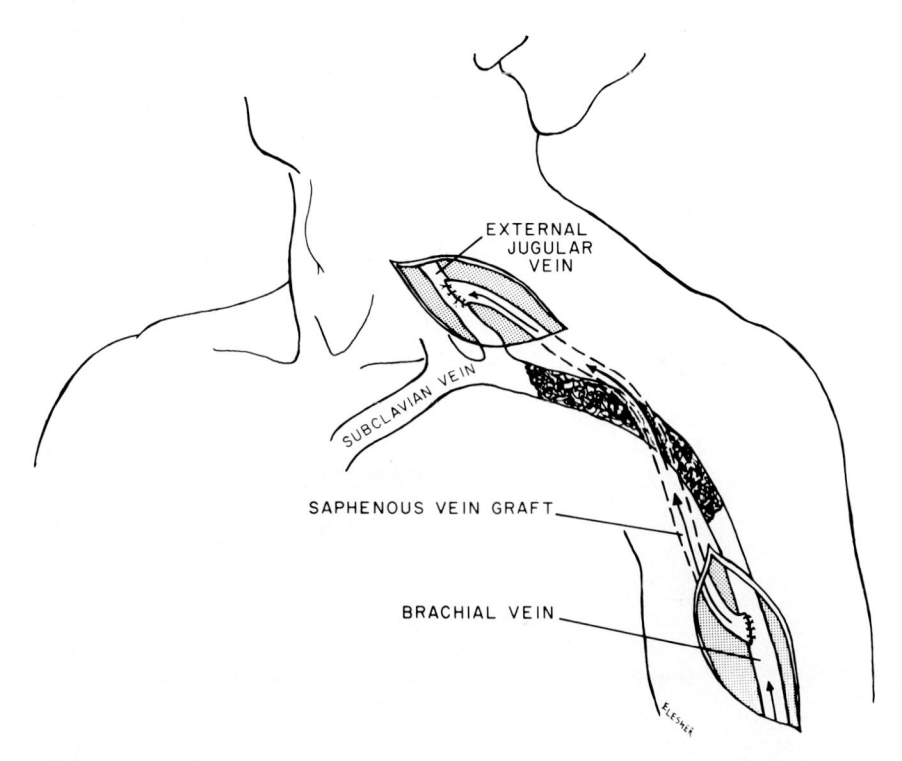

FIGURE 6. A free saphenous vein graft may be used to bypass subclavian or axillary venous thrombosis.

intra-abdominal procedure have usually failed with the exception of the occasional graft replacements for trauma or for a venous resection accompanying tumor dissection. In these latter circumstances, the replacement graft is relatively short, while the segment of abnormal vein in the postphlebitic syndrome is longer and a much longer replacement or bypass graft would be required.

In an effort to provide a feasible solution to the problem we have proposed that a vein be dissected out of the soft tissues of the upper extremity, tunneled inferiorly in the subcutaneous tissue of the chest and abdominal wall and thereafter anastomosed to the femoral vein in the groin. This procedure has been attempted in three patients. In the first patient, the graft failed, perhaps because the arm veins had areas of thrombosis and required resection and anastomoses so that multiple junctions were made. The second patient had inadequate arm veins so the procedure was abandoned. The third patient had a successful replacement with clinical improvement but, at this writing, has not yet had a postoperative phlebogram. Thus, the arm to femoral venous bypass must still be considered a nonestablished operation, which may ultimately be of some use.

Iliac Venotomy for Vein Compression

Occasionally, the aorta and right iliac artery compress the underlying left common iliac vein with resultant fibrosis and/or venous thrombosis. This produces pain and swelling and is diagnosed by venography. Our experience with eight cases and review of the literature indicates that this problem occurs most commonly in females and is sometimes severe enough in terms of edema and discomfort to warrant operation.[2,3,16]

Two different operative treatments may be useful. First, a cross-over saphenofemoral vein graft may be used to shunt blood around the compressed iliac vein. More recently we have come to believe that a direct attack by transabdominal iliac venotomy is preferable. A laparotomy is performed and the intestines are eviscerated to allow exposure of the aortic and caval bifurcation. The aorta and common iliac artery are carefully dissected so that they may be elevated off the underlying iliac veins (Fig. 7). After systemic heparinization and placement of vascular clamps on the cava and iliac veins, an anterior opening is made on the left common iliac vein to allow internal webs and strictures to be removed. The venotomy is then usually closed with a venous patch graft using continuous 6–0 polypropylene sutures. The venous patch may be taken from the dorsum of the hand or forearm rather than disturbing the saphenous vein.

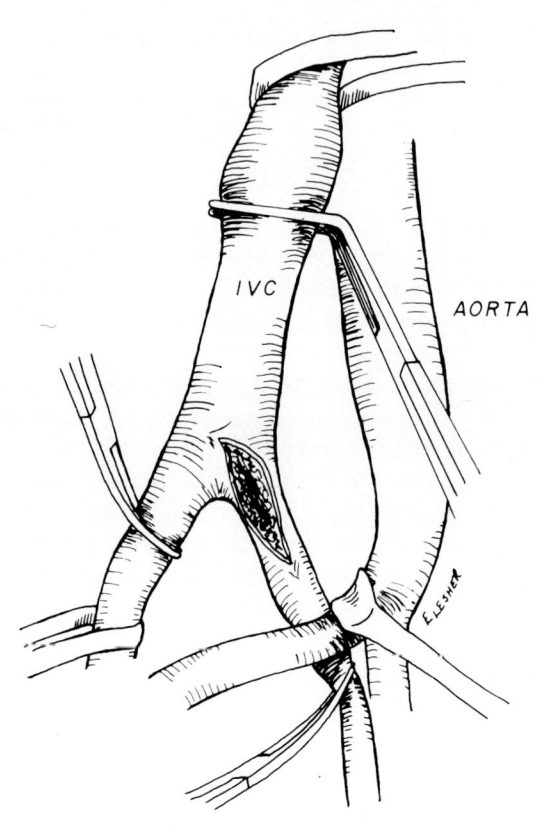

FIGURE 7. The crossing right iliac artery is elevated from the underlying left common iliac vein. An anterior venotomy allows exploration of the lumen and removal of webs and scar. The venotomy is usually closed with a venous patch.

The remaining question is whether to allow the iliac artery simply to lie back on top of the vein and perhaps recreate the original problem, whether to elongate it by interpolating a short segment of synthetic graft, or whether to elevate the artery permanently over a Silastic bridge.[20] In our operative experience with four cases, neither Silastic bridge nor elongation by a graft have been used. From the theroretic standpoint we prefer elongation rather than placement of any firm material in direct contact with an artery where it might provoke erosion and bleeding.

No group has extensive experience with this problem and operative indications are not yet clear. We are currently following four such patients whose symptoms are not severe and for whom operation has not been recommended.

Complications of Reconstructive Venous Surgery

To date, complications have been minimal (Table 5). Earlier we speculated that postoperative venous thrombosis might prove to be an important deterrent, but fortunately this has not occurred. Three instances of phlebitis have occurred with two being in the contralateral extremity and only one in the veins of the leg being operated upon. There have been no infections and only a single instance of wound hematoma and three temporary lymph collections.

POSTOPERATIVE CARE

No discussion of venous reconstruction would be complete without emphasis upon minute attention to the details of postoperative care.[5] The extremity should be elevated when sitting for a period of days and weeks. External compression up to the point of the anastomosis should be provided by Ace bandages or elastic hose for a period of at least 1 year.

Postoperative phlebography is so important in the further development of this field that we have asked each patient undergoing a venous reconstruction to agree to return for this in the postoperative period. Unfortunately this has not always been feasible.

DISCUSSION

How many postphlebitic patients are suitable candidates for venous reconstruction? No accurate data are available but we believe that the percentage of the total number of major venous thromboses who finally have nonreca-

Table 5. Complications in 65 Venous Reconstructions

Mortality	0
Infections	0
Wound seroma or hematoma	
without postoperative heparin	3
with postoperative heparin	1
Deep vein thrombosis	
ipsilateral	1
contralateral	2

nalized venous obstructions that can be satisfactorily bypassed is about 1 or 2 percent. In addition are individuals who develop severe venous occlusion because of malignant tumors as well as the occasional patient with iliac venous obstruction.

Is a temporary arteriovenous fistula useful? This has been reported to increase the patency rate of experimental venous reconstructions by increasing blood flow through the reconstruction.[11,14] On that basis, it has been recommended clinically. Whether the increase in the magnitude of the operation and the necessity for a later secondary corrective procedure will offset a higher patency rate is still unknown. We have had no personal experience in creating such fistulae.

What is the role of intravenous valvular repair? Kistner[13] has emphasized the importance of intact valves in the femoral vein and devised operative methods to repair damaged venous valves. He has also described ingenious methods of transplantation of veins around the root of the thigh to insure valvular compentency at that level. We have searched unsuccessfully to find appropriate patients for these procedures and are unable to comment further upon them.

Is venous reconstruction of practical value in 1981? These operations have proven to be relatively simple and safe and, even when they fail, usually do not worsen the patient's condition. Complications have been infrequent. Particularly notable is the low rate of deep venous thrombosis. We therefore believe that these operations should be recommended to suitably selected patients. While the cross-over saphenofemoral and the saphenopopliteal procedures are fairly well documented and established, the results of the brachial to jugular bypass and use of an arm vein to bypass the inferior vena cava are not yet known.

REFERENCES

1. Chiu CJ, Terzis J, McRae ML: Replacement of superior vena cava with the spiral composite graft. Ann Thorac Surg 17:555, 1974
2. Cockett, FB, Thomas ML: The iliac compression syndrome. Br J Surg 52:816, 1965
3. Connett M: An anatomical basis for unilateral leg edema in adolescent girls. West J Med 121:324, 1974
4. Dale WA: Thrombosis and recanalization of veins used as venous grafts. Angiology 12:603, 1961
5. Dale WA: The swollen leg. Curr Prob Surg 20:1, 1973
6. Dale WA, Allen, TR: Unusual problems of venous thrombosis. Surgery 78:707, 1075
7. Dale WA, Harris J: Cross-over vein grafts for iliac and femoral venous occlusion. Ann Surg 168:319, 1968

8. Dale WA, Scott HW: Grafts of the venous system. Surgery 53:52, 1963
9. Doyen E: Surgical Therapeutics and Operative Techniques, vol. 1. New York, Wm. Wood, 1917, p 363
10. Drapanos T, LoCicero J III, Dowling JB: Hemodynamics of the interposition mesocaval shunt. Ann Surg 181:523, 1975
11. Dumanian AV, Santschi DR, Park K, Walker AP, Frahm CJ: Cross-over saphenous vein graft combined with a temporary femoral arteriovenous fistula. Vasc Surg 2:116, 1968
12. Husni EA: Clinical experience with femoro-popliteal reconstruction. In Bergan JJ, Yao JST (eds): Venous Problems. Chicago, Year Book, 1978, p 485
13. Kistner RL: Transvenous repair of the incompetent femoral vein valve. In Bergan JJ, Yao JST (eds): Venous Problems. Chicago, Year Book. 1978, p 493
14. Krug A, Lehmann K, Zaborsky F: Modified temporary arteriovenous fistula in venous suprapubic cross-over shunt. Chirug 45:389, 1974
15. Lewis MR, Dale WA: Phlebography as a clinical tool. Surg Gynecol Obstet 133:301, 1971
16. McMurrich JP: The occurrence of congenital adhesions in the common iliac veins and their relation to thrombosis of the femoral and iliac veins. Am J Med Sci 135:342, 1908
17. Palma EC, Esperon R: Vein transplants and grafts in the surgical treatment of the post-phlebitic syndrome. J Cardiovasc Surg 1:94, 1960
18. Rigas A, Vamvoyannis A, Trardakas E: Iliac compression syndrome. J Cardiovasc Surg 11:389, 1970
19. Smith DE, Trimble C: Surgical management of obstructive venous diseases of the lower extremity. In Rutherford RB (ed): Vascular Surgery. Philadelphia, Saunders, 1977, p 1247
20. Trimble C, Bernstein EF, Pomerantz M, Eiseman B: A prosthetic bridging device to relieve iliac venous compression. Surg Form 23:249, 1972

Part Four
Difficult Problems with Extremity Ischemia

FOURTEEN

Amputations Below the Knee for Gangrene with Occlusive Disease Below the Inguinal Ligament

Ronald J. Stoney

The traditional indications for amputation in the forefoot and lower leg have been gangrene, intractable ischemic rest pain of the foot, and ischemic ulceration with infection. In the current era of revascularization surgery, a conditional statement must be added, i.e., in circumstances in which arterial revascularization is technically not feasible, or, if feasible, will provide an inadequate or only short-term benefit.

PATHOLOGIC CONSIDERATIONS

Acute occlusion of a major artery in the leg proximal to the popliteal trifurcation usually causes profound ischemia distal to the level of occlusion. If the collateral blood supply is inadequate to maintain viability, ischemia progresses to tissue necrosis. Necrosis begins at a sharply defined level determined by the end-point of functioning collateral blood flow. Beyond this level thrombosis occurs in all segments of the vascular tree and the gangrene that develops involves skin, muscle, and nerve alike. When this point has been reached, attempts at removal of the occluding lesion offer no hope for restoring viability. The systemic reaction from the release of metabolites from the necrotic tissue into the circulation generally makes early amputation necessary.[7] The level of

---

Portions of this work reproduced from Wylie EJ, Ehrenfeld WK, Stoney RJ: Manual of Vascular Surgery, Vol. II. New York, Springer-Verlag, 1980.

amputation is dictated by the vascularity of tissue proximal to the line of demarcation.

When acute occlusion of a single artery in the calf or foot develops, collateral circulation is usually adequate to maintain viability. When gangrene develops from multiple acute occlusion in these arteries, the amputation can be performed adjacent to the demarcation level with anticipation of primary healing.

When chronic occlusion in the major arteries of the leg (usually the result of atherosclerosis) has produced peripheral ischemia in the foot or toes sufficient to produce ischemic gangrene, other factors dictate the required level of amputation. The more distal the level of amputation, the greater the potential for rehabilitation; therefore, a healed pain-free stump at the lowest possible level is the appropriate surgical objective at the time of amputation. The gangrene of a toe is the ultimate manifestation of ischemia at the distal end of the proximally diseased arterial tree. Although demarcation may be evident and the skin on the proximal side is viable, blood perfusion is barely adequate. In the usual situation, perfusion is below the amount required for healing by primary, or even secondary, intention following local amputation. The awareness of this panischemia of the limb at one time led surgeons to advocate the routine use of above-the-knee amputations. Only in recent years has it become evident that carefully performed below-knee amputations and even toe or transmetatarsal amputation in selected cases may be used with high expectations for primary healing.[2] In some situations, patients with lesser degrees of ischemia develop gangrene as a result of trauma to the forefoot or infection of a toe or in an interdigital web space that requires an increase in blood flow that may be impossible to meet. In these cases, amputation at a higher level may be necessary, unless ischemia is reversed and infection controlled.

Chronic occlusive disease of smaller arteries distal to the midcalf or in the foot, although rare, may also produce a degree of ischemia requiring amputation. In most, a local amputation can be performed with or without primary closure and healing can be anticipated. Gangrene of one or more toes from thromboangitis obliterans is the result of segmental local arterial obstructive lesions. Perfusion in adjacent arterial beds is usually unimpaired. The microangiopathy of small arteries in the foot in the diabetic patient with associated but well collateralized occlusions in the proximal arteries is another example. In this disease, toe or transmetatarsal amputation will usually succeed providing Wheelock's[17] four criteria are met: 1) gangrene or infection is localized; 2) the patient is pain-free; 3) rubor of the toes on dependency is minimal or absent; and 4) venous filling time is less than 20 seconds.

INFECTION

Local sepsis in or adjacent to a gangrenous area has a profound influence on the choice of amputation and on the result. Infection may be the precipitating factor to the development of gangrene or may develop as a later complication. Should it occur in the forefoot in situations when local amputation might otherwise be successful, ample bed rest and appropriate antibiotics should precede amputation. If a local purulent collection results, antibiotic therapy and open amputation is required in anticipation of healing by delayed primary closure or by secondary intention. If there is associated cellulitis, the skin flap incision should be made proximal to the inflamed tissue even when a less satisfactory functional result can be expected. Extensive infection and gangrene in the forefoot in a patient who is a candidate for a below-knee amputation is most safely managed by a preliminary guillotine amputation at the ankle. This allows infection in the lymphatic channels in the calf to subside and the primary definitive operation to be performed in 5 to 10 days with primary closure.

MINOR AMPUTATIONS

In the context of the foregoing general considerations, minor amputations are applicable in selective situations for the management of ischemic gangrene confined to the distal portion of one or more digits or the major portion of a single digit. Frequently, debridement by open amputation will control infection present in the gangrenous digit, avoid major amputation, and permit the subsequent amputation to succeed at the lowest possible level. Occasionally, debridement alone will assist in the control and resolution of the infectious process complicating gangrene of the digit and prepare the patient for a successful elective amputation at a more proximal level. Conservation of the majority of the foot is a realistic goal that can be regularly achieved in selected patients. In some circumstances, a proximal arterial reconstructive procedure and/or sympathectomy will increase the probability of local healing. If a successful revascularization operation is performed when necrosis involves only the skin of the toe, new skin may grow beneath the eschar, and the need for minor amputation may disappear.

The Principles of Minor Amputation

Amputation is dependent upon meticulous technique and precise and gentle handling of tissues for success. The skin and subcutaneous tissues must be transected cleanly; fascia, muscle, and bone, as well as nerve, must be sectioned carefully; and hemostasis secured. Wound closure may be possible without drainage when subcutaneous tissue or skin are approximated without tension. Wound approximation with skin tape is preferred by some surgeons, since swelling and tension resulting from sutures may compromise or impair healing.

Transphalangeal digital amputations are applicable when a gangrenous lesion is located distal to the proximal interphalangeal joint of the digit. Lateral and medial based flaps are located at the metatarsophalangeal joint level. After flap elevation, the bone is transected cleanly just distal to the metatarsophalangeal joint. Flap margins are united in a vertically oriented closure (Fig. 1).

Transmetatarsal digital amputations are used when the gangrenous lesion extends to the level of the proximal interphalangeal joint of a digit. A racquet-shaped incision is outlined to surround the base of the digit with extension proximally along the metatarsal head over the dorsum of the foot. The flaps are similar to those of a transphalangeal amputation and are elevated to expose the underlying bone. If the head of the metatarsal bone cannot be easily visualized for transection together with

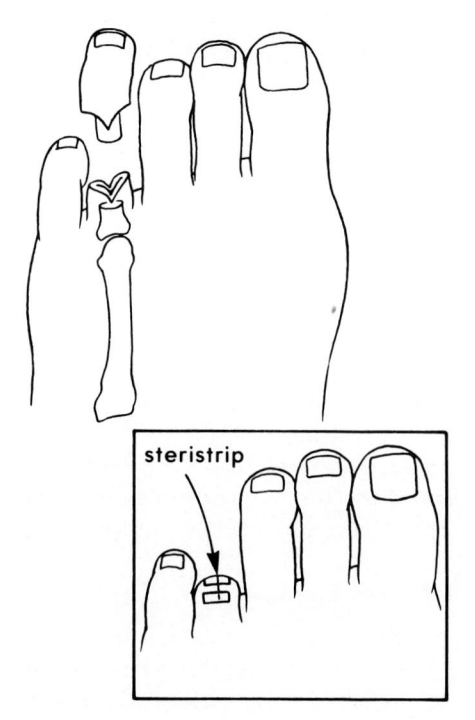

FIGURE 1. Transphalangeal digital amputation.

the flexor and extensor tendons, toe disarticulation at the metatarsal phalangeal joint will facilitate this exposure. Adjacent sesamoid bones are removed, as well as the metatarsal head, so that the level of bone transection is through the osseous cancellus bone itself. Closure is effected in the usual fashion without tension or drainage (Fig. 2).

Transmetatarsal five-digit amputation is used when gangrene and infection are limited to one or more toes but does not extend beyond the proximal interphalangeal joints.

A coronal incision is fashioned across the dorsum of the foot posterior to the heads of the metatarsal bones. The plantar incision extends forward at right angles and then vertically across the forward edge of the plantar surface of the foot proximal to the toes. The dorsal incision is deepened to permit scalpel division of the extensor tendons and atraumatic Gigili saw transection of the metatarsal bones. Bone, interosseous muscle, and tendons are dissected from the thick plantar flap before apposition. After hemostasis is achieved, the wound closure is closed in two layers without tension (Fig. 3).

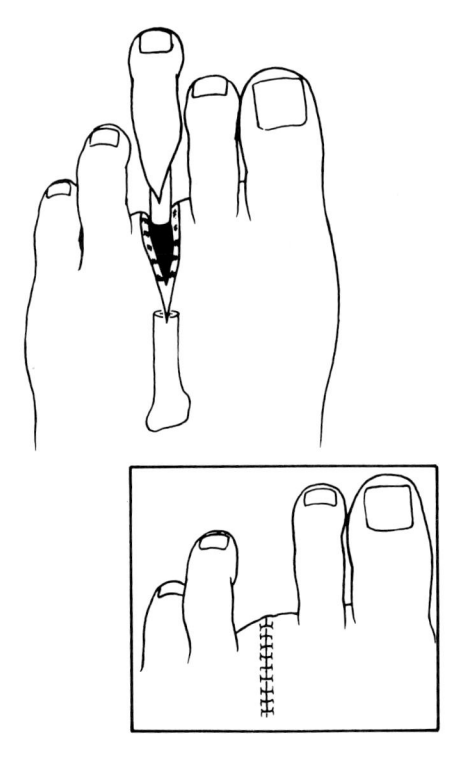

FIGURE 2. Transmetatarsal single-digit amputation.

Rehabilitation following minor amputation of the foot is usually achieved without difficulty. A prosthesis is not required, and balance is possible, since the major portion of the forefoot has been preserved. The fragile and sensitive skin covering minor amputation sites, however, is vulnerable to traumatic injury. Furthermore, associated neuropathy, common in the diabetic, may impair the patient's awareness of local pressure inside close-fitting footwear. It is imperative that a properly designed and fitted shoe be obtained. Soft padding or foam rubber fill is helpful to distribute pressure uniformly as well as to protect exposed prominences from undue wear and eventual skin breakdown as the patient resumes ambulation.

MAJOR AMPUTATIONS

When arterial inflow proximal to the limb is unimpeded and obstructive atherosclerosis is confined to arterial segments beyond the profunda femoris arteries, gangrene is usually localized and can often be controlled

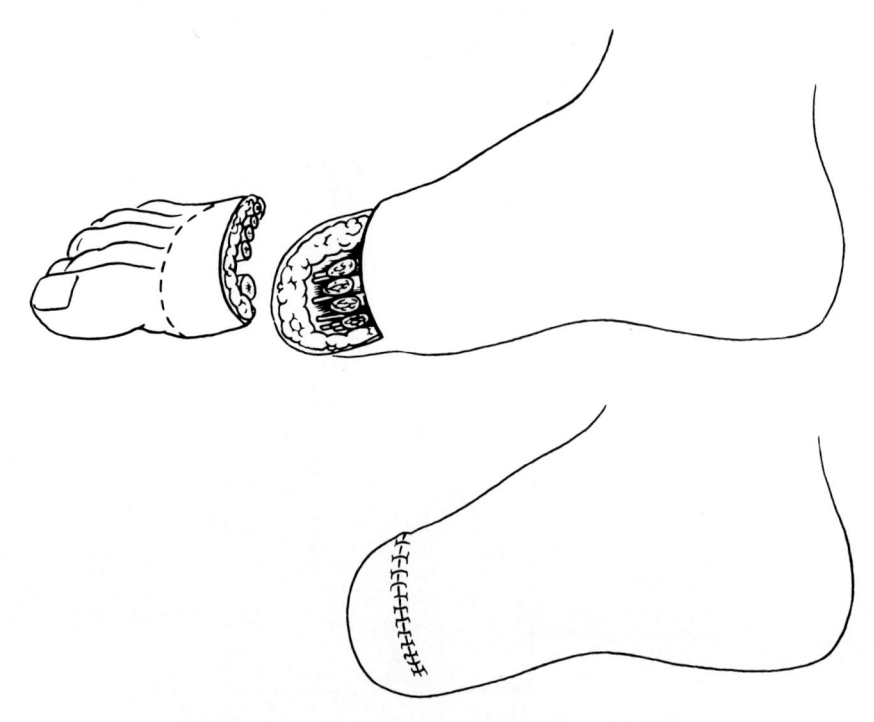

FIGURE 3. Transmetatarsal five-digit amputation.

without a major amputation. For those patients who do require a major amputation under such circumstances, however, healing generally can be anticipated at the below-knee level, since the collateral blood flow through the profunda-geniculate-popliteal/tibial arterial segment will regularly provide adequate skin blood flow for healing at this level. Below-knee amputation is the only alternative when extensive gangrene has destroyed the function of the foot as a weight-bearing unit, when infection is uncontrolled because of distal ischemia, or if the patient is a poor candidate for either extensive limb revascularization or rehabilitation. A limb that would be salvaged by a revascularization procedure but which cannot restore the patient to an ambulatory status because of residual paralysis, joint contracture, or a contralateral above-knee amputation, should be primarily amputated.

Although below-knee amputations are usually accomplished without technical problems, their serious nature cannot be underestimated. A significant mortality and morbidity accompany this procedure, and details of the technique are reviewed in order to emphasize the importance of the precise and meticulous technique required for success (Fig. 4).

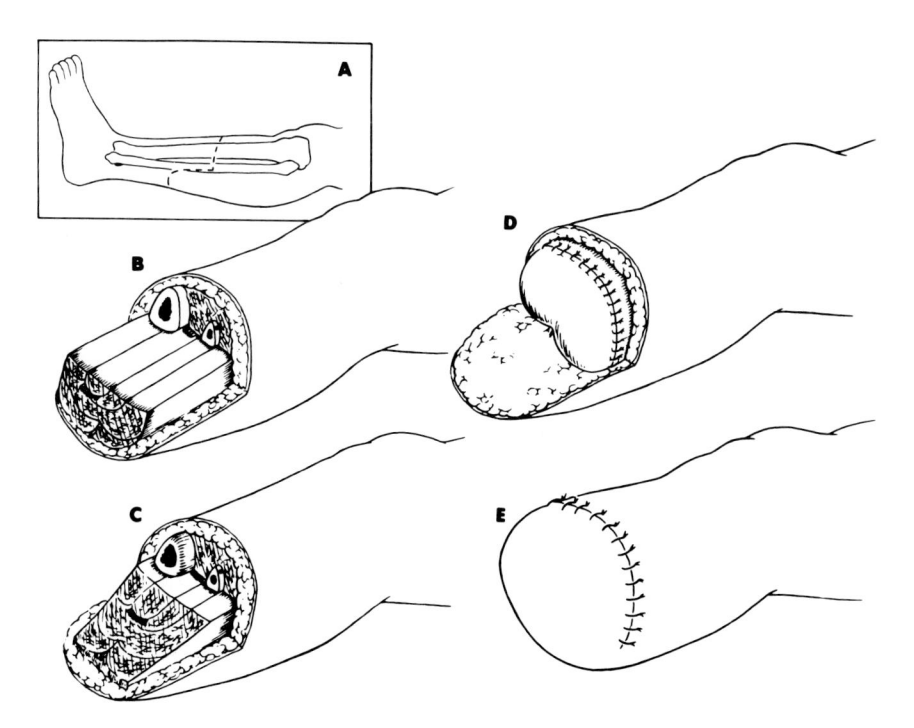

FIGURE 4. Below knee amputation.

The basic principles include the use of a long posterior skin and fascial flap and no anterior flap as advocated by Burgess et al.[2] The tibia is transected 8 cm distal to the inferior border of the tibial tuberosity. A 60° bevel is made on its anterior surface, and the surface is further rounded with a rasp or oscillating saw. The fibula is sectioned 1 cm proximal to the tibial length. Myodesis (fixation of the anterior and posterior musculature to the tibia) has been abandoned by most experienced groups in favor of myoplasty, which requires suturing anterior muscle groups and fascia to the posterior muscular groups over the ends of the tibia in line with the anterior (coronally oriented) incision. Clean transection of muscle, fascia, bone, and nerve must be accomplished and hemostasis secured before myoplasty and skin closure. Because many patients have atrophic subcutaneous tissue that makes careful skin approximation in one layer difficult, closure is often accomplished using a subcutaneous layer to support the skin approximation. The use of suction or other forms of drainage are rarely indicated in our experience.

The rehabilitation potential of the individual below-knee amputee is influenced beneficially by a well-organized team in which surgeon, prosthetist, and rehabilitation therapist each contribute knowledge and skill to the overall rehabilitation program.[18] In major hospitals, an efficient program of this type that can supply the advanced techniques and guidance to such amputees are common. The absence of such programs in smaller community hospitals, where amputations are rarely performed, may result in inadequate care that prolongs or interferes with the ultimate rehabilitation of the dysvascular amputee. Early postoperative care of the lower extremity amputee involves certain principles including improvement in the state of the patient's general health and self-care independence, preparation of the stump for prosthetic fitting as indicated, and minimizing the emotional, social, and economic considerations that follow the amputation. Established rehabilitation goals are set in order to minimize the medical and psychological complications as well as to aid the patient in recovering maximal attainable functional levels of rehabilitation as quickly as possible.

Controversy continues to surround the decision to attempt an extremity revascularization procedure or to proceed directly with primary below-knee amputation in patients with advanced femoral-popliteal-tibial atherosclerosis. Most surgeons would favor femoropopliteal bypass if circumstances permit. DeWeese and Rob's[5,6] results for limb preservation at 5 and 10 years of 69 and 65 percent, respectively, can be anticipated. An extremity bypass grafting operation to the infrapopliteal arteries has a substantially lower 5- and 10-year limb salvage of 46.9 and 42 percent, as reported by Reichle[11] from an extensive experience.

Other authors[1,10] report graft failure rates within 2 years of nearly 50 percent and factual palliation is, of course, less than that. In view of the superb rehabilitative outcome following below-knee amputations, these results raise serious doubt as to the wisdom of considering infrapopliteal bypass an "alternative to primary amputation." Furthermore, reported series of patients undergoing limb salvage bypass include among the indications for operation rest pain and ischemic ulceration, as well as some "disabling" claudication in selected patients. Established gangrene involving the toes or foot, when by infrainguinal obstructive atherosclerosis, remains a most formidable threat to the affected limb and consistently requires an amputation unless a revascularization is possible. Mild ischemic pain may be managed by narcotics, however, and lumbar sympathectomy will suffice for many patients with ulceration.[3,9]

The small group of patients with infrainguinal occlusive disease and established gangrene are of particular interest to discuss regarding management guidelines. The pattern of obstructive disease present in such patients rarely permits a femoropopliteal bypass. If bypass were possible, most surgeons would advocate this procedure rather than a primary amputation. Our own experience showed, however, that only 24 percent of patients were alive with a functioning graft and a salvaged limb one year after a saphenous vein femoropopliteal bypass was performed for foot gangrene (factual palliation).[12]

Usually, a distal bypass to the infrapopliteal arteries will be the only feasible revascularization procedure. No one, however, has reported salvage results with distal bypass in such a subgroup. Reichle[11] reported the operative indications for 164 patients undergoing distal bypass: gangrene, 57 patients (34.8 percent); ischemic ulceration, 44 patients (27.8 percent); rest pain, 54 patients (32.9 percent); and disabling claudication, 9 patients (5.5 percent). In the late follow-up, he does not identify the patients' original ischemic state, but one wonders how many of the 57 patients with established gangrene were among 61 patients followed 5 years and 20 patients available for 10-year review.

My primary concern centers around the proper selection of candidates for revascularization to the infrapopliteal arteries to reverse ischemia, stabilize gangrene, and avoid a major amputation.[13,15] Among the patients meeting the general requirements for an arterial reconstruction, high-quality arteriography that defines the distal tibial arteries and pedal arch integrity is essential. A satisfactory autogenous saphenous vein of at least 4 mm in diameter is ideal, but if not available, synthetic grafts, although having documented inferior results, can occasionally be substituted.[14] Meticulous technique and precise anastomosis to undiseased arterial segments, supplanted by routine intraoperative arteriography, are necessary to define the anatomic repair and the distal runoff of such grafts.

Limb preservation exceeds long-term graft patency in most series, but this observation is not directly applicable to the subgroup of patients with gangrene described in this chapter. A failed graft for these patients will nearly always result in an amputation. Recently, Kassner et al[8] reported a retrospective study of two amputee groups. One group had a previous revascularization procedure to the infrapopliteal arteries that failed, and the other group had no previous vascular procedure. He showed that a failed limb salvage bypass lowered the rate of final healing of below-knee amputation from 87 to 53 percent. This adverse effect of a failed distal bypass on final healing level of amputation should be included among the considerations when selecting patients for the proper management of gangrene with infrainguinal disease.

Major lower extremity amputations number approximately 62,000 annually in the United States and account for nearly 2 percent of all operations performed in Vererans Administration Hospitals throughout the United States.[4,16] The decision to proceed with primary below-knee amputation or a secondary below-knee amputation, if still possible when a distal arterial revascularization procedure fails or gangrene persists despite a functioning graft, demands that the surgeon who undertakes the procedure be aware of 1) the rehabilitation needs of the patient; and 2) the surgical techniques required. The loss of the often functionless, gangrenous part may be a welcome relief from the suffering that the patient has experienced; however, its loss causes grave concern because of the irreparably altered body image. New social, economic, and personal problems are thrust upon the amputee that at times may seem overwhelming. The recovery of independence through rehabilitation with a prosthesis may offer the only hope for the dysvascular amputee in this situation. The far-reaching implications of a major amputation of the limb, therefore, demand a thorough understanding of the problem so that an effective, timely, and safe amputation may result in a well-healed functional stump that will tolerate weight bearing. This should allow the successful application of a prosthetic appliance without pressure necrosis and permit the resumption of independent, bipedal gain for the amputee.

REFERENCES

1. Bernhard VM: Bypass to the infrapopliteal arteries. In Rutherford RB (ed): Vascular Surgery. Philadelphia, Saunders, 1977, pp 541–548

2. Burgess EM, Romano RL, Zetti JH, Schrock RD: Amputations of the leg for peripheral vascular insufficiency. J Bone Joint Surg (Am) 53A:874, 1971
3. Cousins MJ, Reeve TS, Glynn CJ, et al: Neurolytic lumbar sympathetic blockade: Duration of denervation and relief of rest pain. Anaesth Intens Care 7:121, 1979
4. Department of Health, Education and Welfare: Surgical operations in short-stay hospitals, United States, 1973. Vital and Health Statistics, series 13, no. 24. DHEW Publication No. (HRA) 76–1775. Rockville, Md., National Center for Health Statistics, 1973
5. DeWeese JA, Rob CG: Autogenous venous bypass grafts five years later. Ann Surg 174:346, 1971
6. DeWeese JA, Rob CG: Autogenous venous grafts ten years later. Surgery 82:775, 1977
7. Haimovici H: Metabolic complications of acute arterial occlusions. J Thor Cardiovasc Surg 20:349, 1979
8. Kassner M, Satiani B, Evans WE: Amputation level following unsuccessful distal limb salvage operations. Surgery 87:683, 1980
9. Lee BY, Trainor FS, Kavner D, et al: Management of severe ischemia of the foot secondary to occlusive vascular disease. Surg Gynecol Obstet 148:396, 1979
10. Martin CE, Foster JH: Factual palliation with femoropopliteal bypass for salvage. J Surg Res 18:215, 1975
11. Reichle FA, Rankin KP, Tyson RR, et al: Long-term results of 474 arterial reconstructions for severely ischemic limbs: A fourteen year follow-up. Surgery 85:93, 1979
12. Stoney RJ, James DR, Wylie EJ: Surgery for femoropopliteal atherosclerosis. Arch Surg 103:548, 1971
13. Stoney RJ: Ultimate salvage for the patient with limb threatening ischemia. Realistic goals and surgical considerations. Am J Surg 136:228, 1979
14. Szilagyi DE, Hageman JH, Smith RF, et al: Autogenous vein grafting in femoropopliteal atherosclerosis. The limits of its effectiveness. Surgery 86:836, 1979
15. Thompson JE, Garrett WV: The application of distal bypass operations for limb salvage. Surgery 87:717, 1980
16. Warren R, Kihn RB: A survey of lower extremity amputations for ischemia. Surgery 63:107, 1968
17. Wheelock FC Jr: Transmetatarsal amputations and arterial surgery in diabetic patients. N Engl J Med 264:316, 1961
18. Wu Y, Flanigan DP: Rehabilitation of the lower extremity amputee. In Bergan JJ, Yao JST (eds): Gangrene and Severe Ischemia of the Lower Extremities. New York: Grune & Stratton, 1978, pp 435–453

FIFTEEN

Management of Gangrene in Patients Without a Suitable Outflow Tract Below the Inguinal Ligament: Definition of True Unreconstructibility

Wesley S. Moore

Vascular reconstruction to achieve limb salvage is the preferred method for managing patients with limb-threatening ischemia. Amputation is reserved for patients with irreversible, extensive gangrene or for those with an outflow tract unsuitable for successful vascular reconstruction.[7,14-18] This chapter defines unreconstructibility, describes the extent of gangrene that makes an extremity unsalvageable, and outlines an approach for the optimal management of patients who require lower extremity amputation for ischemic gangrene.

DEFINITION OF "TRUE" UNRECONSTRUCTIBILITY

To achieve satisfactory reversal of limb-threatening ischemia, the patient must have an unobstructed proximal arterial tree (inflow) as well as distal arterial reconstitution (outflow) which, if adequately perfused, would provide for the nutritional blood flow requirements of the extremity. If either of these conditions is unfulfilled, particularly the latter, then the arterial system can be defined as being unreconstructible.

"True" unreconstructibility is best described by first outlining the various anatomic outflow patterns that would be suitable for reconstruction; any arterial disease pattern that falls short of this would be defined as unreconstructible. In addition, if the extent of infection or gangrene is such that a major amputation would be required despite successful revascularization, then this would also be included in the definition of true unreconstructibility.

Common Femoral Bifurcation Occlusive Disease

Occlusive disease of the common femoral artery with reconstitution of either or both the superficial femoral and profunda femoris arteries is clearly correctable by vascular reconstruction. The repair is best accomplished by endarterectomy with or without a patch angioplasty of the outflow tract (Fig. 1).

It is not uncommon to have a superficial femoral artery occlusion in combination with an orifice stenosis of the profunda femoris artery, which may occur with or without involvement of the common femoral artery. Beyond the orifice lesion, the profunda femoris artery is usually normal, except in diabetic patients when calcific atheromatous change may involve the greater length of this artery. When there is a good profunda femoris artery distal to an orifice obstruction, profundaplasty alone often sufficiently improves perfusion of the popliteal-tibial system via geniculate collaterals if they are patent and have well established collateral communications with the profunda system (Fig. 2).

Occlusion of the Superficial Femoral Artery

Segmental occlusion of the superficial femoral artery by itself, rarely produces threat of limb loss; however, limb threatening ischemia can occur during the acute phase of superficial femoral artery occlusion or when the collateral connections between the profunda femoris and popliteal arteries are inadequate. In those instances, femoropopliteal bypass grafting yields excellent results and can be expected to provide long-term patency. Before proceeding with femoropopliteal bypass, however, occult proximal occlusive disease of the aortoiliac system must be ruled

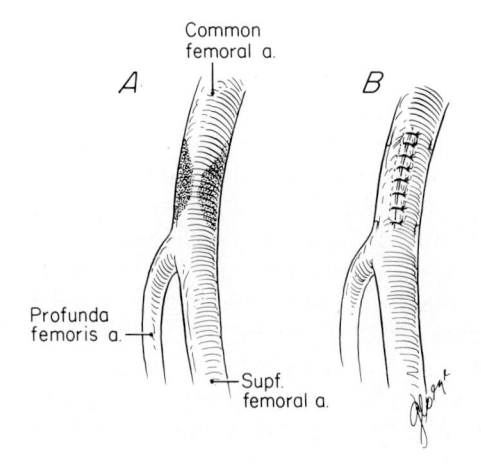

FIGURE 1. Artist's conception of the arteriosclerotic lesion of the common femoral artery treated successfully by localized endarterectomy through a longitudinal arteriotomy.

out. This is best accomplished by obtaining oblique arteriograms to identify occlusive plaques on the posterior aspect of the iliac arteries and to identify lesions involving the orifices of the profunda femoris arteries that may not have been visible on a straight anteroposterior view. Noninvasive studies, using segmental blood pressure measurement, can often suggest the presence of occult occlusive lesions in the iliac system by demonstrating a pressure gradient between the brachial artery and high-thigh measurement. If there is suspicion that an occult iliac lesion is present, this gradient can be amplified by repeating the high-thigh to brachial pressure index after exercise or with reactive hyperemia.

More commonly, a threat of limb loss with superficial femoral artery occlusion would be accompanied by concomitant popliteal or tibial artery occlusive disease. Femoropopliteal bypass grafting is still acceptable under these conditions if there is a suitable site for popliteal anastomosis. Even in the extreme instance of an isolated popliteal segment, many limbs have been salvaged successfully by bypass grafting to this limited outflow segment.[7] Under these conditions, bypass grafting will increase perfusion pressure to the branches of the isolated popliteal artery that have collateral communications with one or more reconstituted tibial branches (Fig. 3). Bypass to the popliteal artery with diseased runoff

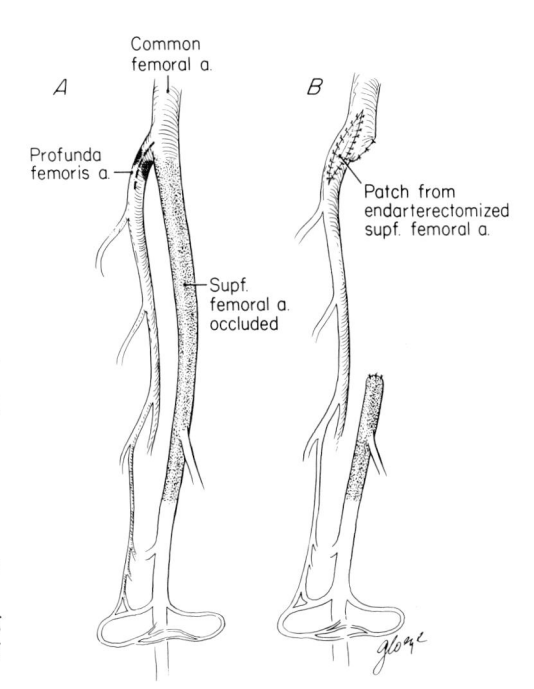

FIGURE 2. A localized lesion of the orifice of the profunda femoris artery can be removed by endarterectomy, and the orifice widened with a patch angioplasty. A chronically occluded superficial femoral artery can serve as a readily available source of autogenous patch material by removing a segment of the artery, opening it longitudinally, and removing the atheromatous content.

232 Critical Problems in Vascular Surgery

will probably not be as durable as one to recipient arteries with normal runoff, but patency is often sufficient to manage an acute ischemic crisis such as a nonhealing ulceration or limited toe-tip gangrene. When the graft ultimately fails months or years later, the limb is not necessarily rethreatened. During the interval of patency, the lesions will have healed, allowing time for development, enlargement, and communication of collateral channels so that the healed extremity often remains viable after late thrombosis of the graft.

Popliteal-Tibial Occlusive Disease

When there is extensive disease or occlusion of the popliteal artery and/or the proximal tibial outflow vessels, the best outflow tract is no longer available for reconstruction, and the conditions for vascular bypass are now marginal. Although the option of bypassing to a distal tibial artery may be available, we must consider the chances of achieving sufficient patency time to heal an ischemic lesion, on the one hand,

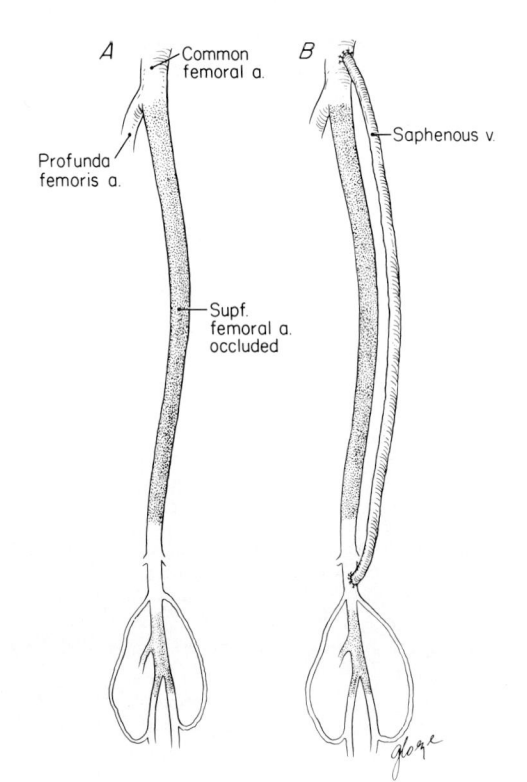

FIGURE 3. Occasionally a reconstituted segment of the popliteal artery can serve as a significant source of blood flow to residual tibial branches via collateral connections. A femoropopliteal bypass to such an isolated segment, using saphenous vein, can often salvage an ischemic limb.

versus the risk of failure leading to amputation at a higher level than would have been required if primary amputation had been performed initially.

Case Report

A 72-year-old woman first presented with bilateral, disabling, intermittent claudication in 1976. She underwent a staged, bilateral femoropopliteal bypass employing autogenous saphenous vein that remained patent for approximately 2 years during which time she was symptom-free. After an occlusion, her symptoms became progressively worse, and in March 1980 she entered UCLA Hospital with profound rest pain in her left foot. Physical examination revealed excellent femoral pulses, with no distal palpable pulses. She had marked blanching on elevation of the left foot and developed intense, dependent rubor. Segmental blood pressures were measured and demonstrated an ankle/brachial pressure index of 0.24 on the left side. A xenon blood flow study was performed at the below-knee level which indicated a flow rate of 4.2 ml/100 g tissue per minute, well above the minimal flow rate required for healing. An aortogram was performed demonstrating nonconclusive disease of the iliac arteries, bilateral superficial femoral artery occlusions, and excellent profunda femoris arteries without plaquing. Although the right popliteal and tibial arteries were reconstituted, the left popliteal artery was occluded. The left anterior tibial and posterior tibial arteries had reconstituted in the calf, however, and there was an intact pedal arch (Fig. 4).

The patient was not a good candidate for vascular reconstruction because she had no available autogenous veins and would require a distal tibial bypass. Nevertheless, she was an excellent candidate for amputation since the procedure could have been performed at the below-knee level with every expectation of rapid rehabilitation on a below-knee prosthesis. These facts were presented to the patient, but she adamantly refused amputation. Therefore, a left femoral-to-posterior tibial bypass was performed with a 6-mm Gore-Tex graft. Operative angiograms demonstrated an excellent technical result, and the patient developed an easily palpable posterior tibial pulse at the ankle upon completion of the operation. That night the graft thrombosed, and the patient was returned to the operating room. Despite a successful thrombectomy, patency could not be maintained in the graft. The patient continued to suffer extreme foot pain, relieved somewhat by sympathetic blockade. A third operation,

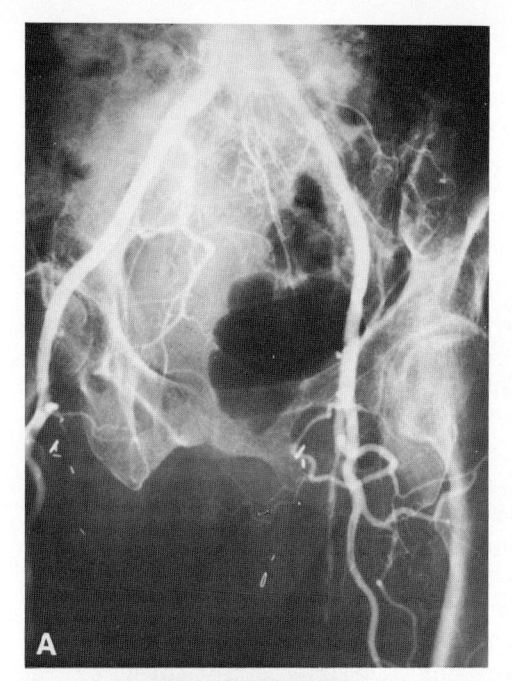

FIGURE 4. **A.** An aortogram demonstrates a good iliac inflow system with excellent outflow through the profunda femoris arteries bilaterally. Both superficial femoral arteries are occluded. **B.** The popliteal arteries are occluded bilaterally, but there was good tibial artery reconstruction bilaterally. **C.** Close-up view of the left malleolar region demonstrating an intact pedal arch with a good anterior tibial and posterior tibial arteries.

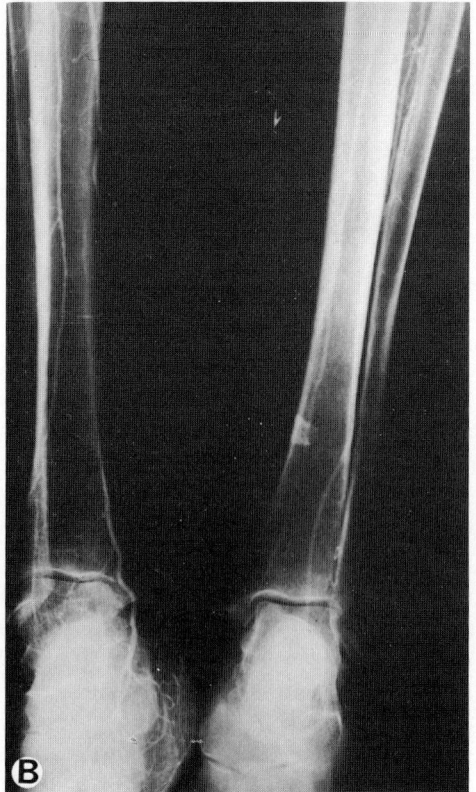

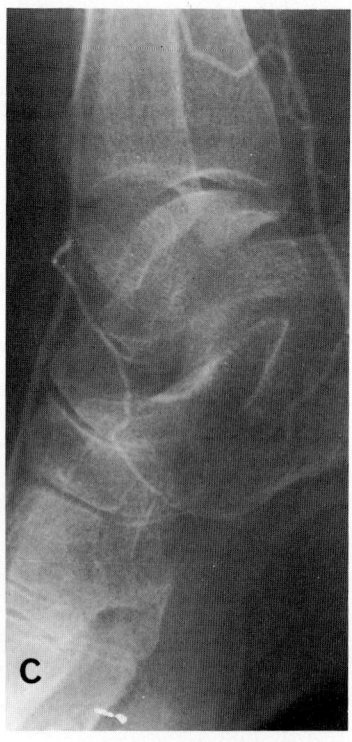

left lumber sympathectomy, was then performed that achieved some improvement in her symptoms. She was ultimately discharged on the 34th hospital day with an estimated hospital and professional expense of $18,000. Two weeks later, she was readmitted for a wound infection over the distal tibial anastomotic site. She was returned to the operating room for incision and drainage where it was found that the graft was involved in the septic process, and this required removal of the entire graft. The wounds were packed open and during the next few days, excellent granulation began to appear. Because of intense rest pain and early forefoot gangrene, however, it was elected to proceed with below-knee amputation. In spite of careful debridement and tailoring of the posterior flap to exclude the previous tibial incision, the below-knee amputation ultimately failed because of a wound infection and an above-knee amputation had to be performed. This healed well and the patient was ultimately discharged some 40 days after her second hospital admission with all wounds healed and pain-free.

While appearing to be extreme, such a case is probably repeated more frequently than we realize. Had the patient consented initially to amputation, she would most likely have had one operation (below-knee amputation), two weeks of hospitalization, and rehabilitation on a below-knee prosthesis. Instead, she underwent six operations culminating in a higher amputation (above-knee), 70 days of hospitalization, enormous medical expense, and immeasurable suffering both for the patient and her family. This experience must be kept in mind when evaluating patients who present with limb-threat and an anatomic condition that is suboptimal for vascular reconstruction.

The availability of precise amputation-level selection employing skin blood measurement with xenon-133 will provide additional information to the preoperative data base, materially benefiting the patient by enabling an informed and rational choice between vascular reconstruction and amputation. If the skin blood flow data indicate that a conservative level such as a transmetatarsal, Syme, or below-knee amputation would heal, then this might be a better option than a tibial bypass. On the other hand, if the skin blood flow data indicate that ischemia is severe enough to require an amputation above the knee, then an attempt at tibial bypass is fully justified. If the bypass is successful, the extremity is salvaged, but if it is unsuccessful, nothing is lost inasmuch as an above-knee amputation was the only available level before the attempted reconstruction.

Tibial bypass can be carried to the anterior tibial, posterior tibial, or peroneal arteries. The level of anastomosis is best performed at the proximal one-third of the vessel, but may extend all the way to the malleolar level. It has been reported that success of tibial bypass is

236 Critical Problems in Vascular Surgery

better if there is an intact pedal arch. It may not be possible, however, to get significant angiographic contrast material past the occlusive lesion to visualize an open arch in the foot. Therefore, failure to obtain preoperative visualization of the pedal arch with an otherwise satisfactory tibial artery should not preclude an appropriately scheduled operation. Inability to visualize a tibial vessel in an otherwise satisfactory arteriogram probably represents the ultimate unreconstructible condition.

Reconstruction As a Function of Extent of Gangrene

Since arterial reconstruction is indicated only when amputation can be prevented or the amputation site lowered to a better functional level, the extent of the gangrenous process will have a significant impact on the decision for or against vascular reconstruction.

Rest pain without gangrene is clearly a reversible process if anatomic conditions are suitable for vascular repair. While gangrene of the toe-tip or of minor toes is not reversible, it will permit salvage of the foot per se, and particularly the metatarsal heads. If skin blood flow is sufficient to heal a toe amputation, vascular reconstruction is not indicated. If skin blood flow is compromised enough to require an amputation at some level proximal to the transmetatarsal region, however, vascular reconstruction, when feasible, is indicated.

If the gangrenous process involves the forefoot, and skin blood flow is sufficient to heal an amputation at the below-knee level, vascular reconstruction is probably not advisable; however, if skin blood flow is so inadequate as to make an above-knee amputation the only available level, vascular reconstruction designed to salvage the knee joint is well-justified.

AMPUTATION LEVEL DETERMINATION

The success or failure of an amputation to heal at a given level depends upon sufficient skin blood flow for primary healing to occur. New techniques now permit precise measurement of skin blood flow in order to assess healing potential at various anatomic amputation levels.

Skin blood flow can be measured by intradermal injection of the isotope xenon-133 dissolved in saline, and monitoring the rate of clearance with a gamma camera. Xenon has the physicochemical properties of being an inert gas that is removed only by crossing the capillary cell membrane and being carried away in the venous effluent. The transfer of xenon across the capillary cell membrane is proportional to the differential concentration of the isotope on either side of the membrane; therefore, the rate of removal of the material, in bolus form, is proportional to the flow rate within the capillary system. These data are entered into the Ketty-Schmidt equation so that a flow rate, calculated in ml/ 100 g tissue/minute, is generated. Initial retrospective and subsequent prospective studies in our laboratory have demonstrated that a critical flow rate for skin healing is 2.4 ml/100 g tissue/minute.[3-6,11-13,20,21] A flow rate approximately equal to or greater than that indicates sufficient blood flow to heal an amputation at the level sampled. Other causes of amputation failure, however, such as skin flap trauma, hematoma, and infection can still lead to failure.

The first amputation level to be sampled is the one most distal on the extremity that corresponds to an amputation level satisfactory for prosthetic fitting while still encompassing the gangrenous process. If skin blood flow is adequate, the amputation can be performed at that level. If the skin blood flow is below the critical level, successive proximal levels are sampled until a level with sufficient blood flow is identified. Information about the most distal level that will heal now forms a part of the data base underlying the decision-making process for or against arterial reconstruction. It also provides the precise statistics necessary for selecting the most conservative level of amputation.

Critical Features of Amputation Surgery

Unlike amputations for trauma or tumor where circulation is normal, amputation for management of ischemic gangrene requires careful attention to detail in order to achieve skin healing and optimum results. For example, a tourniquet should never be employed for amputation in patients with arterial occlusive disease because this could cause trauma or thrombosis of diseased thigh vessels. The amount of bleeding at the time of amputation is usually minimal owing to the primary disease process, and the major vessels can be managed easily by performing a careful anatomic amputation.

The below-knee amputation is the most common level available for primary healing as well as the level that provides the best functional results from the standpoint of prosthetic rehabilitation. Authors have repeatedly noted that use of a long posterior skin flap with no anterior skin flap yields the best healing results. The rationale for using this type of flap is based upon the observation that most failures of amputation healing due to ischemic necrosis of skin usually occur in the anterior midline skin, suggesting that the collateral blood flow to the anterior skin at the below-knee level is not as good as that to the posterior skin.[9,10,19] The delicate handling of skin and skin edges is probably the single most important feature in healing an ischemic amputation. The use of thumb forceps on skin edges is to be condemned because trauma produced with thumb forceps may cause local skin breakdown and ultimate failure of amputation healing. Careful edge-to-edge coaptation with close, carefully placed mattress sutures have provided the best healing results.

Amputation levels that are feasible and yield the best results from the standpoint of rehabilitating the dysvascular amputee include toe amputation, Ray resection, transmetatarsal amputation, Syme's amputation, below-knee amputation, and knee disarticulation. Amputations at the above-knee level are undesirable and should be avoided unless there is no other choice. Elective amputation at the above-knee level is perhaps best applied in the patient who has been bedridden and is obviously not going to walk again. This is also true of the patient with a spastic hemiparesis on the side of the gangrenous extremity.

The precise details of surgical technique for amputation have been covered in other publications, and the reader is referred to those sources.[9,10,20]

Immediate Postoperative Prosthesis

The use of an immediate postoperative prosthesis, applied on the operating table, has been maligned on occasion by some authors. I submit, however, that this technique has been the single most important contribution to modern amputation management. It has now been repeatedly demonstrated that this method of postoperative management reduces postoperative mortality.[1,2,9,10,20] The use of immediate postoperative prosthesis, however, is an exacting technique that requires a skilled prosthetist with whom the surgeon has a good working relationship. It also requires cooperation from the physical therapist. Use of limited weight bearing with immediate or early ambulation must be cautious so that the patient does not introduce excessive vertical loading and traumatize the amputation stump. In the case of an amputation at the below-knee level, no more than 10 to 20 pounds of vertical load is permitted for the duration of the first cast. This cast, applied in the operating room, usually remains in place for about 10 to 14 days. When the second cast is applied and wound healing is observed to be satisfactory, then increased weight bearing can be permitted.

Results of the Team Approach to Amputation

We recently reviewed the results of 142 consecutive amputations using the team approach. This included amputation level selection with the xenon-133 clearance, meticulous surgical technique, application of immediate postoperative prosthesis, and aggressive physical therapy with progressive weight-bearing ambulation. There were no postoperative deaths in this group of patients, in contrast to an average 7 percent mortality in reported series using conventional techniques. There was an overall 89 percent primary healing rate with 100 percent healing of the last 58 consecutive amputations in which xenon data were used prospectively to select the amputation level. One hundred percent of the patients achieved bipedal ambulation on a prosthesis in contrast to a 64 percent rehabilitation reported in the literature with conventional techniques. The average time interval between amputation and the fitting of the final (permanent) prosthesis was 32 days compared with an average of 125 days between amputation and prosthetic ambulation when conventional techniques were employed.

When amputations are performed in an institutional setting like the Veterans Administration, the time between amputation and fitting of a permanent prosthesis inevitably means hospital time. Using the interval between amputation and prosthetic fitting achieved with the team approach as opposed to the interval required for conventional postoperative management, a theoretical cost-effectiveness analysis was projected for the total amputation experience in the Veterans Administration system of 172 hospitals. A review of the Veterans Administration records reveals that there are more than 4000 lower extremity amputations performed each year. If consideration is given to the start-up costs for personnel, supplies, equipment, and facilities to utilize immediate postoperative prostheses, amputation level selection, team coordination, and stay, the technique we advise would achieve a savings to the system of approximately $80 million over a 5-year period in contrast to the hospitalization required for conventional amputation technique. Clearly, the concept of the team approach is not only therapeutically beneficial but also cost-effective.[8]

REFERENCES

1. Burgess EM, Romano RL: The management of lower extremity amputees using immediate postsurgical prostheses. Clin Orthop 57:137, 1968
2. Burgess EM, Romano RL, Zettl JH, et al: Amputation of the leg for peripheral vascular insufficiency. J Bone Joint Surg 53A:874, 1971
3. Bohr H: Measurement of the blood flow in the skin with radioactive Xenon. Scand J Clin Lab Invest (suppl) 93:60, 1967
4. Chimoskey JE: Skin blood flow by ^{133}Xe disappearance validated by venous occlusion plethysmograph. J Appl Physiol 32:432, 1972
5. Daly MJ, Henry RE, Patton DD: Measurement of skin perfusion with Xenon[133]. J Nucl Med 19:709, 1978
6. Lassen NA, Lindjurg J, Munck O: Measurement of blood flow through

skeletal muscle by intramuscular injection of Xenon-133. Lancet 1:686, 1964
7. Maini BS, Mannick JA: Effect of arterial reconstruction on limb salvage. Arch Surg 113:1247, 1978
8. Malone JM, Moore WS, Goldstone J, et al: Therapeutic and economic impact of a modern amputation program. Ann Surg 189:798, 1979
9. Moore WS, Hall AD, Wylie EJ: Below knee amputation for vascular insufficiency; Experience with immediate postoperative fitting with prostheses. Arch Surg 97:886, 1968
10. Moore WS, Hall AD, Lim RD Jr: Below knee amputation for ischemic gangrene. Am J Surg 124:127, 1972
11. Moore WS: Determination of amputation level. Measurement of skin blood flow with Xenon Xe 133. Arch Surg 107:798, 1973
12. Moore WS, Malone JM, Henry RE, et al: Amputation level determination using Xenon[133] clearance. Scand J Clin Lab Invest, in press
13. Moore WS, Henry RE, Malone JM, et al: Prospective use of Xenon [133] clearance for amputation level selection. Arch Surg (in press)
14. O'Donnell JA, Brener BJ, Brief DK, Alpert J, Parsonnet V: Realistic expectation for patients having lower extremity bypass surgery for limb salvage. Arch Surg 112:1356, 1977
15. Perdue GD, Smith RB III, Veazey CR, Ansley JD: Revascularization for severe limb ischemia. Arch Surg 115:168, 1980
16. Ramsburgh SR, Lindenauer SM, Weber TR, et al: Femoropopliteal bypass for limb salvage. Surgery 81:453, 1977
17. Reichle FA, Rankin KP, Tyson RR, Finestone AJ, Shuman C: Long-term results of 474 arterial reconstructions for severely ischemic limbs: A fourteen-year follow-up. Surgery 85:93, 1979
18. Reichle FA, Rankin KP, Tyson RR, Shuman CR, Finestone AJ: The elderly patient with severe arterial insufficiency of the lower extremity. Cardiovasc Surg (suppl 1), Circulation 60:124, 1979
19. Robinson K: Long posterior flap myoplastic below-knee amputation in ischemic disease: Review of experience. Lancet 1:193, 1972
20. Roon AJ, Moore WS, Goldstone J: Below knee amputation: A modern approach. Am J Surg 134:153, 1977
21. Sjersen P: Cutaneous blood flow in man studied by freely diffusible radioactive indicators. Scand J Clin Lab Invest 19 (suppl 99):52, 1967

SIXTEEN

Fate of Patients with a Blind Popliteal Artery Segment: Limb Loss with a Patent Femoropopliteal Graft

Sushil K. Gupta and Frank J. Veith

Although controversy exists about the indications and long-term effectiveness of femoropopliteal bypass, this procedure continues to be one of the most commonly performed arterial reconstructions. During the past 4 years, we have performed femoropopliteal bypass surgery for limb salvage in more than 300 patients, and have used expanded polytetrafluoroethylene (PTFE) grafts whenever ipsilateral saphenous vein was unavailable or unsuitable or when life expectancy was deemed to be less than 1 or 2 years.[14,27] Our approach to limb salvage has generally been aggressive, and we have occasionally performed femoropopliteal reconstructions despite deterrents such as recent myocardial infarction, the presence of infection or extensive gangrene in the foot, or poor runoff from an isolated popliteal artery segment.[26,28] In some patients, however, patent femoropopliteal bypasses and appropriate systemic and local care, including several local debridements, failed to result in a healed foot, and the limb remained threatened. In this chapter, we will analyze the factors that may have contributed to this situation, and we will present a possible plan of management to avert or treat it.

To investigate the question of limb loss in the presence of a patent femoropopliteal bypass, we have reviewed our experience with 220 PTFE femoropopliteal bypasses performed for limb salvage. In the group of patients that underwent such operations, there were 23 cases (9.5 percent) in whom a healed foot could not be achieved even with a functioning femoropopliteal graft. These cases were evaluated with regard to the quality of the runoff from the popliteal artery as seen on angiography, the hemodynamic improvement obtained postoperatively, and local and systemic risk factors.

RADIOGRAPHIC EVALUATION OF THE POPLITEAL ARTERY

Outflow from the popliteal artery can be measured radiographically in terms of the number of patent tibial arteries present and in continuity with the popliteal artery. An isolated or blind popliteal segment is defined as that situation in which there is complete occlusion of the superficial femoral artery, reconstitution of a segment of the popliteal artery, and then complete occlusion of either the distal popliteal artery or all the tibial branches immediately beyond (0–5 cm) their origin. In some patients, one or more tibial arteries may then reconstitute distally in the leg or foot. The true incidence of the occurrence of an isolated popliteal segment in patients whose limbs are threatened cannot be estimated correctly, since many investigators may consider some or all of these patients unreconstructible. In our series, as well as in those of other authors who have reported the use of an isolated popliteal segment for femoropopliteal bypass, the incidence of this condition is approximately 20 to 25 percent of the total population undergoing such reconstructive surgery.[17,28]

Several studies have shown that the results of femoropopliteal bypass depend on the quality of the popliteal and tibial runoff beds.[3,7,9,18] It is thought that reconstructions with the highest proportion of patent leg arteries will provide increased graft flow rates and, therefore, result in higher patency rates.

RESULTS ACHIEVED WITH AUTOLOGOUS SAPHENOUS VEIN BYPASS GRAFTS

Some groups have achieved good results in poor outflow situations by using autologous saphenous vein as a vascular prosthesis.[5,16,17,19,20] In 1967, Mannick and his colleagues[17] reported successful results in 31 patients with autologous saphenous vein grafts to isolated popliteal artery segments and a patency rate of 65 percent over a period of 9 months to 4½ years.[17] Kaminski and his associates[16] achieved 90 percent patency at 48 months in their patients with grade III (poorest) popliteal outflow, and they concluded that graft patency was not dependent upon the status of the outflow tract. Darling[4] reported his experience in 51 patients having saphenous vein femoropopliteal bypasses to an isolated popliteal segment, with a 61 percent patency rate at 5 years.

In several studies determining the intraoperative graft flow rates in femoropopliteal saphenous vein bypasses and their correlation with the radiographic appearance of the popliteal outflow tract, no consistent relationship was noted between graft patency, intraoperative graft flow rates, and distal arterial outflow as determined by arteriography.[1,17,19] Surprisingly, grafts with flow rates as low as 15 ml/min and pressure gradients of up to 30 mm Hg across the graft remained patent 2 years or longer. In these studies, most failures were ascribed to technical difficulties at the distal anastomosis and inadequate saphenous vein. The magnitude of graft flow and the quality of the angiographic outflow tract were considered the least significant factors in predicting success.

RESULTS ACHIEVED WITH SYNTHETIC VASCULAR PROSTHESES

None of the available synthetic grafts has been reported by others to be successful in femoropopliteal bypasses to poor outflow vessels.[23] In our series of 220 femoropopliteal bypasses performed with PTFE grafts, there were 48 patients who had an isolated popliteal segment on preoperative arteriograms. These patients included those with a totally occluded distal popliteal artery or those with runoff only into a single tibial artery that was patent for a distance of less than 5 cm. All bypasses were performed because the limb was threatened by ischemic necrosis (75 percent), a nonhealing ulcer (11 percent), or severe ischemic rest pain with pregangrenous changes (14 percent). An aggressive policy of reoperation was employed for early and late graft closures.[25]

At 47 months, a life table patency rate of 84 percent was achieved in the 48 PTFE femoropopliteal bypasses to an isolated popliteal artery segment. This patency rate was not significantly different from that of 172 PTFE femoropopliteal bypasses to popliteal arteries with angiographically better runoff (Fig. 1). However, 15 of the 48 patients (31 percent) with isolated popliteal segments had threatened limbs despite a patent bypass graft, while in only 8 of 172 patients (5 percent) with nonisolated popliteal arteries was a healed foot not obtained when the femoropopliteal bypass was patent. The etiology of limb loss with a patent graft was further analyzed by assessing the hemodynamic improvement brought about by the arterial reconstruction and by assessing systemic and local risk factors.

HEMODYNAMIC DATA

Mannick and his colleagues[17] have suggested that increased pressure applied to even a diseased popliteal outflow tract may result in the dilation of collaterals resulting in significantly increased perfusion of the

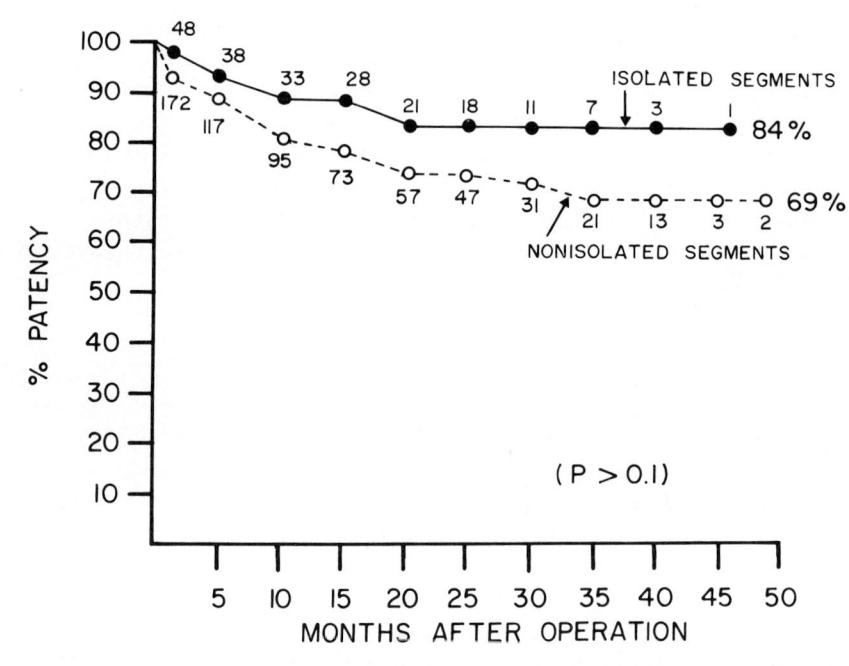

FIGURE 1. Cumulative life table patency rates of 48 PTFE femoropopliteal bypasses to isolated popliteal artery segments and 172 PTFE femoropopliteal bypasses to popliteal arteries with direct runoff into one or more major leg arteries. These patency rates are based on calculations in which a graft is considered patent even if one or more operations was required to maintain that patency.

ischemic foot. This may or may not, however, result in a healed foot.

We have measured the preoperative and postoperative ankle systolic pressure and ankle systolic pressure index (ASPI) (ankle systolic pressure/brachial systolic pressure) in all patients undergoing femoropopliteal bypasses and our results are summarized in Table 1. There was

Table 1. Results of Patients Undergoing Femoropopliteal Bypasses

	Preoperative		Postoperative	
	Ankle Systolic Pressure	*ASPI*	*Ankle Systolic Pressure*	*ASPI*
Isolated popliteal segment	50 ±22	.30 ±.15	97 ±35	.70 ±.21
Nonisolated popliteal segment	52 ±27	.33 ±.18	108 ±37	.89 ±.22
Threatened limbs with open bypass grafts	54 ±23	.29 ±.16	81 ±32	.58 ±.18

no difference in the preoperative ankle pressures and ASPI between patients who had bypasses to the isolated popliteal segment or to the nonisolated popliteal artery or those patients whose limbs remained threatened in the presence of a patent bypass. The postoperative elevation of ankle systolic pressure and ASPI, however, was significantly lower in the isolated popliteal segment group as compared to the nonisolated popliteal artery group ($p < .05$). Postoperative improvement was least in the 23 patients with nonhealing foot lesions despite an open bypass graft confirmed by angiography. Most of these patients also had a flat or poor pulse volume tracing at the forefoot level.

Yao and Dean and their colleagues have shown that the preoperative ankle systolic pressure and ASPI correlate with the severity of limb ischemia.[7,29] These authors have suggested that patients with a preoperative ASPI of less than 0.20 represent the poorest distal outflow and have the worst results in their series of femoropopliteal bypasses. This observation, however, is not consistent with our findings as well as those of others.[24] In 32 patients in our series of 220 femoropopliteal bypasses, the preoperative ASPI was less than 0.20. Cumulative 4-year life table patency in this group of patients was 71 percent which is not significantly different from our overall patency rate of 73 percent for the entire series.

SYSTEMIC AND LOCAL RISK FACTORS

We evaluated various systemic and local risk factors that might have contributed to poor healing in our 23 patients with nonhealing foot lesions despite a patent femoropopliteal bypass. The results of this analysis are summarized in Table 2. There was a higher incidence of diabetes, previous arterial reconstruction, or contralateral major amputation in this group of patients as compared to either the isolated popliteal segment group or the nonisolated popliteal artery group. Local risk factors seemed to be even more important than systemic risk factors in their association with the nonhealing of foot lesions. Almost all of the 23 patients had ischemic necrosis (i.e., gangrene) as an indication for surgery, and half of these patients had extensive necrosis defined by involvement of multiple toes, extension into the forefoot, or extensive involvement of the heel. Infection of the foot was a complicating factor present in 11 or 48 percent of these patients.

AMPUTATION

Twelve of our 23 patients that were threatened with limb loss despite a patent femoropopliteal bypass did not have or were not suitable for a distal graft extension and required a below-knee amputation for non-

Table 2. Systemic and Local Risk Factors Contributing to Poor Healing in Patients with Nonhealing Foot Lesions Despite a Patent Femoropopliteal Bypass

Risk Factor	Isolated Popliteal Segment* (%)	Nonisolated Popliteal Artery† (%)	Threatened Limbs‡ (%)
Diabetes	74	61	81
Previous operation/amputation	20	12	26
Necrosis (gangrene)	75	64	95
Extensive necrosis (gangrene)	24	10	52
Infection	22	12	48

* 48 patients; average age, 73 years.
† 172 patients; average age, 71 years.
‡ 23 patients; average age, 71 years.

healing foot lesions. This frustrating situation has also been reported by other groups.[4,21] The below-knee amputations healed without difficulty in all our cases. We presume that some of these patients may have required above-knee amputations had they not had a functioning femoropopliteal bypass. Thus, the bypass in these cases failed to salvage the foot but saved the knee.

EXTENSION OF GRAFT TO DISTAL LIMB ARTERIES

Preoperative, intraoperative, or postoperative arteriograms were evaluated in some of the 23 patients whose limbs remained threatened despite a patent femoropopliteal bypass to determine whether a secondary bypass to a more distal leg artery could be performed. A reconstituted distal leg artery extending without obstruction into the foot was available in 11 patients, and these patients underwent a secondary bypass from the femoropopliteal graft to that artery. One of these extensions was carried to a distal segment of the popliteal artery, six extended to the distal anterior tibial or dorsalis pedis arteries, three to the posterior tibial artery, and one to the peroneal artery. One patient died postoperatively, but in the 10 remaining patients, the limb was salvaged and remained intact 3 to 43 months later (mean, 20 months). Although three patients had thrombosis of their distal graft extensions after the foot had healed, these limbs have remained viable on the basis of the functioning proximal femoropopliteal bypass. One patient who had closure of both the femoropopliteal bypass and the distal extension due to myocardial infarction 17 months postoperatively required a below-knee amputation.

In 1971, DeLaurentis and Friedman[8] first reported the use of secondary distal graft extensions to distal leg arteries to augment femoropopliteal bypass flow. Since then, several other groups have reported good results using such graft extensions,[2,11,12] as well as sequential grafts inserted into multiple tibial arteries.[10,11,13,15] Indeed, when a patient presents with an angiographic picture of an isolated popliteal segment and a patent distal tibial artery, a dilemma exists as to which of the vessels to use as outflow. Davis and his associates[6] compared their results of bypasses to isolated popliteal segments with direct tibial reconstruction. These investigators favored the use of an isolated popliteal segment. The reasons given for this preference included better long-term patency rates, the need for a shorter length of saphenous vein, and easier anastomosis to a larger popliteal artery. We generally concur with this recommendation, except in circumstances to be detailed below.

Recently, Flinn and his associates,[12] using PTFE and a combination of PTFE and saphenous vein grafts, reported the use of sequential femoropopliteal-tibial bypasses in 40 patients for limb salvage. In most cases, the more proximal outflow anastomosis was to an isolated popliteal segment. The graft was then carried down to a tibial or peroneal artery. Significant hemodynamic improvement was noted, and an early limb salvage rate of 76 percent was achieved in their series.

DISCUSSION

It is generally believed that outflow from the popliteal artery is an important determinant of the results after all femoropopliteal bypasses, although several groups have observed that saphenous vein bypass to an isolated or blind popliteal artery segment can be an effective operation and some authors consider such procedures justified to salvage limbs. There is also a general belief that femoropopliteal bypasses performed to an isolated popliteal segment with prosthetic grafts have poor results.

Our 4-year results with PTFE femoropopliteal bypass grafts to an isolated popliteal artery segment have been surprisingly good (84 percent) and are not statistically different from those to the nonisolated popliteal artery. These results are unexpected in view of other results with the use of prosthetic materials in poor outflow situations. It is possible that PTFE grafts may, like saphenous veins, be capable of maintaining patency at lower flow rates than other prosthetic materials, although experimental evidence by Sauvage and his co-workers[22] suggests that PTFE grafts have a tendency to thrombose at higher flow rates than autologous veins. Another explanation for the good results with PTFE femoropopliteal bypasses in probable low flow circumstances might be the fact that high flow rates could produce pathologic changes that predispose to thrombosis. Intimal hyperplasia and distal atherosclerosis have been shown to occur with certain abnormal or high arterial flow patterns that could produce local vessel injury (see Chap. 8). Mismatch in the compliance of the graft and host artery may also increase the development of intimal hyperplasia. It is possible that the compliance of the PTFE material may be more similar to the more diseased popliteal artery associated with a distal occlusion than to a more normal artery. This might explain a higher incidence of intimal hyperplasia and associated failure in bypasses to more normal popliteal arteries associated with good runoff.

Although graft patency rates of PTFE bypasses to isolated popliteal artery segments were no worse than those to nonisolated segments, one clear disadvantage of bypasses to such isolated popliteal segments was the greater risk of limb loss despite a patent arterial reconstruction (31 percent vs 5 percent). This was particularly common if the bypass to the isolated popliteal artery was performed in a diabetic patient in the presence of extensive necrosis (gangrene) or infection in the foot (see Table 2). In such circumstances, the limited hemodynamic improvement brought about by the bypass was often not sufficient to heal the foot lesion. A secondary extension of the bypass to a more distal leg artery, however, was able to improve the circulation to the foot in 11 such patients with resulting limb salvage in 10.

On the basis of these observations, we recommend presently that patients who have an isolated popliteal artery segment and extensive foot infection or gangrene undergo a sequential femoral-to-popliteal-to-distal artery bypass as the initial operation, and we have performed several such one-stage operations and obtained healing of extensively infected or necrotic feet. If such a patient has a poor quality isolated popliteal segment, that is, less than 7 cm in length,[28] and a good quality leg or foot artery, we recommend a primary small vessel bypass to the distal vessel. If a patient has only ischemic rest pain or minimal necrosis and an isolated popliteal artery segment at least 7 cm in length, or a nonisolated popliteal artery,[28] irrespective of the condition of the foot, we presently would perform a femoropopliteal bypass as the initial procedure. Only if a healed foot cannot be obtained in these circumstances by appropriate local procedures such as debridement with or without skin grafting would we add an extension of the femoropopliteal bypass to a distal artery that communicates directly with the foot. We believe that this approach will minimize the number of patients that lose their limbs despite a functioning femoropopliteal bypass graft.

REFERENCES

1. Barner HB, Judd DR, Kaiser GC, et al: Blood flow in femoropopliteal bypass vein grafts. Arch Surg 96:619, 1968
2. Bliss BP, Fonseka N: "Hitch-hike" grafts for limb salvage in peripheral arterial disease. Br J Surg 63:562, 1976
3. Cutler BS, Thompson JE, Kleinsasser LJ, Hempel GK: Autologous saphenous vein femoropopliteal bypass: Analysis of 298 cases. Surgery 79:325, 1976
4. Darling RC: In discussion of bypass vein grafts in patients with distal popliteal artery occlusion. Am J Surg 129:421, 1975
5. Darling RC, Linton RR, Razzuk, MA: Saphenous vein bypass grafts for femoral-popliteal occlusive disease: A reappraisal. Surgery 61:31, 1967
6. Davis RC, Davies WT, Mannick JA: Bypass vein grafts in patients with distal popliteal artery occlusion. Am J Surg 129:421, 1975
7. Dean, RH, Yao JST, Stanton PE, Bergan JJ: Prognostic indicators in femoropopliteal reconstructions. Arch Surg 110:1287, 1975
8. DeLaurentis DA, Friedman P: Arterial reconstruction about and below the knee. Another look. Am J Surg 121:392, 1971
9. DeWeese JA, Rob CG: Autogenous venous grafts ten years later. Surgery 82:775, 1977
10. Edwards WS, Gerety E, Larkin J, Hoyt TW: Multiple sequential femoral tibial grafting for severe ischemia. Surgery 80:722, 1976
11. Edwards WS, Wright R: Tibial and peroneal bypass in severe occlusive disease of the lower extremities. Ann Surg 183:710, 1976
12. Flinn WR, Flanigan DP, Verta MJ Jr, et al: Sequential femoral-tibial bypass for severe limb ischemia. Surgery, 88:357, 1980
13. Friedman P, DeLaurentis DA, Rhee SW: The sequential femoropopliteal bypass graft: A five year experience. Am J Surg 131:452, 1976
14. Gupta SK, Veith FJ: Three year experience with expanded polytetrafluoroethylene arterial grafts for limb salvage. Am J Surg 140:214, 1980
15. Jarrett F, Berkoff HA, Crummy AB: Sequential femoral-tibial bypass grafting for limb salvage. Ann Surg 188:685, 1978
16. Kaminski DL, Barner HB, Dorighi JA, Kaiser GC, Willman VL: Femoropopliteal bypass with reversed autogenous vein. Ann Surg 177:232, 1972
17. Mannick JA, Jackson BT, Coffman JD, Hume DM: Success of bypass vein grafts in patients with isolated popliteal artery segments. Surgery 61:17, 1967
18. McCurdy JR, Lain KC, Allgood RJ, et al: Angiographic determinants of femoropopliteal bypass graft patency. Am J Surg 124:789, 1972
19. Mundth ED, Darling RC, Moran JM, et al: Quantitative correlation of distal arterial outflow and patency of femoropopliteal reversed saphenous vein grafts with intraoperative flow and pressure measurements. Surgery 65:197, 1969
20. Purdy RT, Bole P, Makanja W, Munda R: Salvage of the ischemic lower extremity in patients with poor runoff. Arch Surg 109:784, 1974

21. Reichle FA, Tyson R: Comparison of long-term results of 364 femoropopliteal or femorotibial bypasses for revascularization of severely ischemic lower extremities. Ann Surg 182:449, 1975
22. Sauvage LR, Walker MW, Berger K, et al: Current arterial prosthesis. Experimental evaluation by implantation in the carotid and circumflex coronary arteries of the dog. Arch Surg 114:687, 1979
23. Sauvage LR, Wood SJ, Davis CC, Mansfield PB: The USCI-Sauvage filamentous vascular prosthesis: Rationale, clinical results, and healing in man. In Sawyer PN, Kaplitt MJ (eds): Vascular Grafts. New York, Appleton-Century-Crofts, 1978, p 185
24. Sumner DS, Strandness DE: Hemodynamic studies before and after extended bypass grafts to the tibial and peroneal arteries. Surgery 86:442, 1979
25. Veith FJ, Gupta S, Daly V: Management of early and late thrombosis of expanded polytetrafluoroethylene (PTFE) femoropopliteal bypass grafts: Favorable prognosis with appropriate reoperation. Surgery 87:581, 1980
26. Veith FJ, Moss CM, Daly V, et al: New approaches to limb salvage by extended extra-anatomic bypasses and prosthetic reconstructions to foot arteries. Surgery, 84:764, 1978
27. Veith FJ, Moss CM, Fell SC, et al: Comparison of expanded polytetrafluoroethylene and autologous saphenous vein grafts in high risk arterial reconstructions for limb salvage. Surg Gynecol Obstet 147:749, 1978
28. Veith FJ, Gupta SK, Daly VR: Femoropopliteal bypass to the isolated popliteal segment: Is polytetrafluoroethylene graft acceptable? Surgery (In press).
29. Yao JST, Hobbs JT, Irvine WT: Ankle systolic pressure measurements in arterial disease affecting the lower extremities. Br J Surg 56:676, 1969

SEVENTEEN
Limitations of Profunda Femoris Revascularization

Victor M. Bernhard

The importance of the profunda femoris artery was recognized in 1961 by Morris[17] and Leeds.[12] Their experience and subsequent reports by others[3,4,13] demonstrated that this artery could provide adequate runoff for aortofemoral bypass and improve limb perfusion when the superficial femoral was occluded. Physiologic data were contributed by Waibel,[23] who noted a significant fall in popliteal pressure below a chronic superficial femoral obstruction when the profunda femoris artery was temporarily occluded. Operative measurements revealed that volume flow through the repaired profunda was twice the amount provided by a femoropopliteal bypass and was equal to the volume of flow through the common femoral when both superficial and profunda branches were patent.[4]

The importance of this vessel as a significant collateral bypassing superficial femoral and popliteal obstruction depends upon two factors: 1) the demonstrated ability of the profunda femoris artery to dilate in response to the increased demand for blood flow by the distal arterial bed, and 2) the capacity to develop a rich plexus of collateral connections to the popliteal artery through the geniculate branches and to the calf through the tibial recurrent vessels. In patients with isolated obstruction of the superficial femoral artery, calf claudication will frequently recede in proportion to the ability of the profunda collateral system to be recruited as a natural bypass. When this prime collateral is also obstructed, however, mild claudication becomes incapacitating and symptoms of ischemia at rest may appear. Relief of profunda obstruction under these circumstances has been shown to alleviate rest pain, permit healing of necrotic foot lesions, and to at least partially relieve claudication.[2,3,5-8,10,11,13,15,22]

Unfortunately, repair of a profunda stenosis alone or even in conjunction with an inflow procedure is not universally accompanied by improved calf and foot circulation. Relief of claudication by such procedures has been variously reported to occur in 60 to 95 percent of patients.[4-7,13] Strandness[21] was the first to demonstrate that subjective relief of claudication was substantiated objectively by lengthened treadmill walking tolerance in only four of seven patients. Limb salvage in patients with rest pain or ischemic necrosis has been achieved in only 40 to 85 percent of limbs subjected to reperfusion of the profunda system.[4-7,11,18,19,24]

The purpose of this chapter is to identify and explain those factors that bear on the success or failure of profundaplasty to provide significant improvement in arterial perfusion to the distal portion of the extremity. Technical factors at the time of surgery and subsequent degenerative changes in the repair or in the proximal and distal arteries may erase potential or temporarily achieved physiologic gains. Although important to immediate and long-term success, they are not germane to the selection of patients who might benefit from profunda repair.

The following have been identified as significant determinants of success or failure of profunda femoris angioplasty: 1) obstruction in the aortoiliac inflow segment, 2) the severity of profunda stenosis, 3) the extent and pattern of disease in the profunda femoris artery itself, 4) the presence or potential for collateral development between the profunda and the popliteal-tibial run-off system, 5) the patency of the popliteal-tibial-pedal run-off system, 6) the presence of distal gangrene, and 7) associated diabetes mellitus. The status of these factors or the ability to alter them must be evaluated before profundaplasty can be considered as the method of choice for revascularization of an ischemic leg.

AORTOILIAC INFLOW

Unrelieved inflow obstruction will limit the effectiveness of a repair of a deep femoral artery stenosis or occlusion or may cause early postoperative thrombosis. Hemodynamically, significant atherosclerotic disease in the iliac arteries may be overlooked on preoperative arteriograms because plaques tend to layer out on the dorsal wall of the artery where they may be undetected in the standard anteroposterior angiographic view. Lateral views of these vessels will identify such lesions, and whenever possible, these should be obtained before vascular repair below the inguinal ligament is undertaken. The presence of a good femoral pulse suggests unimpaired inflow, but may be misleading due to severe obstruction of run-off into the major branches of the common femoral artery. On the other hand, the presence of an iliac bruit does not prove the presence of a hemodynamically significant obstructive lesion above the inguinal ligament.

Direct pressure measurement at the common femoral level is a more reliable method for identifying an inflow pressure gradient.[16] This can be accomplished at the time of arteriography by connecting the angiographic catheter to a pressure transducer and recording aortic, iliac, and then femoral pressures during withdrawal. Alternatively, this can be accomplished at surgery by comparing the femoral pressure with the radial artery pressure monitor. Injection of 15 mg of papaverine directly into the femoral artery augments flow by reducing peripheral resistance in the limb and is used to identify a more subtle stenosis. A resting gradient of more than 10 mm Hg or a papaverine-augmented gradient of greater than 30 mm Hg identifies the presence of a hemodynamically significant inflow obstruction. Proximal bypass or endarterectomy will be required to insure maximum improvement in profunda flow. The presence of a vigorous "gush" during transient release of the proximal clamp after femoral arteriotomy and easy passage of a 6-mm dilator through the iliac system give further assurance that inflow is normal.

An inflow procedure was performed in 70 percent (169 of 232) of the limbs subjected to profundaplasty at our center.[5] A similar incidence of combined procedures versus profundaplasty alone has been noted by others.[13]

SEVERITY OF PROFUNDA FEMORIS STENOSIS

This issue has enjoyed extensive debate. Early investigators assumed that a tight stenosis or occlusion, best demonstrated on an oblique arteriogram, was a primary factor in selecting patients for profunda repair.[1] A report by Beurger, Higgins, and Cotton,[2] however, suggested that the normal profunda in the presence of superficial femoral occlusion presented a relative outflow stenosis to the common femoral artery and that even minimal encroachment produced by a plaque in the vicinity of the profunda orifice would reduce flow significantly. Subsequently, Cotton and Roberts[6] have indicated that the degree of stenosis is unrelated to the outcome of profundaplasty. The initial reports of Morris-Jones and Jones[18] and subsequently of Ward and Morris-Jones[24] supported that point of view.

The value of profundaplasty in the absence of a significant stenosis, however, has recently been challenged. Sladen and Burgess[19] noted that four of five limbs without stenosis were not improved. Mitchell and his associates[14] reported that 60 percent (12 of 20) of their patients with greater than 50 percent stenosis of the profunda and 88 percent (7 of 8) of those with combined common femoral and profunda stenosis obtained a satisfactory result. When profunda stenosis was minimal, however, the operation failed to improve limb perfusion.

In most reports profundaplasty is performed only when significant stenosis (i.e., > 50 percent) or occlusion of the vessel is identified either angiographically or at surgery by direct assessment of the profunda orifice through the femoral arteriotomy. Comparison of results between these series and those in which profundaplasty is performed without regard for the degree of orifice obstruction would not be valid in view of the many other variables that influence the outcome. Nevertheless, it has been the policy at our center to perform this operation only when a stenosis greater than 50 percent of the diameter is present. This is determined by comparing the measurement at the narrowest point of the stenosis with the diameter of the main trunk of the profunda femoris artery beyond the point of poststenotic dilatation on an oblique arteriographic view of the femoral region.

EXTENT AND PATTERN OF DISEASE IN THE PROFUNDA FEMORIS ARTERY

Stenosis may be limited to the profunda orifice because of extension of the atherosclerotic plaque, which is almost always present on the posterior wall of the common femoral artery. More often, however, the plaque extends down to the orifice of the lateral circumflex femoral artery or to a point just beyond the first perforating branch of the profunda. Occasionally, atherosclerosis extends to the second or even the third perforating branch or is confined to the midportion of the profunda femoris artery. In 74 percent of limbs with profunda atherosclerosis the distal segment of the artery is patent and relatively free of disease and able to provide collateral connection to the popliteal-tibial run-off system.[1] It is important, therefore, that profunda reconstruction be carried through the full length of the diseased artery into the distal patent segment to insure unobstructed flow into the collateral bed of the lower thigh. Excellent results have been reported following extension of the repair even to the third perforator.[5,7,10,11] Furthermore, results following extended profundaplasty have been consistently as good as those following more limited procedures.[5] Therefore, extent of profunda disease per se does not adversely affect the results of profundaplasty if the full length of the obstruction is relieved and the distal third of the artery is patent.

Approximately one-fourth of limbs with profunda involvement have obstruction throughout the length of this vessel or have disease that is confined to its distal portion.[1] Profundaplasty is usually not feasible in these patients. The lateral circumflex femoral artery and its large descending branch, however, may occasionally serve as a parallel collateral to the main profunda trunk. Endarterectomy and patch angioplasty through the proximal profunda into this branch may provide sufficient relief of ischemia to permit limb salvage under these circumstances.[9]

It is generally agreed, that all branches of the profunda should be carefully identified and patency of their orifices maintained during profunda endarterectomy so that the full collateral capability of this system can be utilized.[4,7,10] Because major branches, usually of profunda origin, may frequently arise from the common and superficial femoral arteries, these variations should be searched for on arteriograms and verified anatomically at surgery in order to devise a repair that will revascularize all of these branches. Thorough removal of the atherosclerotic plaque from the profunda femoris artery will usually relieve branch obstruction because the obstructing extension of the plaque into the branch is generally confined to its orifice and seldom extends more than a few millimeters into the branch itself.

PROFUNDA-POPLITEAL-TIBIAL COLLATERAL ANASTOMOSES

The ability of the profunda to carry out its function as a collateral bypass for an obstructed superficial femoral artery depends upon its connections with geniculate and recurrent tibial branches. These will generally enlarge in response to the pressure gradient caused by the superficial femoral obstruction and the peripheral vasodilatation produced by the demands of exercise and by the resting hypoxia and acidosis in patients with rest pain and necrosis. These collaterals may be inadequate due to congenital absence or, more likely, as a result of obstruction from atherosclerosis at their junctions with the popliteal and tibial arteries. The availability of these collaterals can be identified by arteriography.[20] The timing of film exposure and the presence of proximal obstructive disease, however, may be such that satisfactory visualization is not achieved.

A hemodynamic guide to the availability and function of these connections provides a more reliable estimate. This can be derived by noninvasively measuring segmental systolic pressures above and below the knee by the Doppler and pneumatic cuff technique.[5] These data permit calculation of a pressure gradient index utilizing the following formula:

$$\frac{AKP - BKP}{AKP} = PPCI$$

where AKP = above knee pressure, BKP = below knee pressure, PPCI = profunda-popliteal collateral index. The index is directly proportional to the pressure gradient so that poor collateralization across the knee is identified by a large gradient and a high index. This concept was tested in a series of patients in whom profundaplasty was performed for limb salvage.[5] No limbs were salvaged when the index was greater than 0.5, whereas salvage was achieved in 55 percent of limbs with an index of 0.25 to 0.5 and in 67 percent of those between 0.00 and 0.25. This simple noninvasive technique can be used to establish guidelines for patient selection for isolated profundaplasty. Severe iliac inflow disease, however, may obscure the pressure relationships across the knee, and data derived from Dopper pressure measurements are subject to errors inherent in the technique. For these reasons, calculation of the PPCI should be considered as a useful adjunct and not relied upon as the sole criterion for patient selection for profundaplasty.

PATENCY OF THE POPLITEAL-TIBIAL RUN-OFF SYSTEM

The success of any arterial reconstruction is related directly to the availability of an adequate run-off bed to accept augmented flow. This principle is no less valid in selection of patients for profundaplasty than it is for femoropopliteal or femorotibial bypass. The absence of an effective terminal delivery system precludes improved perfusion of the pedal tissues so that necrotic lesions and minor amputations may not heal and limb salvage will not be achieved.

The quality of the popliteal-tibial run-off estimated from preoperative arteriography correlated well with the relief of rest pain and the healing of necrotic lesions or minor amputations in a series of patients previously reported from this institution.[4] Limb salvage was achieved in 100 percent of limbs when the distal popliteal artery and at least two of the calf vessels were widely patent. Success fell to 85 percent when the popliteal artery was severely diseased and the tibial run-off reduced to one vessel. Limbs were retained in only 46 percent when the popliteal artery was occluded and only collateral twigs filled the distal tibial vessels. Although angiographic assessment of the popliteal run-off is only semiquantitative, this correlation merits consideration in selecting patients for profundaplasty rather than distal bypass to prevent major amputation. Although Ward and Morris-Jones[24] found no difference in uniformly poor results regardless of the quality of run-off, and Leather and his co-workers[11] and David and Dresner[7] noted good results despite poor run-off, the majority opinion supports our experience in regard to the importance of the run-off bed. Cotton and Roberts[6] noted an 85 percent success rate following profundaplasty when the popliteal was considered suitable for a femoropopliteal bypass, but only 33.3 percent when the popliteal artery was not satisfactory by arteriography. Mitchell and associates[14] and Sladen and Burgess[19] made similar observations.

The presence of a pressure gradient across the tibial vessels as determined by the noninvasive Doppler method, can also be expressed as an index:

$$\frac{BKP - AP}{BKP} = TG$$

where BKP = below knee pressure, AP = ankle pressure, TG = tibial gradient. This gradient was significantly higher in patients undergoing profundaplasty alone than in those in whom both an inflow procedure and a profundaplasty were performed for limb salvage (0.29 vs 0.18, $p < 0.02$). A similar trend that was not statistically significant (0.29 vs 0.18, $p = 0.09$) was also noted in patients with claudication. This difference suggests that in limbs with superficial femoral and profunda obstruction, there is a reciprocal relationship between inflow and outflow disease, that is, with greater aortoiliac inflow obstruction, there will be less popliteal and tibial run-off disease for any given degree of ischemia. There was no difference, however, in the tibial gradient between successful and unsuccessful profundaplasty in patients treated by profundaplasty alone or by inflow and profundaplasty. The tibial gradient index, therefore, in contrast to the profunda-popliteal collateral index, cannot be used to select patients for profundaplasty.[5]

PERIPHERAL GANGRENE

The presence of ischemic necrosis has generally been regarded as a poor prognostic sign in patients who require any form of revascularization for limb salvage, and patients subjected to profundaplasty are no exception. Modgill and his colleagues[15] noted a 54 percent limb salvage rate when necrosis was present, whereas 83 percent of limbs with rest pain alone were saved. David and Dresner[7] recorded 54.5 percent and 95 percent success rates, respectively, in these categories and similar experiences were noted by others.[8,14,19] The poor prognosis for limbs with digital gangrene may be a reflection of more severe disease at the tibial level. This is consistent with our findings that overall results for limb salvage were better with inflow plus profundaplasty (83 percent) than for profundaplasty alone (48 percent). Although the presence of gangrene is discouraging, it is not a contraindication to profundaplasty but this should be considered with other factors in patient selection.

DIABETES

Several reports have noted that the presence of diabetes has an adverse effect upon the results of profunda femoris revascularization for limb salvage.[6,11,14] A similar trend was noted in our experience but the differences were not statistically significant.[5]

DISCUSSION

Selection of patients for profundaplasty requires careful evaluation of the multiple factors just reviewed in relationship to the severity of symptomatology.

Results of Profunda Repair

The usefulness of profundaplasty to relieve ischemic symptoms depends upon many factors among which is whether the procedure was performed to relieve claudication or to salvage a threatened limb because of rest pain, ulceration, or distal gangrene. The immediate response to this operation was evaluated in 232 limbs in 163 patients at the Medical College of Wisconsin.[5] The indication for revascularization was incapacitating claudication in 67 of the limbs subjected to profundaplasty with an inflow procedure and in 10 limbs treated by profundaplasty alone. Nearly all patients were subjectively improved. When postoperative ankle pressure was measured to provide objective assessment, however, only 69 percent of limbs were found to have an increase in ankle/brachial pressure index of more than 0.1, 71 percent for inflow and profundaplasty, and 60 percent for profundaplasty alone. These results are similar to the small group studied by Strandness and Sumner[21] using ankle pressure and treadmill tolerance as objective criteria.

Limb salvage was achieved in 83 percent of limbs subjected to combined inflow and profundaplasty but only in 48 percent of legs in which isolated profundaplasty was performed. These results are similar to those reported by Mitchell and associates,[14] Cotton and Roberts,[6] Hill and Jamieson,[8] and David and Dresner[7] when similar groups of patients were compared. Leather and co-workers[11] reported 90 percent overall limb salvage in 62 patients. One-third of their patients required an inflow procedure, which partially accounts for their outstanding results.

Patients with incapacitating claudication due to combined iliac and superficial femoral obstruction are ideal candidates for an inflow procedure to the common femoral with extension into the profunda to relieve stenosis in the proximal portion of this vessel. The need for profunda femoris repair, either limited or extended, is obvious when a significant stenosis of this vessel is identified angiographically or during surgery. Less severe profunda stenosis should be repaired at the time of aortofemoral bypass to delay progression of disease at this point and to extend the functional life of the inflow graft. Repair of the profunda alone should be chosen to relieve claudication only if a stenosis greater than 50 percent is present. Although claudication will not be totally relieved in most patients, the improvement in limb circulation is usually sufficient to meet the needs of patients with associated medical problems and advanced age. Bypass to the popliteal or tibial vessels can be carried out later if symptoms persist, return, or progress.

Limb salvage is likely to be achieved in 80 to 90 percent of patients who require an inflow procedure in addition to profunda repair.[5] Although residual claudication will persist in most patients, this is usually inconsequential. Profundaplasty should not be considered a failure until sufficient time has elapsed for full development of collaterals through the profunda system. Because this may require several days or weeks, further procedures should be delayed unless progressive or limb-threatening ischemia requires more aggressive intervention.

The area of greatest controversy is the selection of profundaplasty as an alternative to femoropopliteal or femorotibial bypass in patients with unrestricted aortoiliac inflow. The more liberal use of profundaplasty under these circumstances may be preferred, because long-term patency of profunda repair is excellent when autogenous tissue is used, technical results are usually satisfactory, and the danger to the distal circulation is nil (Table 1). All of the factors already discussed in detail should be considered. It is important that the surgeon be assured that inflow is adequate whenever profundaplasty or any other subinguinal procedure is selected.

Profundaplasty alone is probably the ideal approach to limb revascularization when a stenosis greater than 50 percent is limited to the proximal

Table 1. Choice of Operation (Occluded Superficial Femoral, Normal Aortoiliac Inflow)

Criteria						
Profunda Femoral Stenosis > 50%	+	+	+	+	−	−
Collaterals PPCI < 0.5	+	+	−	−	+/−	+/−
Pop-Tib run off Good (+), Poor (−)	+	−	+	−	+	−
Procedure Recommended	P	P	F-P or F-T & P	P (Amp. later?)	F-P, F-T, or SEQ	AMP

P = *Profundaplasty*
F-P = *Femoropopliteal bypass*
F-T = *Femorotibial bypass*
SEQ = *Sequential graft*
AMP = *Amputation (BK or AK)*

profunda in a nondiabetic patient with superficial femoral occlusion, good popliteal-tibial run-off, a low profunda popliteal collateral index (PPCI), and no pedal gangrene (Table 1). Success in this select group should approach 100 percent. If the PPCI is above 0.5 and the popliteal is a reasonable vessel to accept a bypass graft in a patient with gangrene and/or diabetes, femoropopliteal grafting is probably the procedure of choice. When tibial bypass is the only alternative, profundaplasty is probably the better first choice unless the tibial vessel is large with a good pedal run-off, the success of profunda repair is compromised by a high PPCI (> 0.5), and there is questionably significant stenosis of the profunda. A stenosis of less than 50 percent diameter, or the presence of diffuse distal profunda disease are probably categorical contraindications to profundaplasty.

When profunda repair is chosen, the repair should extend distally to a point beyond any significant stenosis. The distal intima should be stabilized with tacking sutures if it is not firmly adherent, branches should be preserved and opened and an autogenous tissue patch should be used to insure an adequate lumen with a wide open funnel into the distal profunda.

Profundaplasty may be performed concomitant with femoropopliteal or femorotibial bypass whenever significant profunda stenosis is present. This will reduce the likelihood of progressive stenosis of this collateral, which may be required to maintain limb circulation subsequently if and when the bypass fails.

Profundaplasty is the only available technique for limb revascularization when neither femoropopliteal or femorotibial bypass is feasible. Limb salvage can be anticipated in less than 50 percent of patients under these circumstances; however, it is the only alternative to amputation. Although the foot may not be saved, there is increased likelihood that profundaplasty will permit successful amputation below rather than above the knee especially if preoperative upper calf arterial pressue is below 60 mm Hg.[5]

Mortality from profundaplasty was 3.5 percent in our center. Operative complications developed in 20 percent of patients; however, most were self-limited or readily managed without long-term sequellae.

REFERENCES

1. Beales JSM, Adcock FA, Frawley JE, et al: The radiologic assessment of disease of the profunda femoris artery. Br J Radiol 44:854, 1971
2. Berguer R, Higgins RF, Cotton LT: Geometry, blood flow, and reconstruction of the deep femoral artery. Am J Surg 130:68, 1975
3. Bernhard VM, Militello JM, Geringer AM: Repair of the profunda femoris artery. Am J Surg 127:676, 1974
4. Bernhard VM, Ray LI, Militello JP: The role of angioplasty of the profunda femoris artery in revascularization of the ischemic limb. Surg Gynecol Obstet 142:840, 1976
5. Boren CH, Towne JB, Bernhard VM, Salles-Cunha S: Profundapopliteal collateral index: A guide to successful profundaplasty. Arch Surg 115:1366, 1980
6. Cotton LT, Roberts VC: Extended deep femoral angioplasty: an alternative to femoropopliteal bypass. Br J Surg 62:340, 1975
7. David TE, Drezner AD: Extended profundaplasty for limb salvage. Surgery 84:758, 1978
8. Hill DA, Jamieson CW: The results of arterial reconstruction utilizing the profunda femoris artery in the treatment of rest pain and pre-gangrene. Br J Surg 64:359, 1977
9. Karmody A: Discussion of David TE, Dresner AD: Extended profundaplasty for limb salvage. Surgery 84:758, 1978
10. Kiely PE, Lumley JSP, Taylor GW: Extended endarterectomy of the profunda femoris artery. Arch Surg 106:605, 1973
11. Leather RP, Shah DM, Karmody AM: The use of extended profundaplasty in limb salvage. Am J Surg 136:359, 1978

12. Leeds FH, Gilfillan RS: Revascularization of the ischemic limb. Arch Surg 82:45/25, 1961
13. Martin P, Renwick S, Stephenson C: On the surgery of the profunda femoris artery. Br J Surg 55(7):539, 1968
14. Mitchell RA, Bone GE, Bridges R, Pomajzl MJ, Fry WJ: Patient selection for isolated profundaplasty: arteriographic correlates of operative results. Am J Surg 138:912, 1979
15. Modgill VK, Humphrey CS, Shoesmith JH, Kester RC: The value of profundaplasty in the management of severe femoropopliteal occlusion. Br J Surg 64:362, 1977
16. Moore WS, Hall AD: Unrecognized aortoiliac stenosis: a physiologic approach to the diagnosis. Arch Surg 103:633, 1971
17. Morris GC, Edwards W, Cooley DA, Crawford ES, DeBakey ME: Surgical importance of profunda femoris artery. Arch Surg 82:52/32, 1961
18. Morris-Jones W, Jones CDP: Profundaplasty in the treatment of femoropopliteal occlusion. Am J Surg 127:680, 1974
19. Sladen JG, Burgess JJ: Profundaplasty: expectations and ominous signs. Am J Surg 140:242, 1980
20. Stoney RJ: Discussion of David TE, Dresner DA: Extended profundaplasty for limb salvage. Surgery 84:758, 1978
21. Strandness DE: Functional results after revascularization of the profunda femoris artery. Am J Surg 119:240, 1970
22. Sugden BA, Sheldon CD: Preoperative flow and pressure measurements in profundaplasty. J Cardiovasc Surg 20:185, 1979
23. Waibel PP, Wolff G: The collateral circulation in occlusions of the femoral artery: an experimental study. Surgery 60(4):912, 1966
24. Ward AS, Morris-Jones W: The long term results of profundaplasty in femoropopliteal arterial occlusion. Br J Surg 64:365, 1977

EIGHTEEN

The Present Role of Lumbar Sympathectomy in the Treatment of Lower Limb Ischemia

James S.T. Yao and William R. Flinn

The release of vascular tone and dilation of blood vessels under control of the sympathetic nervous system, first observed by du Petit in 1727,[10] has served as the rationale for numerous procedures designed to provide sympathetic ablation. For arteriosclerotic occlusive disease, Julio Diez[9] of Argentina first applied lumbar sympathectomy in the treatment of limb ischemia in 1924. At the same time, Royle of Australia[27] advocated the use of lumbar sympathectomy for the alleviation of spastic paralysis. Subsequently, Adson and Brown of the Mayo Clinic[1,2] reported the use of lumbar sympathectomy in the treatment of vasospastic disease. Since then, lumbar sympathectomy enjoyed its greatest popularity in the 1940s and 1950s, before the advent of arterial reconstructive surgery.

Even after 50 years of existence, the role of lumbar sympathectomy in the management of occlusive arterial disease of the lower extremities remains controversial. Although some authors[17] have claimed sympathectomy resulted in successful relief of ischemia, others[14] considered it rarely beneficial. Conflicting results reported by various authors may be due to lack of objective methods for quantitating limb ischemia. In most reported series, moreover, attempts have been made to correlate the results of sympathectomy with subjective symptoms such as claudication, rest pain, ischemic ulcers, or with threatened limb viability. Because of lack of homogeneity in these patients regarding the collateral reserve, the results of lumbar sympathectomy were variable.

Supported in part by the Northwestern University Vascular Research Fund.

There are other factors that may influence the prognosis in sympathectomy. These are regeneration of the nerve or incomplete sympathectomy,[32] anatomic variability of sympathetic ganglia,[6] and, last, the failure of sympathectomy to improve nutrient flow. All these factors have been reported as causes of poor response to sympathetic ablation.

Despite some reservations regarding the role of lumbar sympathectomy in the treatment of arterial ischemia, it is generally considered that the procedure is effective in the treatment of superficial ischemic lesions of the skin, vasospastic disease, causalgia, and hyperhidrosis. This chapter attempts to reassess the effect of sympathectomy on blood flow and the currently available noninvasive techniques that may help in proper selection of patients for lumbar sympathectomy.

SYMPATHETIC INNERVATION OF THE LOWER EXTREMITY

Lumbar sympathetic nerves are efferent fibers that function as vasoconstrictors, pseudomotors, and piloerectors for the lower extremities. The lumbar sympathetic ganglia and nerves arise from the thoracolumbar division of the sympathetic nervous system which has five pairs of lumbar spinal nerves. Contrary to common belief, the distribution of ganglia and their connection with the spinal nerves is extremely variable.[6,32] This anatomic variation helps to explain why lumbar sympathectomy is subject to conflicting results. Considerable anatomic variation is seen, and cross-communications between the right and left sympathetic trunks have also been reported.[32] For denervation of the lower extremity, removal of the L-2, L-3, L-4 ganglia results in satisfactory ablation of activity in the majority of the skin below the knee. Additional denervation of the thigh requires the removal of the L-1 ganglion.

EFFECT OF SYMPATHETIC ABLATION ON BLOOD FLOW

Unlike muscles, the blood vessels in the skin, especially in the terminal portions of the extremity, such as the hands, feet, fingers, and toes, are chiefly supplied by the sympathetic vasoconstrictor fibers. Reflex changes manifested by vasoconstriction of skin vessels may decrease flow to the skin, and this mechanism is essential in the regulation of body temperature. Besides temperature regulation, emotional or mental stimulation may also affect skin blood flow via the sympathetic system.

Vessels within the muscular compartment are under a small degree of vasomotor control as compared with skin vessels. Lumbar denervation produces a reduction in vasoconstrictor tone in skeletal muscle but to a much lesser degree than in the skin. In general, blood vessels in the muscles are predominantly regulated by locally produced metabolites and the vasoconstricting activity of the sympathetic nerves is easily overcome during exercise or ischemia. The rather insignificant increase in muscle flow following ablation of sympathetic tone explains why sympathectomy seldom, if ever, results in relief of intermittent claudication.

An increase of total limb blood flow after sympathectomy may not be sufficient. The selective augmentation of flow to the ischemic tissue is probably essential to the therapeutic outcome from sympathetic ablation. In other words, benefit must be derived from increased nutrient flow rather than an increase of flow through arteriovenous anastomoses. With the development of sophisticated methods, such as microsphere techniques in the measurement of limb blood flow, it is now possible to record arteriovenous shunt flow selectively.[8] This technique uses microspheres of approximately 23 μ, which is equivalent to the size of arteriovenous anastomotic communications. After the administration of these microspheres, increased flow through arteriovenous channels after sympathectomy can be readily detected and quantitated.

Arteriovenous anastomotic shunts are known to be present in the acral skin and subcutaneous tissues of animals and man, and these arteriovenous shunts are not present in muscles. Using the microsphere technique, investigators have found a marked increase of arteriovenous shunt flow after sympathectomy in animals. In fact, most if not all of the flow increase that occurs after lumbar sympathectomy is thought to be due to flow through the nonnutrient arteriovenous pathways, rather than through nutrient pathways that may augment flow to ischemic tissues. This finding casts doubt on the usefulness of sympathectomy in the treatment of tissue ischemia.

This observation was further confirmed by the recent report of Cronenwett and Lindenauer,[7] who found no improvement in nutrient muscle flow in both normal and ischemic canine hind limbs following sympathectomy. They concluded that sympathectomy is probably not useful to increase nutritive muscle blood flow, i.e., it probably is not helpful in patients with intermittent claudication.

SYMPATHETIC ABLATION IN THE TREATMENT OF ARTERIAL OCCLUSIVE DISEASE

Indications for Lumbar Sympathectomy

While lumbar sympathectomy has a clear indication in vasospastic disease and in causalgia, its role in the treatment of arterial occlusive disease remains ill-defined. Sympathectomy has often been performed when reconstructive surgery is said to be not feasible. With the advent of profunda femoris artery reconstruction and extended femoral-distal bypass operations, more patients who would otherwise have been considered for lumbar sympathectomy have become candidates for arterial reconstructive surgery. With better quality arteriography to demonstrate vessels distal to the popliteal artery trifurcation, including the pedal arch, many patients with severe popliteal and trifurcation disease have undergone femorotibial and peroneal bypass with satisfactory results.[37,39] Because of this trend to more aggressive surgical approaches we are now performing fewer lumbar sympathectomies.

In patients with severe ischemia, it is our policy to make every effort to visualize all three leg arteries (posterior tibial, anterior tibial, and peroneal) down to the ankle level for consideration for distal bypass. Even if the preoperative arteriogram fails to visualize these arteries satisfactorily, an intraoperative, prebypass arteriogram is performed. This is done by exposing the common femoral artery as for a bypass from the femoral artery. A needle is then placed in the common femoral artery for administration of contrast media. An x-ray cassette with a sterile cover is placed under the distal limb, including the foot. The common femoral artery is clamped prior to injection of contrast media. Immediately after completion of the injection of contrast media, the clamp is released, and the x ray is then taken about 8 to 10 seconds after the release of the clamp. This maneuver usually allows excellent visualization of distal vessels. In the majority of cases, a patent leg artery (anterior or posterior tibial or peroneal) is identified by this technique, and the femorodistal reconstruction can be undertaken.

With this approach, many patients have been able to have a distal bypass procedure with gratifying results. At present, lumbar sympathectomy is performed only on those patients in whom the preoperative arteriogram clearly demonstrated an unreconstructable anatomic situation and who have superficial skin ischemia. We do not consider lumbar sympathectomy to be indicated for relief of established gangrene or acute ischemia, nor should it be used in an attempt to lower the amputation level.

Selection of Patients for Lumbar Sympathectomy

In addition to arteriography to identify patients for extended femorodistal bypass, noninvasive tests may help to select patients for lumbar sympathectomy. The variability in the reported results of sympathectomy is obviously due to the lack of a method to quantitate ischemia. With the development of noninvasive techniques, it is now possible to grade the degree of ischemia and to assess its response to sympathectomy more objectively. At present, several techniques are useful in predicting the result of lumbar sympathectomy.

Transcutaneous Doppler Flow Detection. The Doppler technique allows the recording of pulsatile flow patterns in accessible arteries including the dorsalis pedis and posterior tibial. At the same time, it can be used as an endpoint to measure systolic pressure at various levels in a limb. Using the brachial systolic pressure as the normal control, the ratio between the ankle and brachial pressure represents the ischemic index (pressure index) or the status of the collateral flow. Recording of systolic pressure and comparison of its level with the brachial artery pressure is, therefore, a useful method to quantitate the degree of ischemia.

In one of our previous reports, we have compared the pressure index recorded by the Doppler technique with a vasodilating technique to predict vascular reactivity relative to sympathetic ablation.[45] The vasodilating technique employs a strain-gauge plethysmograph to record blood flow in the foot before and after the administration of an alpha-blocker. After preoperative measurements were obtained, patients underwent lumbar sympathectomy, and blood flow measurements were repeated 3 to 4 days postoperatively. The overall value of the vasodilating technique as a predictive test was only 40 percent. In contrast, the pressure index, which grades the degree of ischemia, was a better predictor of the response to sympathectomy. All patients with a pressure index greater than 0.35 responded well to sympathectomy. Patients with a pressure index less than 0.25 responded poorly and were faced with subsequent amputation. None of the patients with unrecordable ankle pressure responded well to sympathectomy.

The rationale for the use of the pressure index in predicting the result of sympathectomy is based on the fact that ankle pressure represents the level of collateral flow. Folse and his colleagues[12] have found that a significant increase in blood flow following sympathectomy occurred only in patients with good collateral development. The use of ankle pressure level in predicting the response to lumbar sympathectomy has also been reported by Thulesius, Gjores, and Mandaus.[36] They found that a poor response to sympathectomy, manifested by failure to elevate the skin temperature, was seen in patients with an ankle systolic pressure of less than 60 mm Hg. Seeger and his colleagues[29] also reported a pressure index greater than 0.25 to be associated with a high rate of success in lumbar sympathectomy. Recently, in a study of the effect of lumbar sympathectomy assessed by multiple regression analysis, Walker and Johnston[40] have found that patients with an ankle pressure exceeding 30 mm Hg responded well to sympathetic blockade.

Based on these reports, it would appear that a critical level of ankle pressure, hence, the presence of a reasonable level of collateral circulation, is prognostic for the success of lumbar sympathectomy. The 30 mm Hg level for response to sympathectomy has also been suggested by Nielsen and his colleagues.[24] They found that a drop of toe pressure after sympathetic blockade to a level less than 30 mm Hg is accompanied by a decrease of subcutaneous blood flow measured adjacent to the ischemic area. This finding may explain the so-called paradoxical gangrene, which may have been provoked by aggravation of an already critically low distal pressure.

The use of ankle pressure alone is not helpful in diabetic patients, in whom calcified arteries may cause a falsely high ankle pressure measurement. Because of this, the Doppler flow waveform recording at the posterior tibial or dorsalis pedis artery may be useful. A severely damped flow waveform with poor pulsatile characteristics suggests the presence of severe ischemia. In diabetics or in patients with uremia, it is not uncommon to encounter a spuriously high reading of ankle pressure, often up to the 300 mm Hg level.

Table 1 summarizes the hemodynamic criteria for successful sympathectomy as reported by various investigators.

Plethysmography. A strain-gauge plethysmograph may be used to record pulse waveforms in the first or second toe. Changes in the shape of the waveforms are then observed after a period of cuff-induced ischemia. The presence of reactive hyperemia, manifested by an increase in pulse amplitude, has been reported to be of value in predicting the success of sympathectomy.[5]

Another use of strain-gauge plethysmography is to measure blood flow in the foot. This flow is predominantly to the skin of the foot.[23] An increase of flow following a period of occlusive ischemia again may serve as an indicator that sympathectomy may have a beneficial response. Recently, Shanik and Barnes[30] have reported the use of Doppler ankle pressure and strain-gauge plethysmography to record foot flow. Using these two parameters, the peripheral resistance of the foot was calculated to represent the vasomotor tone of the foot. They have reported that the foot arterial resistance index is useful to predict the response to sympathectomy, especially in patients undergoing concomitant arterial reconstruction.

Concomitant Sympathectomy in Arterial Reconstruction

One of the most controversial issues relating to lumbar sympathectomy is its use during arterial reconstruction. Although increased arterial flow has been observed immediately after lumbar sympathectomy when the

Table 1. Summary of Hemodynamic Criteria in Predicting the Outcome of Lumbar Sympathectomy

Authors	Year	No.	Hemodynamic Criteria of Failure	Result
Thulesius, Gjores, Mandaus	(1973)[36]	16	Ankle pressure less than 60 mm Hg	Paradoxical drop of skin temperature
Nielsen et al.	(1975)[24]	16	Toe pressure less than 30 mm Hg after sympathetic blockage	Decrease of subcutaneous blood flow
Uhrenholdt	(1973)[38]	35	Xenon skin blood pressure less than 22 mm Hg	Decrease of pedal flow by xenon-133 clearance technique
Yao and Bergan	(1973)[45]	84	Doppler pressure index less than 0.205	Amputation required
Seeger, Lazarus, Albo	(1977)[29]	8	Doppler pressure index less than 0.20	All patients with pressure index greater than 0.20 responded to sympathectomy
Walker and Johnston	(1980)[40]	72	Doppler ankle pressure less than 30 mm Hg	Outcome of patients with pressure less than 30 mm Hg was not stated

measurements are made with an electromagnetic flowmeter,[35] the effect of sympathectomy on maintaining long-term patency of bypass grafts remains unclear, and the question of whether or not lumbar sympathectomy should be added to revascularization procedures remains unanswered.

It is generally known that the effect of sympathectomy on blood flow is often transient. Immediately after sympathectomy, there is an increase in limb blood flow, often reaching a maximum 24 to 48 hours following surgery. The blood flow then gradually returns to the preoperative level within 7 to 10 days. The time-sequence effect of sympathetic ablation implies that sympathectomy, though effective in decreasing foot resistance during the immediate postoperative period, is of doubtful value in maintaining the long-term patency of arterial reconstructions. In a randomized trial, Barnes and his colleagues[3] observed a decrease of foot resistance if sympathectomy was added to aortic reconstruction. The procedure was found to have no effect, however, on limb circulation assessed by ankle/arm indices determined by Doppler ultrasound. The absence of a change in the pressure index indicates that lumbar sympathectomy is probably not effective to improve the distal circulation.

Recently, Collins and his co-workers[4] have used intraoperative electromagnetic flow measurement to evaluate the effect of lumbar sympathectomy during aortic reconstruction. In eight patients who underwent aortoiliac reconstruction, intraoperative flow measurements before and after aortofemoral bypass and after the addition of sympathectomy were recorded by an electromagnetic flowmeter. In their report, there was an increase of flow about 1.55 times greater with added sympathectomy than with aortofemoral bypass alone. They reasoned that such an increase of flow is of use in patients with limited outflow. They failed to recognize, however, that the immediate increase in flow following sympathectomy may be due to a release of the abnormally exaggerated vascular tone due to exposure of the foot to the cold operating room environment. Not only is intense vasoconstriction of arterioles present due to environmental temperature, but a depression of venomotor tone caused by halothane may also be a responsible factor. Interference with the sympathetic activation of venous smooth muscle cells by halothane anesthetics, resulting in exaggerated vasomotor tone, has been reported.[22] It is conceivable that sympathectomy may release this exaggerated venomotor response and hence, an increase of flow after sympathetic ablation may occur without any lasting beneficial effect. In a prospective randomized study of concomitant lumbar sympathectomy with aortoiliac reconstruction, Satiani and his colleagues[28] have found no difference in graft patency during a follow-up period of 11 months in 93 patients.

CHEMICAL SYMPATHECTOMY

Recently, chemical sympathectomy has received renewed attention, especially in Europe.[13,16,26,41] Chemical sympathectomy is done by injecting phenol at the level of the third and fourth lumbar vertebrae with the aid of an image intensifying fluoroscope for accurate needle positioning.[26] The correct plane for the phenol injection is achieved by the injection of 5 ml of air and 1.0 ml of contrast media through each needle. Air and contrast media spread along the tissue planes in a characteristic pattern when the needles are in satisfactory position. Afterward, 4 ml of 6 percent phenol in water are injected through each needle. During needle placement, repeated aspiration is done to ensure that there is no inadvertent puncture of blood vessels.

The chief advantage of chemical sympathectomy is that a surgical procedure can be avoided. This approach is attractive in elderly or high-risk patients, in whom surgical sympathectomy is undesirable. On the other hand, chemical sympathectomy, though effective, is not without hazard.[33]

COMMENTS

Even among experienced vascular surgeons, opinion regarding the role of lumbar sympathectomy in the treatment of ischemia in arteriosclerotic occlusive disease remains divergent.[31,42] There is little doubt that sympathectomy is effective in improving skin blood flow in normal limbs or in the experimental animal. Lumbar sympathectomy is less effective in increasing muscle blood flow, and it is generally believed that sympathectomy is rarely of benefit in patients with intermittent claudication. The ineffectiveness of sympathectomy in claudicants is confirmed by the failure to normalize or improve the ankle or calf pressure response to exercise[15,34] in animal model studies[44] and also in microsphere studies[7] in which increased nutrient is seldom seen.

For severe ischemia, selection of patients for lumbar sympathectomy is influenced by the surgeon's ability to determine feasibility of extended distal bypass. Both detailed arteriographic study of distal arteries and transcutaneous Doppler examination are helpful to select patients for distal bypass. When distal bypass is not feasible, the ankle pressure level is helpful in predicting the response to sympathetic ablation. In order for sympathectomy to be effective, an adequate collateral flow is essential. As indicated by Nielsen et al.[24] and Walker and Johnston,[40] a pressure level exceeding 30 mm Hg is necessary to achieve a good response. When proximal flow increases, the distal pressure may drop, and a decrease of pressure distal to an occlusion following sympathectomy has been confirmed by Weale.[43] With an already critically low distal pressure, that is, a pressure below a level of 30 mm Hg, a further drop in pressure may increase the ischemia. This observation has been confirmed by a decrease in the subcutaneous blood flow close to a gangrenous area in the study reported by Nielsen et al.[24] Based on these findings and our experience, we consider sympathectomy not to be advisable in patients with severely depressed ankle pressure.

Recently, Plecha and his colleagues[25] have advocated a distal thigh/arm index as a predictor for the value of lumbar sympathectomy. According to their criteria, patients with a distal thigh/arm index greater than 0.7 have a good response to sympathectomy, even with unrecordable ankle pressure. They theorized that an adequate inflow is the factor responsible for the success. The effect of sympathectomy on collateral vessels in patients with arterial occlusive disease is unknown.[11] Sympathectomy results in peripheral vasodilation of the most distal part of the limb. Whether the five of six patients with unrecordable pressure in the series of Plecha and colleagues[25] represent an increase of collateral resistance by sympathectomy or a spontaneous improvement of collateral flow remains unknown because there was no mention made of the duration of ischemia in their report.

Perhaps the best information derived from noninvasive testing in these patients is that unrecordable flow signals and hence, zero ankle pressure, represents the presence of acute ischemia, in which lumbar sympathectomy is a useless procedure. The finding of zero pressure warns the surgeon that only an arterial reconstruction can restore the circulation. Based on our own data[45] as well as other studies,[24,38,40] sympathectomy should not be contemplated when the ankle or toe pressure is less than 30 mm Hg.

Ankle pressure is obviously not useful in diabetic patients with calcified arteries because of falsely elevated ankle pressure measurements. Pulse recording of posterior tibial or dorsalis pedis arteries may be helpful. A poor pulsatile flow indicates the presence of severe ischemia, in spite of a falsely high or sometimes incomprehensible pressure with readings up to the 300 mm Hg level. In diabetics, autosympathectomy has been cited as a common associated condition. Therefore, sympathectomy may not be effective. Moorhouse et al.[21] have observed that sympathetic denervation almost always accompanied neurologic signs of a peripheral neuropathy in a diabetic patient and that the autonomic nervous system was usually intact in diabetic patients without peripheral neuropathy. The mechanism of failure of sympathectomy in diabetics has been suggested by Kott and his co-workers.[18] In an ultrastructural study of lumbar sympathetic ganglia in diabetic patients and nondiabetics, they have found abnormal morphology in the ganglia of patients with diabetes. Because of these morphologically abnormal cells in the sympathetic ganglia, an unsatisfactory response to sympathetic ablation may be expected in diabetic patients. Even with increased flow after sympathectomy, Moore and Hall[20] have found that only one of five diabetic patients had an increase in nutritional blood flow.

The use of concomitant sympathectomy in reconstructive arterial surgery has been a subject of debate. Enough evidence has shown that flow may increase intraoperatively, but the effect does not persist, and sympathectomy is not effective in prolonging the patency of bypass grafts. The renewed interest in chemical sympathectomy deserves further study before it can be recommended for routine use. Finally, it must be emphasized that in selecting patients for sympathectomy, clinical findings such as the diagnosis of tissue necrosis, infection, and the general condition of the patient must enter into decision making. With proper clinical judgment supplemented by noninvasive testing, there will currently be only a few patients who are candidates for lumbar sympathectomy.

[*Editor's Note:* The authors' last statement is borne out by the decreasing frequency of lumbar sympathectomy as an operative procedure on most major vascular surgical services.]

REFERENCES

1. Adson AW, Brown GE: Treatment of Raynaud's disease by lumbar ramisection and ganglionectomy and perivascular sympathetic neurectomy of the common iliac artery. JAMA 84:1908, 1925
2. Adson AW, Brown GE: Treatment of Raynaud's disease by resection of upper thoracic and lumbar sympathetic ganglia and trunks. Surg Gynecol Obstet 48:577, 1929
3. Barnes RW, Baker WH, Shanik G, et al: Value of concomitant sympathectomy in aortoiliac reconstruction. Arch Surg 112:1325, 1977
4. Collins GJ, Rich NM, Andersen CA, et al: Acute hemodynamic effects of lumbar sympathectomy. Am J Surg 136:714, 1978
5. Courbier R, Reggi M, Jansseran JM: Evaluation of effectiveness of lumbar sympathectomy by noninvasive diagnostic techniques. J Cardiovasc Surg 20:333, 1979
6. Cowley RA, Yeager GH: Anatomic observations on the lumbar sympathetic nervous system. Surgery 25:880, 1949
7. Cronenwett JC, Lindenauer SM: Hemodynamic effects of sympathectomy in ischemic canine hind limbs. Surgery 87:417, 1980
8. Delaney J, Scarpino J: Limb arteriovenous shunting following sympathetic denervation. Surgery 73:202, 1973
9. Diez J: Un nuevo metodo de simpatectomia perfiferica para el tratemiento

de las afecciones troficas y gangrenosas de los miembros. La disociacion fascicular. Bul Soc Cir B Aires 8:792, 1924
10. du Petit FP: Memoire dans lequel il est demonstre que les intercostaux fournessent des rameaux qui portent des espirits dans les yeux. Hist Acad Roy Sci 1727
11. Folkow B: Pathophysiological aspects of blood flow distal to an obliterated main artery with special regard to the possibilities of affecting the collateral resistance and the arterioles in the distal low-pressure system. Scand J Clin Lab Invest 19: (Suppl) 99: 211, 1967
12. Folse R, Mack RM, Cantrell JR: Alterations in femoral blood flow and resistance following sympathectomy blockade. Ann Surg 162:873, 1965
13. Forslund L, Kovamees A, McCarthy G: Sympathetic blocks. Acta Chir Scand (Suppl) 482: 67, 1978
14. Fulton RL, Blakely WR: Lumbar sympathectomy: a procedure of questionable value in the treatment of arteriosclerosis obliterans of the leg. Am J Surg 116:735, 1968
15. Fyfe T, Quinn R: Phenol sympathectomy in the treatment of intermittent claudication. A controlled clinical trial. Br J Surg 62:68, 1975
16. Keane FBV: Phenol lumbar sympathectomy for severe arterial occlusive disease in the elderly. Br J Surg 64:519, 1977
17. Kim GE, Zhrahian AM, Imparato AM: Lumbar sympathectomy in end stage arterial occlusive disease. Ann Surg 183:157, 1976
18. Kott I, Uria Z, Sandbank U: Lumbar sympathetic ganglia in atherosclerotic patients, diabetic and nondiabetic. A comparative morphological and ultrastructure study. Arch Surg 109:787, 1974
19. Masuoka S, Shimonura T: Lumbar sympathectomy and blood flow in the lower extremity. Am J Surg 136:369, 1978
20. Moore WS, Hall AD: Effects of lumbar sympathectomy on skin capillary blood flow in arterial occlusive disease. J Surg Res 14:151, 1973
21. Moorhouse JA, Carter SA, Doupe J: Vascular response in diabetic peripheral neuropathy. Br Med J 1:883, 1966
22. Muldoon SM, Vanhoutte PM, Lorenz RR, Van Dyke RA: Venomotor changes caused by halothane activity on the sympathetic nerves. Anesthesiology 43:41, 1975
23. Myers KA, Irvine WT: An objective study of lumbar sympathectomy. II. Skin ischemia. Br Med J 1:943, 1966
24. Nielsen PE, Bell A, Angustenborg G, Paaske-Hansen O, Lassen NA: Reduction in distal pressure by sympathetic nerve block in patients with occlusive arterial disease. Cardiovasc Res 7: 577, 1973
25. Plecha FR, Bomberger RA, Hoffman M, Macpherson K: A new criterion for predicting response to lumbar sympathectomy in patients with severe arteriosclerotic occlusive disease. Surgery 88:375, 1980
26. Reid W, Kennedy WJ, Gray TA: Phenol injection of the sympathetic chain. Br J Surg 57:45, 1970
27. Royle ND: New operative procedure in treatment of spastic paralysis and its experimental basis. Med J Austr 1:77, 1924

28. Satiani B, Liapis CD, Hayes JP, Kimmins S, Evans WE: A prospective randomized study of concomitant lumbar sympathectomy with aortoiliac reconstruction. Presented to 4th Ann. Mtg. Midwestern Vascular Surg. Soc., Cincinnati, Sept. 26–27, 1980
29. Seeger JM, Lazarus HM, Albo D: Preoperative selection of patients for lumbar sympathectomy by use of Doppler index. Am J Surg 134:749, 1977
30. Shaink G, Barnes RW, Fitzgerald P: Foot vasomotor tone following aortofemoral and femoropopliteal reconstruction for limb ischemia. J Cardiovasc Surg 18:129, 1977
31. Shumacker HB: A place for sympathectomy in arteriosclerotic occlusive disease. Surg Gynecol Obstet 149:72, 1979
32. Simeone FA: The anatomy of lumbar sympathetic trunk in man (with special reference to the question of regeneration after sympathectomy). J Cardiovasc Surg 20:283, 1979
33. Smith RC, Davidson N McD, Ruckley CV: Hazard of chemical sympathectomy. Br J Med 1:552, 1978
34. Strandness DE Jr, Bell JW: Critical evaluation of the results of lumbar sympathectomy. Ann Surg 160:1021, 1964
35. Terry HJ, Allen JS, Taylor GW: The effect of adding lumbar sympathectomy to reconstructive arterial surgery in the lower limb. Br J Surg 57:51, 1970
36. Thulesius O, Gjores JE, Mandaus L: Distal blood flow and blood pressure in vascular occlusion; influence of sympathetic nerves on collateral blood flow. Scand J Clin Lab Invest (Suppl) 128:53, 1973
37. Tyson R, Reichle FA: Femorotibial bypass. Ann Surg 170:429, 1969
38. Uhrenholdt A: Relationship between distal blood flow and blood pressure after abolition of the sympathetic vasomotor tone. Scand J Clin Lab Invest 128: (Suppl):63, 1973
39. Veith FJ, Moss CM, Daly V, Fell SC, Haimovici H: New approaches to limb salvage by extended extra-anatomic bypass and prosthetic reconstructions to foot arteries. Surgery 84:764, 1978
40. Walker PM, Johnston KW: Predicting the success of a sympathectomy: a prospective study using discriminant function and multiple regression analysis. Surgery 87:216, 1980
41. Walker PM, Key JA, Mackay IM, Johnston KW: Phenol sympathectomy for vascular occlusive disease. Surg Gynecol Obstet 146:741, 1978
42. Warden R: Editorial: Sympathectomism. Arch Surg 111:928, 1976
43. Weale FE: The hemodynamic assessment of the arterial tree during reconstructive surgery. Ann Surg 169:489, 1969
44. Weissenhofer W, Schenk WG Jr: Effects of sympathectomy on blood flow through stenotic vessels during exercise. An experimental study in a canine model. Surgery 74:743, 1973
45. Yao JST, Bergan JJ: Predictability of vascular reactivity relative to sympathetic ablation. Arch Surg 107:676, 1973

NINETEEN

Upper Extremity Ischemia: Role of the Vascular Surgeon in Raynaud's Syndrome and Finger Gangrene

John M. Porter

The correction of typical large artery obstruction caused by atherosclerosis, trauma, embolization, and so on has constituted the traditional concern of vascular surgery and vascular surgeons since the evolution of the specialty, an effort that has met with considerable success as attested by other chapters in this volume. At first glance, it may appear that the topics covered in the present section, namely the diagnosis and treatment of Raynaud's syndrome as well as finger gangrene caused by intrinsic small artery occlusive disease, should hardly concern the vascular surgeon at all. Although one may think these diseases should be the proper concern of a variety of medical specialties, including immunology, rheumatology, and dermatology, clinical experience suggests otherwise. Sooner or later a large number of these patients are referred to vascular surgeons for definitive diagnosis and treatment. It is apparent that vascular surgeons must be familiar with the basic principles of the diagnosis and management of these patient groups.

During the past 10 years at the University of Oregon Medical School we have conducted an ongoing program of clinical research in vasospastic and obstructive diseases of the hands and fingers. We have studied over 300 patients with Raynaud's syndrome and have tabulated follow-up data on the first 141 patients. During the same time, we have evaluated and treated 35 patients with finger gangrene caused by intrinsic small

Supported by GCRC Grant #RR-00334 General Clinical Research Centers Branch Division of Research Resources National Institutes of Health.

artery occlusive disease of the hands and fingers. Our experience with the diagnosis and management of these two groups of patients forms the basis for this report.

RAYNAUD'S SYNDROME

The term *Raynaud's syndrome* refers to a condition caused by episodic attacks of severe arterial constriction of the small arteries of the hands and fingers and occasionally the feet in response to cold or emotional stimuli. Attacks classically consist of pallor or cyanosis of the fingers with associated significant numbness, both of which persist as long as the cold exposure continues. When the patient enters a warm area, the pallor gives way to cyanosis as a trickle of blood enters the capillaries and veins; this is followed in time by rubor, which is accompanied by dilatation of the regional arteriolar and capillary nets. The entire recovery phase takes from 10 to 30 minutes. A large number of patients develop only pallor or cyanosis during attacks, and it presently appears that the classic triple color response occurs only in the minority of patients. With increasing experience, we currently recognize some patients who complain only of cold hands without any recognizable color changes and in whom we find identical arteriographic and hemodynamic changes as in patients with triple color response, leading one to speculate whether any color change is essential for diagnosis. For the present, however, I believe that an obvious color change with cold exposure is a minimal requirement for the diagnosis of Raynaud's syndrome.

History and Incidence

A brief review of the history of this condition is essential to an understanding of our current views of Raynaud's syndrome. A detailed historical review is beyond the scope of this report, but will soon be published elsewhere.[7] The condition was first described in 1862 by Maurice Raynaud.[22] He clearly described the episodic digital color changes. Unfortunately, he included cases of advanced arteriosclerosis and digital gangrene despite his belief that the syndrome was caused by vasospasm and sympathetic overactivity without organic arterial occlusions. Many of the inconsistences of Raynaud's work were clearly recognized by Hutchinson[14] who accurately observed that Raynaud's attacks may occur in association with a large group of disease, and proposed that the term *Raynaud's phenomenon* be applied. The suggestions of Hutchinson were further amplified by Allen and Brown in 1932.[1] This remarkably influential publication suggested that Raynaud's condition occurred in two forms: Raynaud's disease and Raynaud's phenomenon. The former occurs in the absence of any associated disease process, is limited to women, and follows a benign course of little clinical consequence. The latter is associated with various disease processes, frequently connective tissue diseases, and may pursue a violent course including digital gangrene. Critical evaluation, however, suggests there is little merit in attempting to separate Raynaud's disease from Raynaud's phenomenon. Allen and Brown's classification was based on clinical observations alone as detailed immunologic testing was unavailable at that time. It is now well recognized that Raynaud's symptoms may precede the development of overt signs of connective tissue disease by years. It appears more reasonable to refer to the condition as Raynaud's syndrome without attempting further semantic separation.

Etiology and Incidence

A Raynaud's attack is caused by vasospasm of the arteries sufficiently severe to arrest blood flow. Abundant evidence suggests that Raynaud's syndrome occurs across a spectrum ranging from the vasospastic type with digital arteries unobstructed to the obstructive type with digital arteries occluded.[19,24] Young female patients tend to be on the vasospastic end of the spectrum while most male and most older patients tend toward the obstructive end. The majority of patients, however, exist on a continuum sharing clear evidence of both arterial spasm and organic luminal obstruction.

The vasospastic type corresponds generally to the "Raynaud's disease" type described by Allen and Brown. These patients have essentially normal arterial pressure at room temperature, but a significant reduction in flow. Arteriography reveals significant resting and cold-exacerbated (cryogenic) vasospasm (Fig. 1).[23] With local cooling pressure declines moderately until a critical temperature of 18 to 20C is reached and pressure and flow decline abruptly to zero. The second type of patient has arterial obstruction from a variety of causes, such as atherosclerosis, Buerger's disease, chronic arteritis associated with connective tissue disease, and so on. These patients show a low digital pressure and flow at all temperatures, and additional precipitous decreases with cooling. As noted above, however, most patients with Raynaud's syndrome show both vasospasm and obstruction. Rösch[23] of our group found that 88 percent of patients undergoing hand angiography for Raynaud's showed vasospasm, while 85 percent showed obstructive arterial disease. An example of obstructive Raynaud's is seen in Figure 2.

Current evidence suggests that the mechanism of the Raynaud's attack in patients with primarily obstructive disease is that of a normal vasocon-

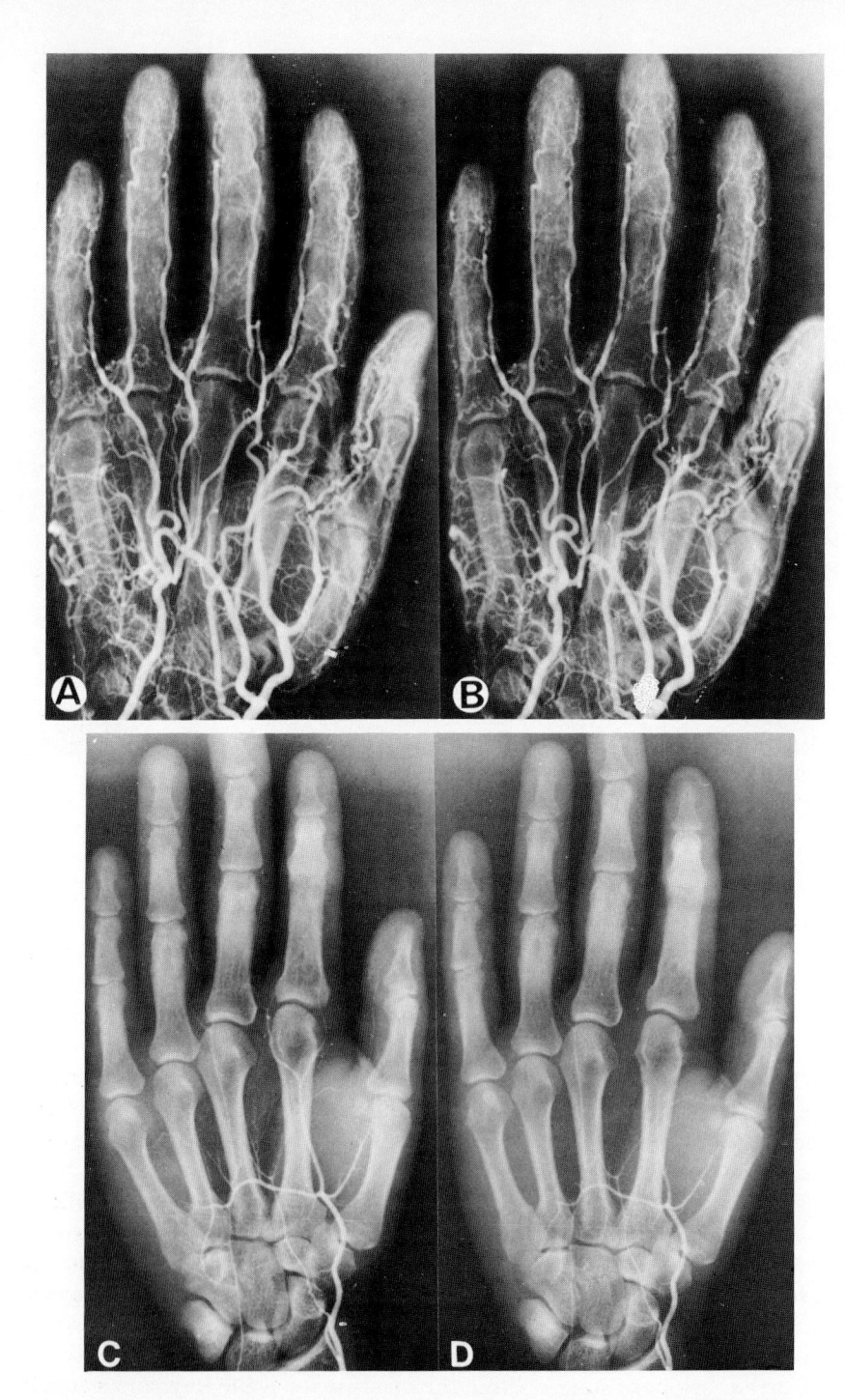

FIGURE 1. Vasospasm. Normal hand angiogram (A) before and (B) 20 minutes after ice water exposure. Young female with Raynaud's shows significant resting vasospasm (C) before ice exposure which is worsened (D) after exposure.

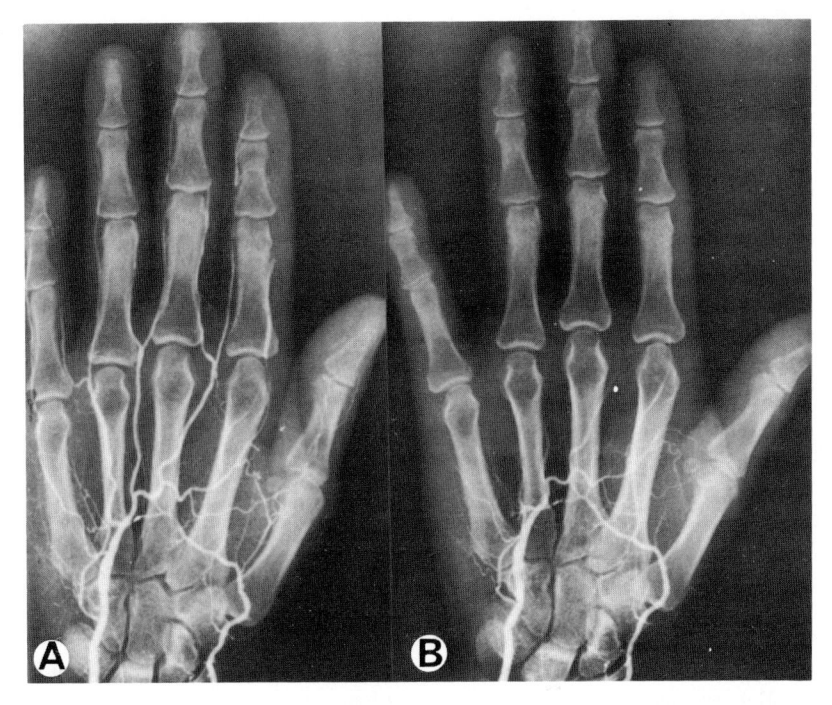

FIGURE 2. Obstruction. **A.** Multiple occlusions of digital arteries with easily visible subocclusive lesions in the palmar arches plus **(B)** significant ice-induced vasospasm in a middle-aged female patient.

strictive response to cold exceeding the reduced intraluminal pressure distal to an area of arterial obstruction; thereby exceeding the critical closure pressure and producing digital artery closure. This theory predicts that every patient with extensive hand and finger arterial obstruction should have some degree of Raynaud's attacks upon cold exposure, and indeed this appears to be the case. An explanation of the mechanism of Raynaud's attacks in patients with the vasospastic type of Raynaud's is more difficult.

Evaluation of our own patient data suggests that the usual arteriographic pattern of young patients with Raynaud's syndrome and connective tissue disease is severe vasospasm with little or no occlusive disease. As the patient gets older, the angiographic picture becomes that of combined spasm and occlusive arterial disease. This suggests to us that some factor present in the plasma of connective tissue disease patients causes vasospasm; possibly this is an immune complex or some other type of autoimmune serologic substance. As the person ages, digital occlusive disease begins to predominate, either as a consequence of the same immunologic event that initially caused vasospasm, which upon prolonged exposure causes arterial damage and occlusions, or else from an associated arteritis that is a recognized component of almost all of the connective tissue diseases. One is left, however, to explain the occurrence of the arteritis only or primarily in the distal extremities. Because this is the coldest part of the body one can speculate that the peripheral vasospasm and subsequent occlusive disease are related to a temperature dependent immune process. Presently there is no evidence to support this speculation.

The true incidence of Raynaud's syndrome in the population at large is totally unknown. We know a great deal about the characteristics of the patients who present for evaluation, but what of the multitude who never are evaluated? Several groups have found an incidence of Raynaud's syndrome of about 20 percent upon questioning apparently healthy asymptomatic individuals selected at random.[7]

Evaluation

A classification of the conditions that may be associated with Raynaud's syndrome appears in Table 1. It is apparent that this table reflects the spectrum ranging from the spastic type to the obstructed type: I is spastic, II is a mixed spastic and obstructive, II-B is obstructive, II-C is obstructive, II-D is spastic, and II-E is a mixture.

The physician treating a patient with Raynaud's syndrome first needs to establish a diagnosis as objectively as possible; next, conduct a methodical search for evidence of any of the diseases described in Table 1 is conducted; and then treatment is recommended.

It is clear at the present time that Raynaud's syndrome usually occurs in association with other recognizable diseases. The largest group of associated diseases is the connective tissue diseases. Raynaud's syndrome is frequently the first sign of collagen vascular disease and may precede other manifestations by years. Raynaud's syndrome occurs at some point in over 90 percent of patients with scleroderma, 85 percent of patients with mixed connective tissue disease, and 25 percent of patients with rheumatoid arthritis.[21] Recent reviews of large numbers of Raynaud's patients point to the diminishing likelihood of Raynaud's syndrome occurring in the absence of any recognized associated disease, confirming the prophetic prediction made by DeTakats in 1961.[8] A summary of these recent series comprising 342 patients with Raynaud's syndrome shows no associated recognizable disease in only 63 patients or 18 percent of the group. Associated autoimmune disease was present or suspected in 195 patients or 57 percent of the group.[21,25,26]

It is currently uncertain how frequently Raynaud's syndrome coexists with another disease process. We are convinced that this frequency re-

Table 1. Classification of Raynaud's Syndrome

I. Idiopathic Raynaud's Syndrome
II. Raynaud's Syndrome with an Associated Disease or Cause
   A. Vasculitides
      1. Undefined immunologic disorder
         Scleroderma
         Dermatomyositis
      2. Immune complex deposition: self-antigen
         Systemic lupus erythematosus
         Rheumatoid disease
         Mixed connective tissue disease
      3. Immune complex deposition: foreign antigen
         Hepatitis B antigen vasculitis
         Drug-induced vasculitis
      4. Cryoglobulinemia
   B. Obstructive Arterial Disease without Immunologic Disturbance
      1. Thromboangiitis obliterans
      2. Arteriosclerosis
      3. Thoracic outlet syndrome
   C. Occupational Raynaud's Syndrome
      1. Vibration
      2. Direct arterial trauma
   D. Drug-induced Raynaud's Syndrome
      1. Ergot
      2. Beta-blocking drugs
      3. Cytotoxic drugs
      4. Birth control pills
   E. Miscellaneous Causes
      1. Vinyl chloride disease
      2. Chronic renal failure
      3. Cold agglutinins
      4. Neoplasia
      5. Cold injury
      6. Neurologic disorders

---

flects the referral basis for the patients. A referral center seeing complicated cases will undoubtedly see more associated disease, especially connective tissue disease, than a primary care physician seeing a group of Raynaud's patients. A tabulation of associated disease found in our most recent 141 patients is listed in Table 2. Presently 30 percent of our patients with Raynaud's syndrome are classified as idiopathic. The slight decrease in our incidence of associated connective tissue disease and the increase in the incidence of idiopathic Raynaud's compared to our previous report is, we feel, related to changing patient referral pattern in our community, as we now receive younger patients earlier in their disease than previously.[21]

Table 2. Associated Diseases Found in 141 Patients with Raynaud's Syndrome

Scleroderma	25
Systemic lupus erythematosus	7
Mixed connective tissue disease	4
Dermatomyositis	1
Undifferentiated connective tissue disease	27
Acute onset vasculitis	9
Thromboangiitis obliterans	5
Arteriosclerosis	13
Vibration associated Raynaud's syndrome	3
Neoplasm (Renal sarcoma)	1
Causalgia	2
Idiopathic Raynaud's syndrome	42
Synchronous onset of Raynaud's syndrome and acromegaly	1
Synchronous onset of Raynaud's syndrome and Addison's disease	1
Total	141

Examination

The essential requirement for the diagnosis of Raynaud's syndrome is the patient's history of color change of his digital extremities upon cold exposure. The diagnosis may be confirmed by a simple digital temperature recovery test, which has a high specificity but a rather low sensitivity.[20] A history should be carefully sought of any condition that may suggest an associated autoimmune disease including arthralgias, dysphagia, skin tightening, xerophthalmia, or xerostomia.

The skin of the hands and fingers should be carefully inspected for any ulcerations or small hyperkeratotic areas suggesting healed ulcers. The skin should be carefully observed for any thinning or tightening suggestive of scleroderma and the fingers should be carefully observed for sclerodactyly. All joints should be examined for synovial thickening, effusion, or other evidence of arthritis. The presence of telangiectasia should be carefully noted, as should the status of the palpable peripheral pulses. Signs of carpal tunnel syndrome should be sought with care. The physical examination is frequently normal in patients with Raynaud's syndrome. The diagnosis is made primarily from the history.

Laboratory Tests

The laboratory tests performed in these patients are shown in Table 3. The specific serologic tests of greatest value in detecting associated diseases include the determination of antinuclear antibody, rheumatoid factor, complete blood count, and HEP-2 ANA. Based on the results of these tests one may subsequently perform extractable nuclear antigen assay, immunoglobulin electrophoresis, or anti-N-DNA antibody assay. Forearm and hand x-rays should be obtained for detection of joint changes, sclerodactyly, or calcinosis. Any clinical suspicion of carpal tunnel syndrome should be confirmed by upper extremity nerve conduction velocity determinations. Carpal tunnel syndrome coexists in a large number of patients with connective tissue disease.[21]

Treatment

The initial treatment of patients with Raynaud's syndrome is cold avoidance and abstinence from tobacco. In patients with mild disease no further therapy is necessary.

Cervicothoracic surgical sympathectomy has been widely used for many years in the treatment of Raynaud's symptoms. Long-term results, however, have not been particularly good. While the procedure appears of lasting benefit in 40 to 60 percent of patients with mild Raynauld's symptoms, it has been of benefit in only 20 to 30 percent or less of

Table 3. Laboratory Tests Used in Evaluating Patients with Raynaud's Syndrome

CBC*
Sed rate
Serum protein electrophoresis
Cold agglutins
Rheumatoid factor (latex particle)*
VDRL
Antinuclear antibody*
Hep-2 ANA*
Antinative DNA antibody
Extractable nuclear antibody
Total hemolytic complement
Complement (C3, C4)
Immunoglobulin electrophoresis
Cryoglobulin (Cryocrit)
Cryofibrinogen
Direct Coomb's test
Hbs Ab-Hepatitis B antibody
Hbs Ag-Hepatitis B antigen
Hand x-ray*
Cine esophagogram
Schirmer's test
Skin biopsy

*Most helpful

patients with more severe symptoms.[11,15] It has been of strikingly little value in patients with Raynaud's syndrome associated with scleroderma. At present we do not use or recommend surgical sympathectomy in the treatment of Raynaud's syndrome.

The best clinical results have been obtained from the use of drugs which decrease sympathetic neuromuscular synaptic transmission. Although a wide variety of agents have been used, the best appear to be reserpine, guanethidine, and phenoxybenzamine.[12,28] The use of the alpha-receptor blocking drug, prazosin, in Raynaud's syndrome has been recently described and appears quite promising.[27] The effect of these drugs in increasing digital blood flow has been confirmed by isotopic, thermographic, and arteriographic studies. Low drug doses daily appear to be effective: 10 mg of guanethidine and phenoxybenzamine and 1 to 2 mg daily of prazosin.

Prognosis

The prognosis for patients with Raynaud's syndrome and an associated disease process is that of the associated disease. It should be remembered that a connective tissue disease is not always inexorably progressive. We have observed a remarkable group of patients with severe associated connective tissue disease in whom the associated disease has remained stationary or has spontaneously improved with time. The prognosis for patients with idiopathic Raynaud's with no associated disease process appears quite good but it is presently unknown how many patients will remain in this category as our diagnostic tests become more sophisticated. A large percentage of such patients have been reported to never develop any associated diseases,[6,9] but it should be noted that these follow-up data date from an era in which sophisticated immunologic screening was not available and many associated disease processes may have gone unrecognized. We are currently following a large number of such patients with detailed annual immunologic testing.

FINGER GANGRENE CAUSED BY INTRINSIC SMALL ARTERY OCCLUSIVE DISEASE

Localized finger and hand gangrene is rarely encountered in clinical practice. Several recent publications suggest that in about two-thirds of such patients the hand and finger gangrene is a manifestation of large artery obstruction proximal to the wrist.[5,18] This obstruction may be due to a variety of causes including cardiac embolization, thoracic outlet syndrome with adjacent arterial damage, trauma, or atherosclerosis. The diagnosis and treatment of these lesions have been well described.

The remaining one-third of patients presenting with localized finger gangrene have an associated systemic condition of which the hand and finger small artery occlusive disease is but one manifestation. We have treated 35 patients presenting in this fashion during the past 10 years.

Patient Presentation

The patient group consisted of 23 females and 12 males with an age range of 12 to 75 years, median 46 years. Twenty-two patients presented with subacute finger gangrene while 13 patients presented with chronic gangrenous finger changes.

The subacute group consisted of 15 females and 7 males, with a median age of 40 years. Thirteen of the patients smoked. None had a history of diabetes or symptomatic systemic atherosclerosis. The patients typically described the sudden onset of pain and cyanosis at the tips of one or more fingers, which over a few days became considerably worse and sharply demarcated from surrounding tissue. Six of these patients had experienced Raynaud's symptoms prior to the onset of the localized gangrene. These patients had been symptomatic for several weeks to several months before presenting to us.

Thirteen patients presented with a history of chronic localized gangrene of multiple fingers with frequent exacerbations and remissions. This patient group included five male and eight females with a median age of 49 years. Eleven of these patients smoked. Six had clear evidence of systemic atherosclerosis, including diminished peripheral pulses. All of these patients had Raynaud's syndrome prior to the onset of finger gangrene, which is in keeping with our thesis that patients with diffuse palmar and digital artery obstruction from any cause will have Raynaud's syndrome. Two patients had undergone prior cervicothoracic sympathectomy without benefit.

Patient Evaluation

All patients were carefully questioned and examined for signs and symptoms of associated connective tissue disease including skin binding and thickening, calcinosis, vasculitic skin rash, sclerodactyly, arthritis, arthralgias, myalgias, dysphagia, and xerophthalmia. Angina pectoris, myocardial infarction, stroke, transient cerebral ischemic attacks, claudication, and absence or decrease of peripheral pulses were sought to document associated systemic atherosclerosis.

Trauma, emboli, thoracic outlet syndrome, and prior cold injury were all carefully excluded. The gangrenous lesions were all sequentially photographed.

The following laboratory examinations were performed in each patient: CBC, sedimentation rate, multichem screen, 24-hour urine for creatine/creatinine ratio, chest x-ray, hand x-ray, upper gastrointestinal series, barium enema, and intravenous urogram. Noninvasive vascular laboratory digital plethysmography was used to confirm arterial obstruction in all patients, and peripheral arterial exams were performed in all patients suspected of systemic atherosclerosis. Skin biopsies were obtained from most. All patients were subject to the same extensive serologic immunologic screening tests as outlined Table 3.

Magnification hand arteriography including all vessels of the upper extremity from the aortic arch to the fingertips was performed in each patient. The arteriograms were done by transfemoral Seldinger technique both before and after ice exposure and before and 48 hours after the intra-arterial injection of resperine as previously described by us in detail.[23] Arteriography remains the single most valuable diagnostic test in evaluation of these patients, providing objective information about the nature, location, and distribution of arterial obstructions, the extent of development of collateral vessels and, when performed with ice and reserpine exposure, quantification of the degree of vasospasm present in addition to the underlying occlusive disease. Response to vasodilating agents can also be noted.

A representative hand angiogram of one of these patients is shown in Figure 3. The angiograms all showed severe occlusive disease of the palmar and digital arteries with variable amounts of associated vasospasm. The diagnosis established on these patients are listed in Table 4. Hypersensitivity angiitis as a cause of digital gangrene was first described by us from this group of patients.[4] The patients with scleroderma-CREST were diagnosed using the criteria of Barnett.[3] Five patients were diagnosed as having diffuse arteriosclerotic obstruction of the digital and palmar circulation. All were heavy smokers and had significant peripheral atherosclerosis, and none had any evidence of associated autoimmune disease. All presented with Raynaud's syndrome and localized finger gangrene characteristically random in distribution. The single patient with lupus met the ARA criteria for diagnosis. The patient with Sjögren's syndrome, in addition to xerophthalmia and xerostomia, had a minor salivary gland biopsy substantiating the diagnosis. An excellent review of this increasingly important syndrome has been published recently.[13] A single patient each was diagnosed as having myeloid metaplasia, calciphylaxis,[10] and a globulin producing renal carcinoma.[2] A

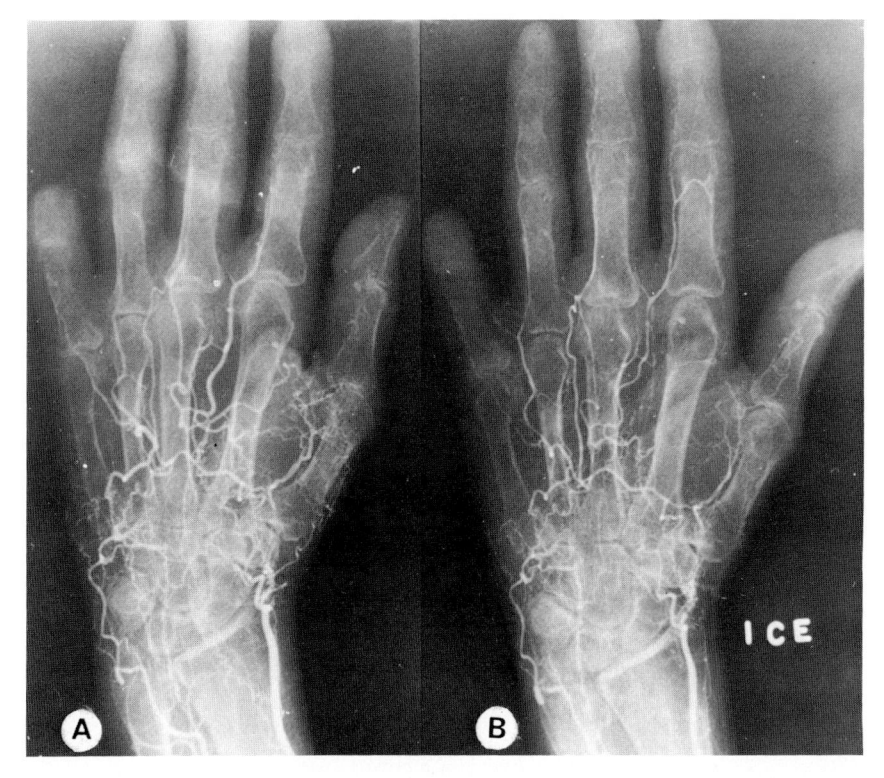

FIGURE 3. **A.** Severe extensive palmar and digital occlusions in a young female with hypersensitivity angiitis with **(B)** little additional cold induced vasospasm.

list of the recognized diseases that may present with localized finger gangrene caused by intrinsic small artery occlusive disease is shown in Table 5.

Treatment and Results

All patients are counseled to avoid cold and tobacco. The underlying principle of therapy is simple wound care. Gangrenous ulcers are scrubbed with plain soap and water twice daily and covered with plain dry gauze bandages. Extremely conservative local debridement of necrotic tissue is performed as required, including local rongeuring of protruding phalangeal tips. All debridement is delayed weeks to several months if possible to allow maximal collateral circulation to develop. Formal phalangeal amputation is performed only when an entire digital segment

Table 4. Final Diagnoses of 35 Patients with Finger Gangrene from Intrinsic Small Artery Occlusive Disease

Hypersensitivity angiitis	13
Scleroderma-CREST	7
Arteriosclerosis	5
Undifferentiated connective tissue disease	3
Mixed connective tissue disease	2
Systemic lupus erythematosus	1
Sjögren's syndrome	1
Myeloid metaplasia	1
Calciphylaxis	1
Carcinoma	1

Table 5. Possible Causes of Intrinsic Small Artery Disease of the Palmar and Digital Arteries

I. Connective Tissue Diseases and Other Arteritidies
   A. Scleroderma-CREST
   B. Rheumatoid arthritis
   C. Sjögren's syndrome
   D. Systemic lupus erythematosus
   E. Polyarteritis nodosa
   F. Mixed connective tissue disease
   G. Undifferentiated connective tissue disease
   H. Wegener's granulomatosis
   I. Allergic granulomatosis
   J. Henoch-Schönlein purpura
   K. Hypersensitivity angiitis
II. Myeloproliferative disorders
   A. Polycythemia rubra vera
   B. Thrombocytosis
   C. Leukemia
III. Immunoglobulin abnormalities
   A. Mixed cryoglobulinemia
   B. Myeloma or benign monoclonal gammopathy
   C. Macroglobulinemia
   D. Cold agglutinin disease
   E. Tumor-produced globulins
   F. Myeloid metaplasia
IV. Miscellaneous
   A. Systemic malignancy
   B. Disseminated intravascular coagulation
   C. Chronic renal failure (calciphylaxis)
   D. Arteriosclerosis
   E. Buerger's disease

is necrotic. There is no benefit from the topical application of antiseptic, antibiotic, or debriding ointments, and these are not used.

Because the angiograms of most of these patients have showed some associated vasospasm, we use the same oral medications as in the treatment of Raynaud's syndrome, including guanethidine, 10 mg/day, phenoxybenzamine, 10 mg/day, or prazosin, 2 mg/day.

On this treatment program, 24 patients have healed completely without any recurrence, although most have had persistent Raynaud's symptoms. Photographs of one such patient are seen in Figure 4. Five additional patients have experienced a single recurrent episode of localized finger gangrene after initial healing. The recurrent gangrene has subsequently healed and all five patients have done well. The remaining six patients have all had nonhealing of gangrenous finger ulcers and have required partial finger amputation. One had subsequently healed, while five remain symptomatic. Good results were obtained in 30 of the 35 patients, or 83 percent. All patients with recurring digital gangrene after amputation have been heavy cigarette smokers who were unable to stop smoking.

We are uncertain to what degree our therapeutic program of local wound care and low dose oral vasodilators has been responsible for the good results obtained in 83 percent of these patients. We suspect this outcome, in significant part, reflects the natural history of localized finger gangrene. Beneficial results obtained in the treatment of localized finger gangrene that are attributed to a certain type of therapeutic intervention should be accepted with extreme caution. This is especially true of cervicothoracic sympathectomy that has been recommended by others as the treatment of choice in this condition. Thus, Laroche reported 78 percent of 64 patients improved by sympathectomy, most of whom had symptoms far less severe than those of our patients, while Machleder, again in patients with less severe disease than ours, reported good results following sympathectomy in 81 percent of patients.[16,17] These results are obviously no different from those obtained in our patients without sympathectomy. We are aware of absolutely no persuasive evidence that cervicothoracic sympathectomy has any beneficial effect in the treatment of upper extremity ischemia from small artery disease.

OVERVIEW

Raynaud's Syndrome

The objective of therapy in this condition is to ascertain the presence of any associated diseases and to prescribe symptomatic therapy for

292 Critical Problems in Vascular Surgery

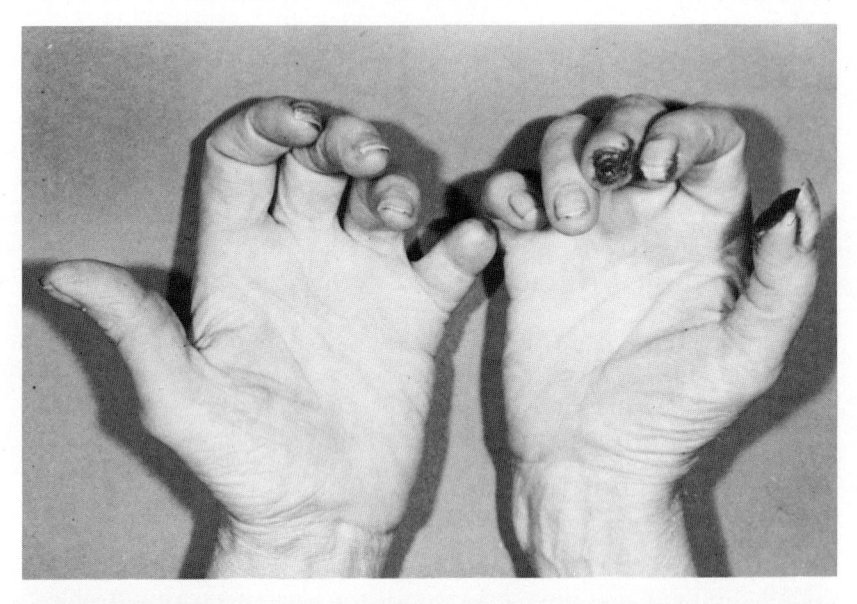

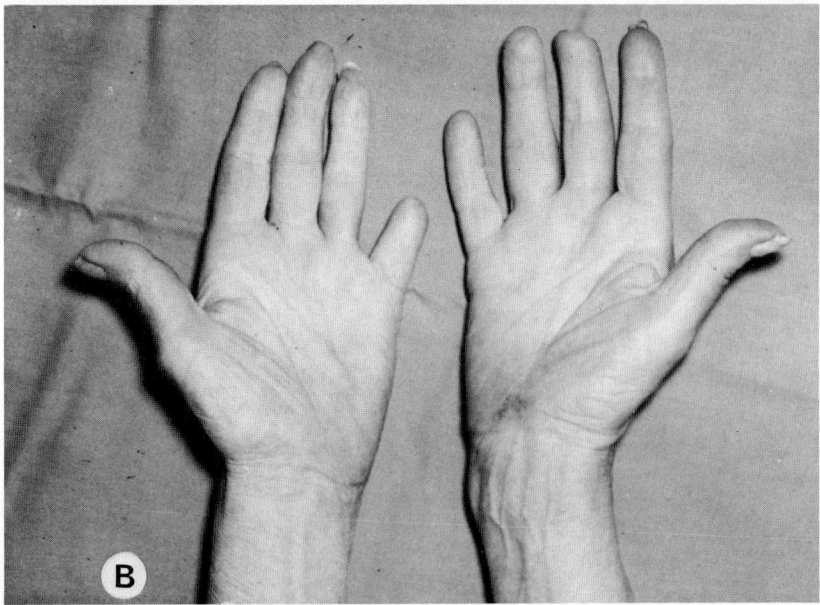

FIGURE 4. **A.** Original multiple gangrenous fingertip lesions in a patient with arteriosclerosis. **B.** Complete healing after 3 months conservative therapy.

the Raynaud's event itself. Referral to an immunologist or internist would seem appropriate for any associated disease process that may be found.

The hallmark of diagnosis is a history of digital color change upon cold exposure. Diagnosis may be confirmed by determining digital temperatures recovery time after cold exposure, but this test has relatively low sensitivity. The serologic tests outlined in Table 3 should be obtained along with the other tests mentioned in the text. Digital plethysmography is most helpful but the fingers must be above 32C for this test to be interpretable. Angiography is not required for the evaluation of these patients.

Once these data have returned the patient should be classifiable as outlined in Table 2. Additional medical therapy for systemic diseases may be required at this point. The patient should be strongly urged to avoid cold exposure and tobacco use. If the Raynaud's symptoms are sufficiently severe one may recommend oral vasodilators. The most effective ones have been guanethidine, phenoxybenzamine, and prazosin.

Finger Gangrene Caused by Small Artery Occlusion

The initial objective is, of course, to establish the etiology of the finger gangrene. Because the majority of these patients will have potentially treatable large artery obstruction proximal to the wrist, we feel an angiogram should be obtained with complete visualization from the arch to the fingertips. If proximal disease is ruled out, one conducts a methodical search for disease processes that may cause digital artery occlusions (Table 5). All patients should ultimately be categorizable. If the patient is found to have severe hand artery occlusion without any associated systemic disease, he should be placed in the "hypersensitivity angiitis" category, admittedly a relatively nonspecific category but it does appear to serve a purpose similar to "idiopathic Raynaud's syndrome."

Therapy is directed toward cold and tobacco avoidance, local wound care, and conservative surgical debridement. There appears to be no benefit from the use of cervicothoracic sympathectomy in the treatment of this condition.

REFERENCES

1. Allen EV, Brown GE: Raynaud's Disease: A critical review of minor requisites for diagnosis. Am J Med Sci 183:187, 1932
2. Andrasch RH, Bardana EJ, Porter JM, Pirofsky B: Digital ischemia and

gangrene preceeding renal neoplasm—as association with sarcomatoid adenocarcinoma of the kidney. Arch Intern Med 136:486, 1976
3. Barnett AJ: Scleroderma (Progressive Systemic Sclerosis). Springfield, Ill., Thomas, 1974
4. Baur GM, Porter JM, Bardana EH, Wesche DH, Rösch J: Rapid onset of hand ischemia of unknown etiology. Ann Surg 186:184, 1977
5. Bergan JJ, Conn J, Trippel OH: Severe ischemia of the hand. Ann Surg 173:301, 1971
6. Blain A, Coller FA, Carger GB: Raynaud's disease: A study of criteria for prognosis. Surg 29:387, 1951
7. Blunt RJ, Porter JM: Raynaud's syndrome. Semin Rheumatol (in press)
8. DeTakats G, Fowler DF: The neurogenic factor in Raynaud's phenomenon. Surg 51:9, 1962
9. Gifford RW, Hines EA: Raynaud's disease among women and girls. Circulation 16:1012, 1957
10. Gipstein RM, Coburn JW, Adams DA, et al.: Calciphylaxis in man. Arch Intern Med 136:1273, 1976
11. Hall DV, Hillestad LK: Raynaud's phenomenon treated with sympathectomy. Angiology 11:186, 1960
12. Halperin JL: Pathophysiology of Raynaud's disease. Arch Intern Med 139:89, 1979
13. Haralampos MM (Moderator), Chused TM, Mann DL, et al: Sjögren's syndrome (Sicca syndrome): Current Issues. Ann Intern Med 92:212, 1980
14. Hutchinson J: Inherited liability to Raynaud's phenomenon, with great proneness to chilblains—gradual increase of liability to paroxysmal local asphyxia-acrosphacelus with scleroderma—cheeks affected. Arch Surg 4:312; 1893
15. Johnston ENM, Symmerly R, Birnstingl M: Prognosis in Raynaud's phenomenon after sympathectomy. Br Med J 1:962, 1965
16. Laroche GP, Bernatz PE, Joyce JW, McCarty CS: Chronic arterial insufficiency of the upper extremity. Mayo Clinic Proc 51:180, 1976
17. Machleder HI, Wheeler E, Barker WF: Treatment of upper extremity ischemia by cervico-dorsal sympathectomy. Vasc Surg 13:399, 1979
18. McNamara MF, Takali HS, Yao JST, Bergan JJ: A systematic approach to severe hand ischemia. Surg 83:1, 1978
19. Mendlowitz M, Naftchi N: The digital circulation in Raynaud's disease. Am J Cardiol 4:580, 1959
20. Porter JM: The diagnosis and treatment of Raynaud's phenomenon. Surg 77:11, 1975
21. Porter JM, Bardana EJ, Baur GM, et al.: The clinical significance of Raynaud's syndrome. Surg 80:756, 1976
22. Raynaud M: On Local Asphyxia and Symmetrical Gangrene of the Extremities. Selected Monographs. London, New Sydenham Society, 1888
23. Rösch J, Porter JM, Gralino BJ: Cryodynamic hand arteriography in the diagnosis and management of Raynaud's syndrome. Circulation 55:807, 1977

24. Strandness DE, Sumner DS: Hemodynamics for Surgeons. New York, Grune & Stratton, 1975, p 543
25. Sumner DS, Strandness DE Jr: An abnormal finger pulse associated with cold sensitivity. Ann Surg 175:294, 1972
26. Velayos EE, Robinson H, Porciuncula FV, et al: Clinical correlation analysis of 137 patients with Raynaud's phenomenon. Am J Med Sci 262:347, 1971
27. Walso R: Prazosin relieves Raynaud's vasospasm. JAMA 241:1037, 1979
28. Willerson JT, Decker JL: Raynaud's disease and phenomenon, a medical approach. Am Heart J 82:572, 1971

Part Five
Miscellaneous Topics

TWENTY

New Developments in Surgery of the Visceral Circulation

Scott J. Boley and Lawrence J. Brandt

During the past decade, new concepts concerning the pathophysiology and treatment of intestinal ischemia and renovascular hypertension have provided a broader selection of approaches to these conditions with improved therapeutic results. Recognition of the important role of persistent vasoconstriction in acute renal and mesenteric ischemia has stimulated investigations of vasodilator therapy in the kidney and bowel, while transluminal angioplasty has provided a less formidable treatment for chronic visceral ischemic syndromes. Microsurgical techniques and the application of autotransplantation have provided new methods for correcting abnormalities of small vessels.

THE ROLE OF VASOCONSTRICTION IN VISCERAL ISCHEMIA

Vasoconstriction in response to shock, decreased cardiac output, or various toxins has long been recognized as a cause of acute renal or intestinal ischemia. The occurrence of persistent or sustained vasoconstriction after the initiating cause is corrected, however, has only recently been identified. Hollenberg and his co-investigators[19] demonstrated persistent renal cortical vasoconstriction in patients with acute renal insufficiency and in transplanted kidneys exposed to prolonged ischemia. They attributed the maintenance of the oliguria to sustained vasoconstriction and suggested the possible use of local infusions of suitable vasodilators. While the latter approach has not been applied in the treatment of acute renal insufficiency, injections of vasodilators into the renal artery have been employed effectively for relief of vasoconstriction seen after renal transplantation and during revascularization procedures for correction of renovascular hypertension.

Case Report

A 5-year-old boy with neurofibromatosis involving both renal arteries had hypertension uncontrolled by medication. Bilateral renal vein renin levels were markedly elevated in samples from both renal veins. Prior attempts at revascularization of the left kidney, including parenchymal implantation of the gastroepiploic artery were unsuccessful because of stenoses of tertiary renal artery branches. At operation the left kidney was removed and rearterialization of the right kidney was performed by anastomosing the right internal iliac artery end-to-end to the main renal artery. Renal ischemic time was 20 minutes. Following an uncomplicated anastomosis, pulsations in the renal artery disappeared over a 5-minute period. The anastomosis was opened, clot removed, and the vessels reapproximated; again the renal artery clotted. After removing the clot, 60 mg of papaverine hydrochloride were injected into the renal artery and the arteries resutured. A much stronger pulse was noted and the color of the kidney was markedly improved. The anastomosis has remained open, and the patient is normotensive.

In this patient, persistent renal vasoconstriction resulted in such low renal arterial blood flow that the anastomosis thrombosed repeatedly. After relieving the vascular spasm, the flow was sufficient to maintain patency of the vessel.

Acute ischemia of all or major segments of the intestine supplied by the superior mesenteric artery (SMA) has been diagnosed with increasing frequency during the past 25 years, yet this intra-abdominal catastrophe remains as lethal today[21,28] as in 1933, when Hibbard et al.[18] reported a mortality rate of 70 percent. The lack of improvement in the outcome of these vascular accidents, in spite of the advances in roentgenologic and surgical techniques used to diagnose and treat them, can be attributed to three major factors: 1) inability to make the diagnosis before intestinal gangrene develops; 2) progression of the bowel infarction after the primary initiating vascular or systemic cause has been corrected; and 3) the increasing frequency of nonocclusive mesenteric ischemia (the "low flow" syndrome) with its reported mortality rate of over 90 percent.

Nonocclusive mesenteric ischemia (NMI) and superior mesenteric artery emboli are each responsible for approximately 25 to 50 percent of these vascular accidents in recent series.[6,21] The pathogenesis of nonocclusive mesenteric ischemia is presently believed to be splanchnic vasoconstriction that occurs in response to a decrease in cardiac output and that persists even after the initial cause is corrected. Such episodes of vasoconstriction have been associated with myocardial infarctions, congestive heart failure, hypovolemia, hypotension, or the use of vasopressor drugs. That persistent vasoconstriction may develop following a controlled decrease in mesenteric blood flow has been demonstrated by our group in a series of experiments performed on more than 200 anesthesized dogs.[7,8,12] These investigations showed that when the SMA blood flow is decreased 50 percent with a hydraulic occluder, the mesenteric arterial pressure in the peripheral bed immediately falls proportionately, and blood flow through the sources of collateral blood supply, i.e., the celiac and inferior mesenteric arteries, rises. A decreased SMA flow of several hours duration, however, results in mesenteric vasoconstriction with the pressure in the mesenteric bed rising to the level of the systemic arterial pressure and blood flow through the arteries supplying collateral flow returning to normal. Initially, the mesenteric vasoconstriction is reversible with release of the SMA occlusion, but after it is present for several hours the vasoconstriction persists even after the occlusion is removed. Thus, a low SMA flow initially produces mesenteric vascular responses that tend to maintain adequate intestinal blood flow, but if the diminished flow is prolonged, active vasoconstriction develops and may persist even after the primary cause of mesenteric ischemia is corrected.

Further studies showed that this persistent mesenteric vasoconstriction can be reversed by the selective injection of papaverine, a vasodilator, into the SMA. Such injections, therefore, could interrupt the vicious cycle that might result in persistent mesenteric ischemia following a transient fall in cardiac output or other temporary local or systemic causes of decreased mesenteric blood flow. This persistent mesenteric vasoconstriction could account for the delayed appearance of intestinal ischemia after low flow states, and the progression of infarction after removal of an arterial occlusion such as an SMA embolus.

In the past, no reliable method for diagnosing acute mesenteric ischemia before intestinal infarction has been available. Although mesenteric angiography has been employed in suspected cases of acute mesenteric ischemia, until recently its role has been limited to the exclusion of emboli or acute thromboses, both of which might be treated successfully by prompt operation. Experimental and clinical studies of low perfusion states from our own and other institutions, however, have now established angiographic criteria for diagnosing mesenteric vasoconstriction.[1,4,10,25] Thus, if angiography is performed sufficiently early in their course, patients with acute mesenteric ischemia of a nonocclusive origin as well as those with surgically correctable occlusive lesions can be identified before bowel infarction occurs.

MANAGEMENT OF ACUTE MESENTERIC ISCHEMIA

Our clinical and experimental experiences have led us to conclude that:

1. The mortality rate of all forms of acute mesenteric ischemia will remain at its present high level unless the diagnosis is established and therapy instituted before intestinal necrosis develops.
2. Early diagnosis only can be accomplished if all patients suspected of having acute mesenteric ischemia are subjected to prompt roentgenologic studies.
3. Reluctance to subject these severely ill patients to the rigors of angiography because of its previously limited value (only to exclude embolus or thrombosis) is no longer valid, as the angiographic diagnosis of occlusive *and* nonocclusive mesenteric ischemia is now possible and active therapeutic measures are available for both.
4. Persistent vasoconstriction is a major factor in both nonocclusive and occlusive mesenteric ischemia and can be relieved or prevented by direct intra-arterial infusion of papaverine.

In 1972, based upon these conclusions, we proposed an aggressive approach to the management of acute mesenteric ischemia with the hope of preventing intestinal gangrene and decreasing the extremely high mortality rate reported with this entity.[5] The essential features in this approach are the earlier and more extensive use of angiography to diagnose mesenteric ischemia and to determine its cause, and the intra-arterial infusion of papaverine to interrupt the splanchnic vasoconstriction persisting after successful management of the underlying local or systemic cardiovascular etiology. The proper incorporation of these concepts in a comprehensive radiologic and therapeutic plan for the management of patients with suspected acute mesenteric ischemia has resulted in an impressive improvement in both patient survival and salvage of compromised bowel.

Plan for Diagnosis and Therapy

All patients suspected of having acute mesenteric ischemia are promptly treated for associated cardiovascular problems and sent for plain radiographic studies of the abdomen. Subsequent abdominal angiography is always performed unless some other intra-abdominal condition is diagnosed on the plain film examination. Based on the angiographic findings and the presence or absence of signs of peritoneal irritation on physical examination, the patient is then treated according to the schema outlined in Figure 1.

Selection of Patients. Acute mesenteric ischemia is most likely to develop in patients over 50 years of age with either 1) valvular or arteriosclerotic heart disease; 2) long-standing congestive heart failure, especially with unsatisfactory control of digitalis therapy or prolonged use of diuretics; 3) cardiac arrhythmias; 4) hypovolemia or hypotension of any origin such as burns, pancreatitis, and gastrointestinal or postoperative hemorrhage; or 5) recent myocardial infarction.

Patients in any of these high-risk categories who develop sudden onset of abdominal pain lasting more than 2 or 3 hours are started on the management protocol. Less absolute indications for an aggressive investigation are unexplained abdominal distension or gastrointestinal bleeding. Because the presence of more extensive and specific signs and symptoms usually signifies irreversible intestinal damage, these broad selection criteria are essential if early diagnosis and treatment are to be achieved.

Even when the decision to operate has been made, an angiogram must be obtained to manage the patient properly at operation. Of equal importance is the utilization of the angiography catheter for the intra-arterial infusion of papaverine to relieve mesenteric vasoconstriction. Relief of this mesenteric vasoconstriction is an integral part of the therapy for SMA emboli and thromboses, as well as for low flow states.

Initial Preparation and Resuscitation. Initial treatment is directed toward correction of predisposing or precipitating causes of the mesenteric ischemia. Relief of acute congestive heart failure, correction of cardiac arrhythmias, and replacement of blood volume precede any diagnostic studies. In general, efforts at increasing intestinal blood flow will be futile if low cardiac output, hypotension, or hypovolemia persist. On rare occasions, we have combined dopamine administered intravenously into a peripheral vein with papaverine administered intra-arterially into the SMA, and have been able to improve both systemic and mesenteric blood flow.

We have also studied the use of combinations of systemically administered ionotropic agents and vasodilators in animals in cardiogenic shock produced by ligation and mercury embolization of the coronary arteries. With administration of combinations of intravenous levarterenol and phentolamine, cardiac output rose from −44 percent to +36 percent and SMA flow rose from −42 percent to +34 percent.

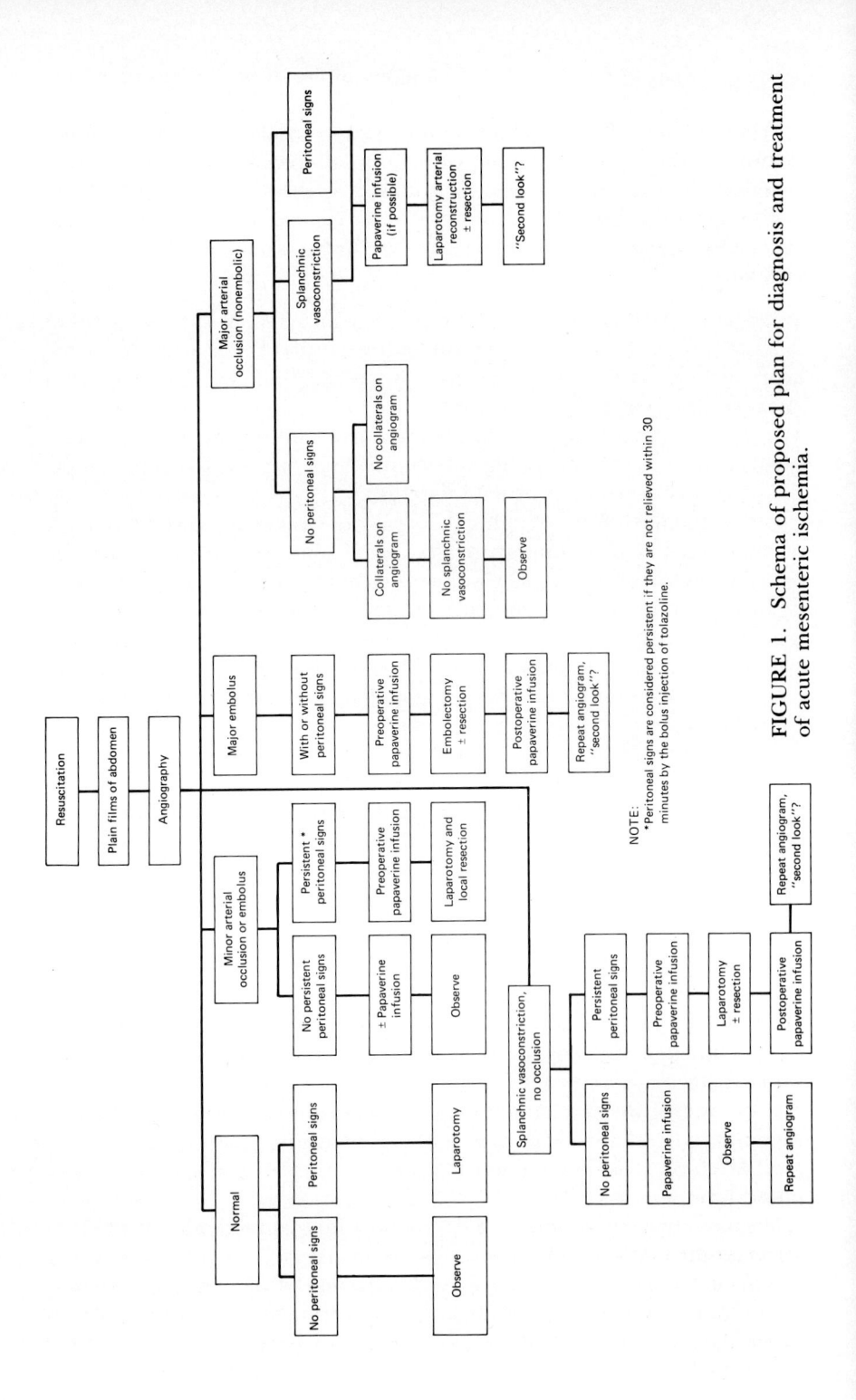

FIGURE 1. Schema of proposed plan for diagnosis and treatment of acute mesenteric ischemia.

Recently, it has been recognized that systemic administration of vasodilators to patients with congestive heart failure and myocardial infarction increases cardiac output and decreases myocardial ischemia.[11,22] A variety of vasodilators have been used systemically primarily to diminish afterload or arterial impedance, (e.g., hydralazine), diminish preload by producing venodilitation (e.g., nitroglycerin), or to diminish both afterload and preload (e.g., prazosin and nitroprusside). Those agents that reduce arterial impedance thereby increase the cardiac output and theoretically are ideal agents to treat the low flow mesenteric syndromes associated with congestive heart failure. They achieve the same goal of increased cardiac output and vasodilitation as does combination therapy with an inotropic agent and a vasodilator.

Patients in shock should not have angiography as mesenteric vasoconstriction will always be evident even without intestinal ischemia. Such patients should not be given papaverine intra-arterially because this will increase the size of the vascular bed and aggravate the hypovolemia (Fig. 2). The management of congestive heart failure or shock when complicated by mesenteric ischemia is especially difficult as utilization of digitalis or vasopressors may further aggravate the diminished intestinal blood flow. It is in just such a situation, however, that systemic vasodilator therapy for the congestive heart failure may be particularly effective. All digitalis preparations have a direct vasoconstrictor action on SMA smooth muscle, especially with the blood levels observed during rapid digitalization or with digitalis toxicity. The decision to discontinue digitalis is often difficult because the drug may be required to control rapid ventricular rates associated with atrial fibrillation or to manage severe congestive heart failure. Vasopressors are contraindicated in the treatment of shock if mesenteric ischemia is suspected.

When intestinal ischemia has progressed to the extent that systemic alterations associated with bowel infarction are present, appropriate correction of plasma volume deficits and fluid loss, gastrointestinal decompression and parenteral antibiotics are included in the preparation before roentgenologic studies. After the initial corrective and supportive measures have been completed, roentgenographic studies are undertaken irrespective of the abdominal physical finding or the surgeon's decision to operate.

Plain Film Studies. The initial examination includes a chest roentgenogram and roentgenograms of the abdomen with the patient in the supine, erect, and both lateral decubitus positions. Signs of intestinal ischemia on plain film studies occur late and usually indicate bowel infarction. In cases in which a significant portion of the patients have had such signs, the mortality has been discouragingly high.[13,17,27]

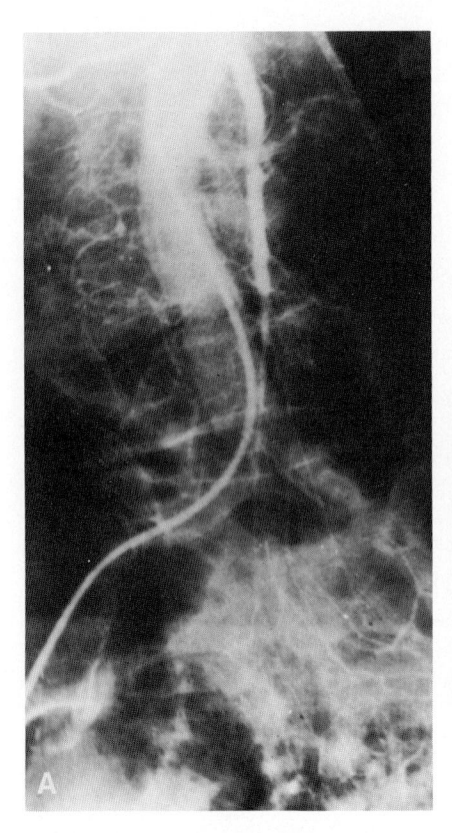

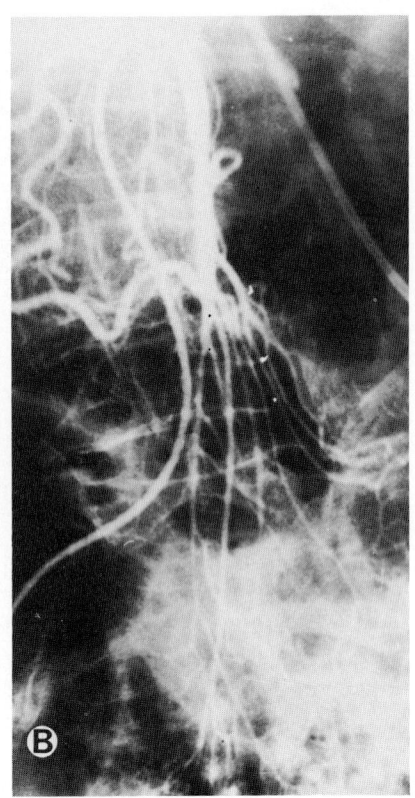

FIGURE 2. A. Superior mesenteric arteriogram in a patient with moderate hypovolemic hypotension. Marked vasoconstriction is apparent. **B.** Repeat angiogram after bolus infusion of papaverine shows relief of the mesenteric vasoconstriction. In the absence of correction of the hypovolemia, the relief of the vasoconstriction was accompanied by a further fall in the blood pressure. This sequence of events emphasizes the importance of adequate resuscitation before performing angiography for suspected mesenteric ischemia. (From, Boley SJ, Brandt LJ, Sprayregen S: Mesenteric ischemia. In Abrams HL (ed): Angiography. Boston, Little, Brown, 1980.)

A normal plain film of the abdomen does not exclude acute mesenteric ischemia, and ideally all patients should be studied before roentgenographic signs of ischemia develop. Thus, *the primary pupose of these plain film studies is not to help in the diagnosis of acute mesenteric ischemia, but to exclude other radiographically diagnosable causes of abdominal pain,* for example, a perforated viscus or intestinal obstruction. If no other acute abdominal condition is detected, angiography is performed.

Therapeutic Papaverine Infusion. When the therapeutic regimen includes the use of papaverine, the drug is infused through the angiography catheter, which is left in the SMA. To prevent dislodgement, the catheter is sutured to the skin at its point of entry in the thigh. The papaverine is administered at a constant rate of 30 to 60 mg/hour using an infusion pump. The drug is usually diluted in saline to a concentration of 1.0 mg/ml, but this may be varied with the fluid limitations or requirements of the patient. Continuous monitoring of systemic arterial pressure and cardiac rate and rhythm is indicated as these amounts of papaverine theoretically could have systemic effects. We have not observed such problems in either our experimental or clinical studies probably because the drug is metabolized in the liver before it reaches the general circulation. Infusion at these rates has been used clinically for as long as 5 days without untoward systemic changes.

Heparin is not added to the infusion as it is not compatible with papaverine hydrochloride, and we have not found it necessary to prevent thrombus formation within the SMA. No other medications or fluids should be administered through the arterial catheter, and the patient must be observed carefully for evidence of dislodgement of the catheter.

The duration of the papaverine infusion varies with both the purpose for its use and the response of the patient. In conjunction with an embolectomy or arterial reconstruction, the infusion is continued for 12 to 24 hours if no "second look" is planned. At that time the angiogram is repeated and, unless some specific indication for more prolonged vasodilator therapy is demonstrated, the infusion is discontinued. When a second look operation is to be performed, the papaverine is continued until the abdomen is reopened, but a repeat angiogram is obtained before operation. The need for an additional period of infusion is assessed intraoperatively, depending on the state of the bowel and the results of the preoperative angiogram.

When papaverine infusion is used as the primary treatment for nonocclusive mesenteric ischemia, it is continued for approximately 24 hours and then a repeat angiogram is performed 30 minutes after changing the infusion to isotonic saline without papaverine. Based on the clinical course of the patient (i.e., abdominal distension, bowel function, abdominal findings, and evidence of blood in the stools) and the response of the vasoconstriction to therapy as noted on the angiogram, the infusion is discontinued or maintained for another 24 hours; the patient is then re-evaluated (Fig. 3). Infusions have been continued for up to 5 days, but usually can be stopped after 24 hours. When papaverine is used in conjunction with laparotomy for nonocclusive disease, a "second look" is frequently necessary. In such cases, the infusion is continued as de-

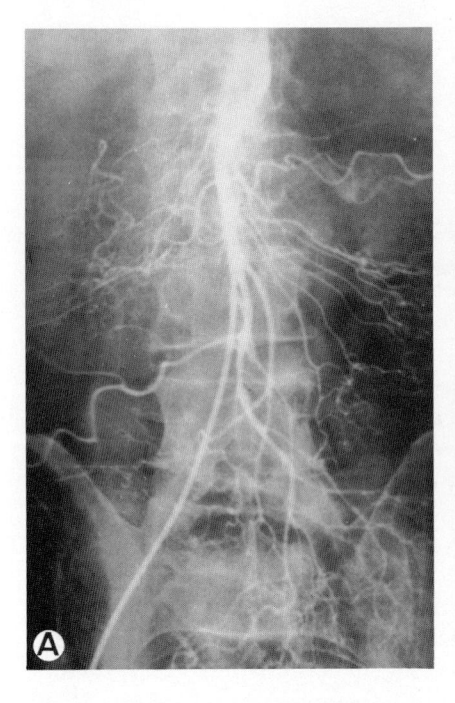

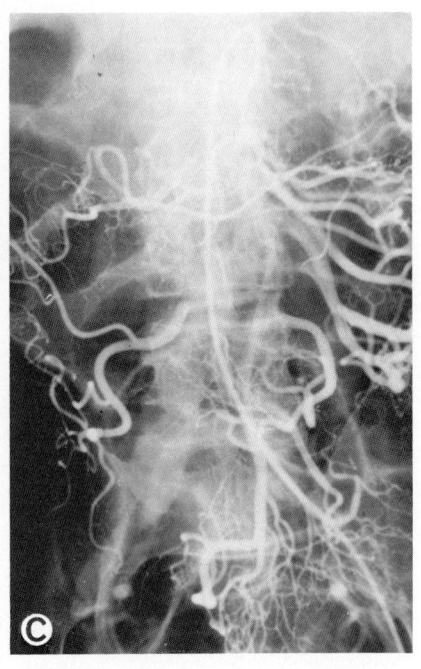

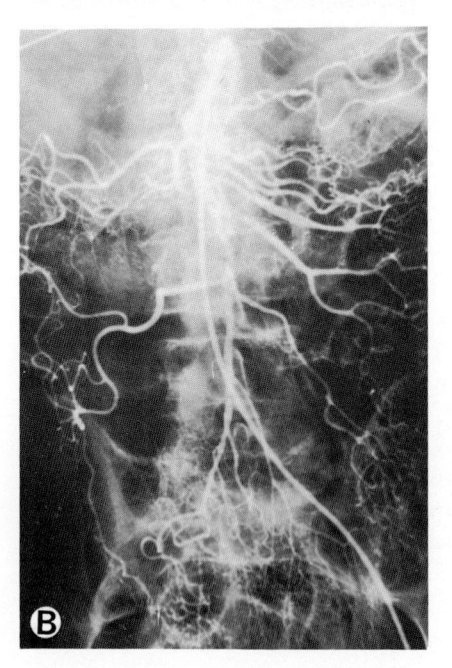

FIGURE 3. Patient with nonocclusive mesenteric ischemia following episode of gastrointestinal hemorrhage and shock. **A.** Initial superior mesenteric anteriogram showing diffuse vasoconstriction. **B.** Repeat angiogram after papaverine infusion for 24 hours shows partial but not complete relief of vasoconstriction. **C.** Angiogram performed after 48 hours of papaverine infusion shows dilatation of all vessels. Patient was asymptomatic at that time. (Courtesy of Dr. Leon Schultz, Peninsula General Hospital, Far Rockaway, N.Y.)

scribed previously for second look operations following embolectomy. The papaverine infusion is discontinued when no signs of vasoconstriction remain on an angiogram that is obtained 30 minutes after the vasodilator infusion is temporarily replaced by saline alone. The SMA catheter is removed promptly when the intra-arterial infusion is stopped.

Supportive Therapy. An essential aspect of the supportive therapy of patients with acute mesenteric ischemia is the maintenance of an adequate plasma volume. Just as massive losses of protein-rich fluids occur with early bowel infarction, so can they occur following revascularization of ischemic bowel. Hence, it is important to correct continually for losses before undertaking treatment, during papaverine infusions, and following surgical relief of arterial occlusions. The use of low-molecular-weight dextran may serve a dual purpose because of its effect as a plasma expander and because of its potential value in decreasing sludging in the microcirculation.

The value of both systemic and locally administered antibiotics in improving the viability of compromised bowel is well accepted. For this reason, and because of the high incidence of positive blood cultures with acute mesenteric ischemia, systemic antibiotics are started as soon as the diagnosis is established.

Intestinal decompression by nasogastric suction, the use of furosemide and mannitol to maintain urinary output, and specific therapy for the cardiac problems all play a role in the management of most patients. Digitalis, as previously mentioned, must be used cautiously, and vasopressors should be avoided. Anticoagulant therapy is avoided specifically, except in patients with venous thrombosis, because of the danger of intestinal hemorrhage. Early in our experience, we had two patients who bled massively as a result of heparin administered after successful embolectomy.

Prognosis

The outlook for patients with acute mesenteric ischemia is improving. Although mortalities of 70 to 90 percent have been reported through 1979 using traditional methods of diagnosis and therapy, the aggressive approach described above can reduce these catastrophic figures.[6] Of the first 50 patients managed by this approach, 35 (70 percent) proved to have acute mesenteric ischemia; 33 had angiographic signs of nonocclusive or occlusive ischemia; the remaining 2 patients had normal angiograms. Fifteen patients (30 percent) did not have mesenteric ischemia, but in 8 of these the correct diagnosis was made from the angiographic study. Of the 35 patients with AMI, 19 (54 percent) survived, including 9 of 15 patients with nonocclusive mesenteric ischemia, 7 of 16 with SMA embolus, 2 of 3 patients with SMA thrombosis, and 1 patient with mesenteric venous thrombosis; 17 of the 19 survivors did not lose any bowel or had excision of less than 3 feet of small intestine.[6]

Of special interest were the three patients with emboli managed initially with papaverine infusions for 24, 36, and 54 hours, respectively. Two were subsequently operated on and the bowel was found to be normal; the third survived without operation. Future studies may justify wider use of this nonoperative management of SMA emboli.

Complications

The complications of the angiographic studies and prolonged infusions of vasodilator drugs have not been excessive. Three of the first 50 patients developed transient acute tubular necrosis following angiography and treatment of their mesenteric ischemia. One patient developed arterial occlusions in both lower extremities during a papaverine infusion for an SMA embolus. These probably represented other emboli from his primary source of embolization, but the SMA catheter could not be excluded as a factor. There were several instances of local hematomas at the arterial puncture site, but no other major problems with blood flow to the lower extremities were encountered.

Problems with prolonged papaverine infusions have been minimal. Infusions for more than 5 days have been used without significant systemic effects. Because more than 90 percent of the drug is inactivated with each circulation through the liver, large doses can be safely infused into the mesenteric circulation. Fibrin clots on the arterial catheter have been observed commonly, but have not caused any difficulty. Three catheters clotted and had to be removed, but this complication can be avoided if a continuous infusion pump is used. Catheter dislodgement occurred several times and required replacement under fluoroscopy.

The 54 percent survival rate in our series is encouraging and represents a marked improvement over the 20 to 30 percent survival previously reported. Equally gratifying is the preservation of the normally functioning gastrointestinal tract in 85 percent of the surviving patients.

The survival of 9 of the 10 patients with acute mesenteric ischemia who had angiography in the absence of physical signs of peritonitis demonstrates the potential value of early diagnosis. Ideally, all patients with acute mesenteric ischemia should be studied before physical signs develop, at a time when the plain films of the abdomen are normal. Physical signs and plain film abnormalities usually indicate the presence of bowel necrosis; to await the development of these is to wait for ischemia to progress to infarction, and to accept the high mortality that accompanies this progression.

Case Report

A 70-year-old woman had an episode of upper gastrointestinal hemorrhage attributed to gastritis. The bleeding was not severe enough to produce hypotension. Two days after the bleeding stopped, the patient developed severe generalized abdominal pain with minimal physical findings. This pain persisted for 6 hours at which time an angiogram demonstrated mesenteric vasoconstriction (Fig. 3). A bolus injection of papaverine produced some relief of the spasm, and an SMA infusion of papaverine was started at a rate of 60 mg/per hour. A repeat angiogram 24 hours later showed marked improvement in the vasoconstriction, but clinically the patient still had some abdominal pain. Forty-eight hours after the original study the patient was free of pain, and an angiogram performed 30 minutes after stopping the papaverine showed marked dilatation of the mesenteric bed. The catheter was removed and the patient had an uneventful recovery.

In this instance, an episode of nonocclusive mesenteric ischemia responded to early use of intra-arterial vasodilator therapy. Prompt angiography in a patient at risk led to the correct diagnosis and treatment.

Thrombolytic Therapy

Two fibrinolytic drugs, streptokinase (SK) and urokinase (UK) have undergone extensive clinical evaluations in the treatment of venous thrombosis and arterial thromboembolism with inconclusive results. Isolated reports of the successful use of these agents in patients with acute SMA embolus, however, have prompted suggestions that they be used more often in the mesenteric circulation.[15,20] Gurll and his associates[16] studied the potential vasodilator and thrombolytic effects of UK infused into the SMA of dogs after they previously showed the drug to be a vasodilator in the femoral circulation. Although they demonstrated both vasodilator and thrombolytic effects in the SMA, the dose of UK required to produce vasodilation was greater than that required to lyse thromboses.

We have compared the effects of papaverine, SK, and the two drugs together in maintaining intestinal viability in dogs with experimentally produced SMA emboli. The intestines of animals infused with intra-arterial papaverine alone were normal after 4 hours while those dogs infused with SK were cyanotic and had a large amount of intraluminal bleeding. Dogs receiving both drugs had healthy bowel but also had intraluminal bleeding. Our study suggests that vasodilation is more important than thrombolysis in maintaining intestinal viability in the early postocclusion period. The complication of intestinal bleeding may be a major deterrent to the use of these agents in the SMA, although a more purified form of UK may prove safer.

Since many SMA emboli originate from long-standing clots within the heart, the relative resistance of such older thrombi to lysis is another factor militating against the effectiveness of thrombolytic agents.

While the concept of combining the effects of intra-arterial vasodilator and thrombolytic drugs to prevent the need for operation in acute SMA occlusions remains very attractive, further investigations are necessary before this approach is employed clinically.

PERCUTANEOUS TRANSLUMINAL ANGIOPLASTY

The rapidly increasing experience with percutaneous transluminal angioplasty (PTA) has been reviewed in a previous chapter. In the visceral circulation the technique has been employed primarily for renal artery disease, but the nature and location of the lesions producing chronic mesenteric ischemia would appear to make them ideal candidates for dilatation.

The term *chronic intestinal ischemia* (CMI) includes a host of conditions in which blood flow is insufficient to satisfy the demands of increased motility, secretion, and absorption that develop after meals. These disorders manifest themselves either by ischemic visceral pain or abnormalities in gastrointestinal absorption or motility. Patients with CMI are actually experiencing recurrent acute episodes of insufficient blood flow during periods of maximal intestinal workload. The pain is similar, therefore, to that arising in the myocardium with angina pectoris, or in the calf muscles with intermittent claudication.

Atherosclerosis commonly involves the splanchnic arteries in persons over 45 years of age, and in 88 adult patients studied by Reiner, Jiminez, and Rodriguez, 77 percent had some evidence of atherosclerosis of the splanchnic vessels.[23] Some degree of luminal stenosis was observed in 72 percent of those with atherosclerosis, and in 65 percent the SMA, celiacaxis, and inferior mesenteric artery were involved. Narrowing of the major vessels was almost always due to a plaque at the aortic ostium or in the proximal 1 to 2 cm of the artery. Severe stenoses were uniformly associated with marked aortic atherosclerosis, and as expected patients with severe mesenteric involvement had a higher incidence of coronary artery disease and diabetes mellitus. Little correlation occurred between the degree of mesenteric atherosclerosis and the clinical course of the patients.

No specific reliable diagnostic test for abdominal angina exists at this time. The diagnosis must be based on the clinical symptoms, the arteriographic demonstration of an occlusive process of the splachnic arteries, and, to a great measure, on the exclusion of other gastrointestinal disease. The one essential clinical symptom of CMI is abdominal pain, which is usually postprandial, progressive, and associated with weight loss. Physical findings are limited and nonspecific. A systolic bruit is heard in the upper abdomen in approximately one-half of the patients although even when present its diagnostic significance must be questioned since similar bruits have been reported in 6.5 to 15.9 percent of healthy patients.[9]

Conventional roentgenographic examinations of the gastrointestinal tract are usually unremarkable, or nonspecifically abnormal. Demonstration of extrinsic pressure defects along the medial border of the descending duodenum may indicate the presence of large collaterals between the SMA and celiacaxis. Abnormalities in absorption studies or in small bowel biopsies may be present but are not specific for disease due to ischemia.

In the past, the only treatment for CMI was some form of operative arterial reconstruction. Today, transluminal angioplasty might be an alternative approach of lesser magnitude and risk in some patients. Several patients have already been managed by transluminal dilatations with good short-term responses (Fig. 4).[2,14,24] In the absence of a method for measuring intestinal blood flow, precise criteria to define the need for operative arterial reconstruction have been lacking. There is agreement that a patient with classic abdominal angina and unexplained weight loss, whose diagnostic evaluation has excluded other gastrointestinal disease and whose angiogram shows occlusive involvement of at least two of the three major arteries should be treated. The issue has been much less clear if only one major vessel is involved or if the nature of the clinical presentation is atypical. With the availability of transluminal angioplasty, dilatation of stenoses of the SMA and celiacaxis at the time of the original angiography is possible, and thus the indications for treatment may be liberalized. Further experience and follow-up will reveal if this method will be as helpful in the management of patients with CMI as it has been in those with iliac artery stenosis and renovascular hypertension.

There is one special situation in which reconstruction or dilatation of obstructed splanchnic arteries is indicated in the absence of abdominal

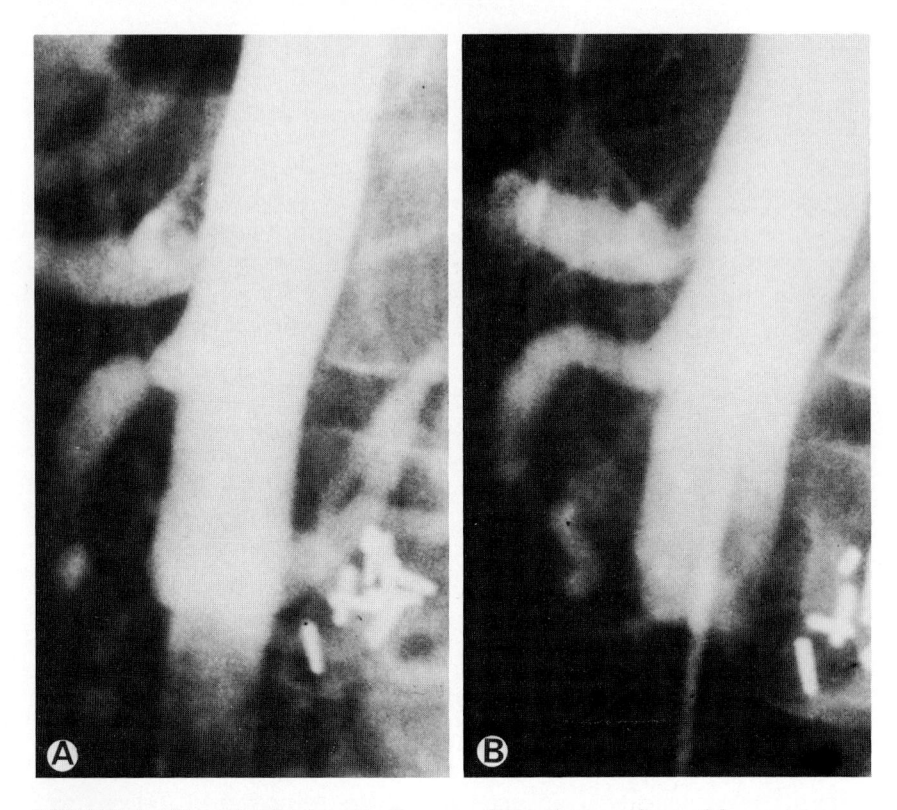

FIGURE 4. Transluminal angioplasty performed on patient with symptoms of chronic intestinal ischemia. **A.** Aortogram prior to dilatation shows stenosis and poststenotic dilatation of both celiac and superior mesenteric arteries. **B.** Aortogram performed after dilatation of SMA shows correction of SMA stenosis. Patient was relieved of her symptoms. (Courtesy of Dr. Christos Athanasoulis, Massachusetts General Hospital, Boston, Mass.)

complaints. This indication arises in a patient who is undergoing an aortic operation for peripheral vascular disease and in whom aortography has demonstrated occlusive involvement of the SMA and/or CA and the presence of a large "meandering artery." In such patients, the latter artery is supplying most of the blood flow to the splanchnic circulation from the IMA. Because the IMA may be compromised during the aortic procedure, it is advisable to provide another source of blood flow as part of this operation. The occurrence of acute intestinal ischemia resulting from "aortoiliac steal syndromes" has also been described in this situation after successful restoration of blood flow to the legs, but when no reconstructive procedure has been performed on the visceral vessels.

Although the question arises whether or not the acute intestinal ischemia in these reports represents a true "steal," the occurrence of this complication indicates the need for prophylactic revascularization.

"Bench Surgery" and Autotransplantation

Involvement of secondary and tertiary renal artery branches has often precluded successful revascularization of ischemic kidneys in patients with renovascular hypertension, and nephrectomy has ultimately been required. These smaller arterial lesions cannot be corrected by angioplasty (direct or by percutaneous transluminal techniques), endarterectomy, or with bypass grafts. "Bench surgery" during isolated perfusion of the kidney was made possible by preservation techniques developed for donor kidneys. In this method, the renal arteries and veins are transected and the kidney perfused with cold solutions while small vessel stenoses and aneurysms are corrected, often using the operating microscope. The ureter is usually left intact and the kidney either reimplanted or autotransplanted after completion of the "bench surgery." This use of this technique has generally been limited to operations on the kidney and, when combined with bypass grafts or preoperative PTA, has been used successfully on patients with extensive renal artery disease.[3,26]

Case Report

A 6-year-old girl with neurofibromatosis was admitted with persistent hypertension and elevated renin levels in samples from the right renal vein. Angiograms revealed a stenosis of a branch of the right renal artery with a poststenotic aneurysmal dilatation involving secondary and tertiary branches (Fig. 5). At operation, the involved vessels were not accessible with the kidney it situ. The renal artery and vein were transected and the kidney was flushed with a cold balanced salt solution (Collins solution) outside the abdomen. The ureter was left intact. One wall in the area of the aneurysmal dilatation was excised and a venous patch graft was placed so as to correct the stenosis and to cover the arterial wall defect (Fig. 6). The kidney was then autotransplanted to the right iliac fossa anastomosing the renal vessels to the internal iliac vessels. Postoperatively, the child has been normotensive, and the right kidney has normal function.

In this patient, the ability to operate upon the kidney ex vivo enabled us to correct small vessel lesions with relative ease and thus salvage

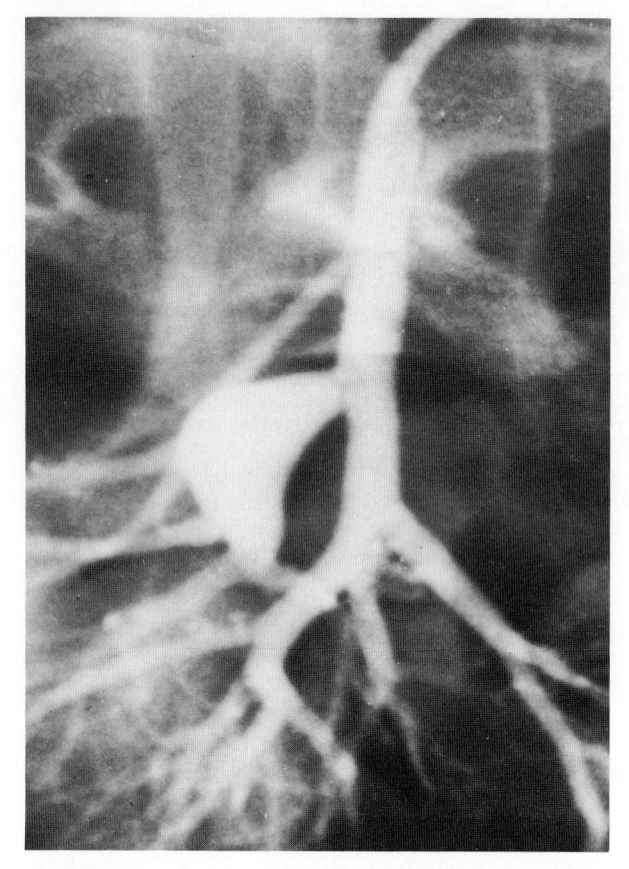

FIGURE 5. Right renal angiogram from 6-year-old girl with neurofibromatosis and renal hypertension. A stenosis and poststenotic aneurysmal dilatation involving secondary and tertiary branches of the renal artery.

the kidney. With these techniques, renal ischemic time can be extended to permit prolonged vascular reconstructions.

CONCLUSIONS

Some of the advances described in this chapter are supplemental to traditional modes of therapy while others offer alternative approaches in selected situations. All provide an opportunity for better results in the treatment of visceral ischemia. It is both a challenge to, and the responsibility of, surgeons managing patients with visceral ischemia to become conversant and comfortable with these new techniques.

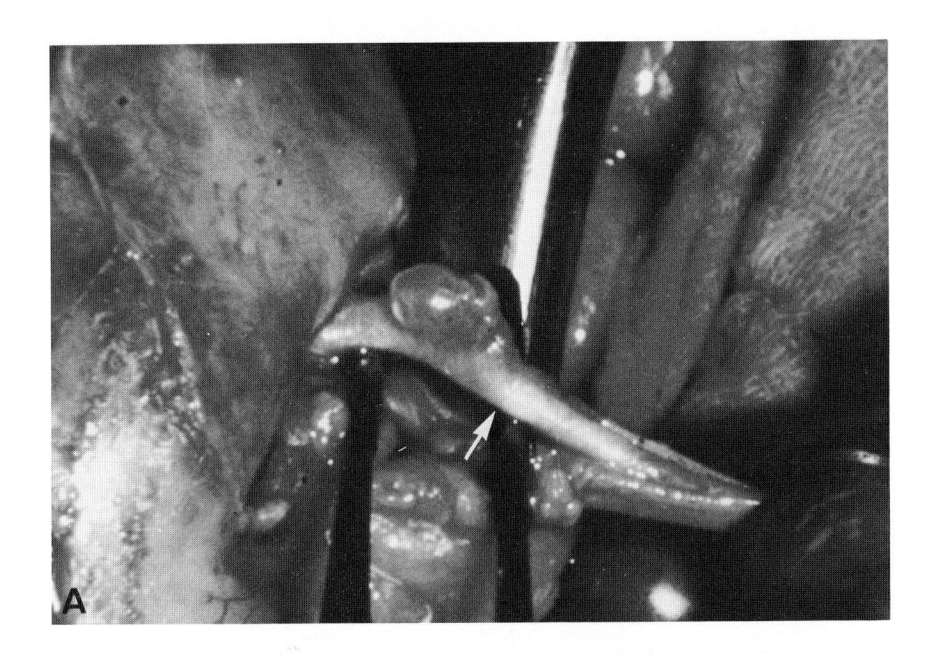

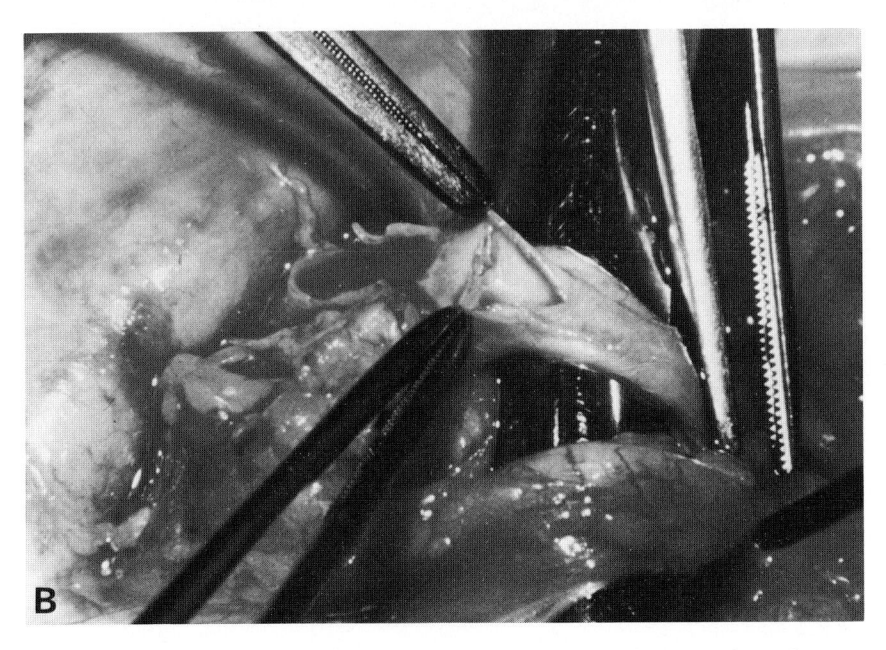

FIGURE 6. **A.** Operative view of aneurysm of secondary branch of renal artery demonstrated in Figure 5. The kidney has been removed from the body leaving the ureter intact and is being repaired after flushing of the renal vessels. Stenosis is present proximal to the aneurysm (arrow). **B.** Dilated portion of artery has been excised and the artery opened through the area of stenosis (seen between the forceps). (Continued.)

318 Critical Problems in Vascular Surgery

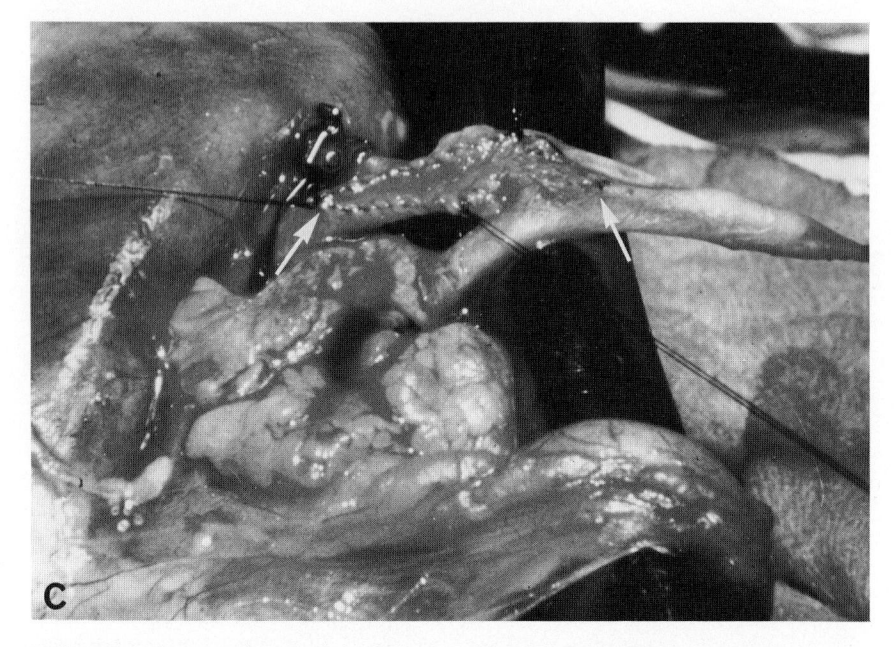

FIGURE 6. C. A vein patch has been applied to the defect, repairing arterial continuity and correcting the stenosis. The graft extends from the tertiary branch on to the secondary branch of the artery (arrows). After repair the kidney was transplanted to the right iliac fossa.

REFERENCES

1. Aakhus T, Brabrand G: Angiography in acute superior mesenteric arterial insufficiency. Acta Radiol (Diagn) 6:1, 1967
2. Athanasoulis C: Personal communication
3. Belzer FO, Salvatierra O, Palubinskas A, Stoney RJ: Ex vivo renal artery reconstruction. Ann Surg 182:456, 1975
4. Boley SJ, Siegelman SS: Experimental and clinical nonocclusive mesenteric ischemia: Pathophysiology, diagnosis and management. In Hilal SK (ed): Small Vessel Angiography. St. Louis, Mosby, 1973
5. Boley SJ, Sprayregen S, Veith FJ, Siegelman SS: An aggressive roentgenologic and surgical approach to acute mesenteric ischemia. In Nyhus LM (ed): Surgery Annual. New York, Appleton-Century-Crofts, 1973
6. Boley SJ, Sprayregen S, Siegelman SS, Veith FJ: Initial results from an aggressive roentgenogical and surgical approach to acute mesenteric ischemia. Surgery 82:848, 1977
7. Boley SJ, Treiber W, Winslow PR, Gliedman ML, Veith FJ: Circulatory response to acute reduction of superior mesenteric arterial blood flow. Physiologist 12:180, 1969
8. Boley SJ, Regan JA, Tunick PA, et al: Persistent vasoconstriction—A major

factor in nonocclusive mesenteric ischemia. Curr Top Surg Res 3:425, 1971
9. Brandt LJ, Boley SJ: Celiac axis compression syndrome: A critical review. Am J Dig Dis 23:633, 1978
10. Britt LG, Cheek RC: Nonocclusive mesenteric vascular disease. Ann Surg 169:704, 1969
11. Cohn JN, Francisiosa JA: Vasodilator therapy of cardiac failure. N Engl J Med 297:27, 254, 1977
12. Everhard ME, Regan JA, Veith FJ, Boley SJ: Mesenteric vasomotor response to reduced mesenteric blood flow. Physiologist 13:191, 1970
13. Frimman-Dahl J: Roentgen examination in mesenteric thrombosis. Am J Roentgenol 64:610, 1950
14. Furrer J, Gruntzig A, Kugelmeier J, Goebel N: Treatment of abdominal angina with percutaneous dilatation of an arteria mesenterica superior stenosis. Cardiovasc Intervent Radiol 3:43, 1980
15. Griffen WO: In discussion of Boley SJ, Sprayregen S, Siegelman SS, Veith FJ: Initial results from an aggressive roentgenological and surgical approach to acute mesenteric ischemia. Surgery 82:848, 1977
16. Gurll N, Zinner MJ, Turtinen L, Reynolds DG: Vasodilation, fibrinolysis, and thrombolysis with intraarterial infusion of urokinase in the canine superior mesenteric artery. Gastroenterology 75:425, 1978
17. Hessen I: Roentgen examination in cases of occlusion of the mesenteric vessels. Acta Radiol 44:293, 1955
18. Hibbard JS, Swenson JC, Levin AG: Roentgenology of experimental mesenteric vascular occlusion. Arch Surg 26:20, 1933
19. Hollenberg NK, Epstein M, Rosen SM, et al: Acute oliguric renal failure in man: Evidence of preferential renal cortical ischemia. Medicine 47:455, 1968
20. Jamieson AC, Thomas RJS, Cade JF: Lysis of a superior mesenteric artery embolus following local infusion of streptokinase and heparin. Aust NZ J Surg 49:355, 1979
21. Ottinger LW, Austen WG: A study of 136 patients with mesenteric infarction. Surg Gynecol Obstet 124:251, 1967
22. Packer M, Mellor J: Vasodilator therapy of acute congestive heart failure: A plea for caution. Am J Cardiol 42:686, 1978
23. Reiner L, Jiminez FA, Rodriguez FL: Atherosclerosis in the mesenteric circulation: Observations and correlations with aortic and coronary atherosclerosis. Am Heart J 66:200, 1963
24. Ring E: Personal communication.
25. Siegelman SS, Sprayregen S, Boley SJ: Angiographic diagnosis of mesenteric arterial vasoconstriction. Radiology 112:533, 1974
26. Stewart BH, Banowsky LH, Hewitt CB, Straffon RA: Renal autotransplantation: Current perspective. J Urol 118:363, 1977
27. Tomchik FS, Wittenberg J, Ottinger LW: The roentgenographic spectrum of bowel infarction. Radiology, 96:249, 1970
28. Vellar ID, Doyle JC: Acute mesenteric ischemia. Aust NZ J Surg 47: 54, 1977

TWENTY-ONE

Management of Posttraumatic Pain Syndromes: Causalgia and Reflex Sympathetic Dystrophy

Jesse E. Thompson and R. Don Patman

The expected response to trauma in an extremity after proper treatment is orderly and predictable healing of the wound, return of function and circulatory dynamics, and gradual cessation of pain. Occasionally this predictable response is altered in a bizarre fashion despite adequate treatment and the absence of any obvious factors detrimental to prompt healing. Pain may become severe and unrelenting, with a marked disparity between severity and the apparent injury. Sympathetic dysfunction, usually overactivity, becomes evident. Trophic changes ensue to varying degrees, and, if the process is left unattended for any length of time, they may become irreversible.

Two major categories of posttraumatic syndromes have the aforementioned characteristics: causalgia and mimocausalgia states, or, as frequently termed, *reflex sympathetic dystrophy*. In 1864, Mitchell, Morehouse, and Keen[11] described a syndrome of burning pain in the extremities of American Civil War soldiers suffering from gunshot wounds of the peripheral nerves. Their description of this entity was so accurate that it remains a classic today. Not until 1867, however, did Mitchell first term his condition *causalgia*.[12]

> *Causalgia—there is, however, one species of pain arising out of nerve wounds which have never been described except by my colleagues and myself, although the state of skin which is usually found with it had been spoken of by Mr. Paget, who seems to have seen it only in association with common neurologic pain. In writing of this peculiar kind of suffering, I felt that it would be well to give it some more convenient name than merely "burning pain," and, in*

accordance with the suggestion of my friend, Professor Robley Dunglison, I have therefore adopted the term causalgia as being both descriptive and convenient.

The word *causalgia,* from the Greek, means literally "burning pain." It is clear that Professor Robley Dunglison, a distinguished professor of medicine, coined the term. Thus, causalgia should be strictly used to designate that syndrome which may develop following a major peripheral nerve injury.

Homans[4] used the term *minor causalgia* in an effort to show a relationship between Mitchell's causalgia and similar conditions arising from trauma other than direct nerve injuries. Over the ensuing years, a number of similar syndromes have been observed to occur following extremity trauma of almost any variety and severity. Many terms have been used to describe these entities: minor causalgia, posttraumatic sympathetic dystrophy, reflex dystrophy, Sudeck's atrophy, posttraumatic dystrophy, shoulder-hand syndrome, traumatic edema, posttraumatic pain syndrome, sympathetic neurovascular dystrophy, causalgia-state, posttraumatic vasomotor disorder, painful osteoporosis, chronic segmental arterial spasm, posttraumatic sympathetic dysfunction, posttraumatic painful osteoporosis, posttraumatic spreading neuralgia, sympathalgia, acute atrophy of bone, traumatic angiospasm, chronic traumatic edema, and peripheral trophoneurosis.[6,13,14] These confusing terms all relate to similar syndromes that form one large category similar to but distinct from the true major causalgia of Mitchell, Morehouse, and Keen. They may be grouped together under a single designation, *mimocausalgia states.*[13] "Mimo" in Greek means an attempt to re-create or imitate. Therefore, the term *mimocausalgia* will be used throughout this chapter to designate all of the posttraumatic pain syndromes except causalgia.

CLINICAL MANIFESTATIONS

In causalgia, the injury is to a major mixed nerve in the proximal part of the extremity. In the upper extremity, the nerve most commonly involved is the median nerve, while in the lower extremity the sciatic and tibial nerves are usually responsible. Causalgia ordinarily results from a partial severance of the nerve, but cases have been seen with complete division. Patients complain of a sensation of burning pain in the peripheral portion of the extremity. The cutaneous dyesthesias may be so intense that the patient cannot tolerate contact with clothing. Vasomotor dysfunction is almost always present and is usually vasoconstriction. Because of the pain there is limitation of motion of the extremity followed by delay in functional recovery over and above that caused by any nerve injury. As trophic changes occur, the extremity may become disabled permanently. Pain and disability from this condition may be so profound as to cause serious emotional problems.

A similar syndrome may occur in mimocausalgia. Variations are quite common, but in most patients one finds pain, sympathetic dysfunction, usually overactivity, delayed or abnormal functional recovery, and trophic changes with limitation of motion and stiffness. Hyperesthesia is common and such alterations as edema, cyanosis, coldness, and hyperhidrosis occur. Because of the pain, motion is limited and one may find stiffness of the fingers, hands, wrists, elbows, shoulders, and of the ankle joints. If allowed to go untreated for any period of time, these trophic changes may become irreversible, and, in spite of relief of pain after treatment, the patient may have a disabled extremity. Ofter a great disparity exists between the apparent trauma and the physical findings and the severity of pain. This point should be strongly emphasized if the diagnosis is to be made early, and proper treatment instituted.

For mimocausalgia to occur, three factors must be present at the same time: a painful lesion, the diathesis or susceptibility of the patient, and an abnormal autonomic reflex. All observers have noted the diathesis in these patients.[8] They are frequently emotionally labile, are in poor health, avoid responsibility, have a low pain threshold, have an unstable personality, are chronic complainers and are looking for a crutch or secondary monetary gain. Thus, a vicious cycle is established. In an individual with the diathesis, a traumatic painful lesion leads to vasospasm, immobility, edema, tissue reaction, and finally a stiff, nonfunctional dystrophic extremity.

ETIOLOGY OF POSTTRAUMATIC PAIN SYNDROMES

A number of theories have been proposed to explain the etiology of posttraumatic pain syndromes; however all have shortcomings and none has been accepted universally. A simple explanation is that the sympathetic nerve fibers themselves transmit the pain impulses to the central nervous system.[2] Unfortunately, there is no good evidence that afferent fibers are in the sympathetic pathways to the extremities. A popular theory is that proposed by Doupe et al.[1] in which artificial synapses occur at the site of injury. A "short circuit" occurs at the point of partial nerve interruption or demyelinization that allows efferent sympathetic impulses to be relayed back along afferent somatic fibers.

Livingston[9] suggested a cycle of reflexes to explain the pain with three main components consisting of 1) increased production and release of afferent impulses in a periphral sensory nerve following injury or irritation from any cause; 2) abnormal activity or increased stimulation of the internuncial pool located in the anterior horn of the spinal cord; 3) subsequent increase in sympathetic efferent activity.

Melzak and Wall[10] suggested a theory similar to Livingston's to explain pain transmission. They suggest that certain cells in the substantia gelatinosa of the dorsal horn of the spinal cord act as a computer or gate control system that direct the incoming afferent sensory impulses. These cells on a highly sophisticated basis interpret the type, number, and frequency of afferent sensory impulses, and then relay these patterns of impulses to the brain for the perception of pain. The authors propose that impulses along large myelinated fibers inhibit this control system or "gate" and impulses transmitted along small fibers tend to stimulate or "open the gate," and thus increase the number of impulses transmitted centrally via the neurons in the spinal center.

Although the basic etiology remains obscure, the one common denominator in most cases is the sympathetic nervous system, since interruption of the sympathetic fibers to both the upper and lower extremities relieves the pain and allows for an orderly return of normal function in most cases.

TREATMENT

In the past when no effective treatment was known, causalgia frequently resulted in chronic invalidism, mental deterioration, drug addiction, and all too often self-destruction. In the years before 1930, many different procedures were attempted to abort the severe pain in the extremities, but none gave consistently good results.

In 1930, Spurling[15] reported a case of true causalgia in peacetime. A bootlegger sustained a gunshot wound of the brachial plexus that was dramatically cured by cervical thoracic sympathetic ganglionectomy after several local procedures including periarterial sympathectomy had failed. In 1935 Kwan[7] reported a similar case. These isolated instances brought about a dramatic change in the management of this bizarre syndrome.

Experiences during World War II demonstrated clearly and dramatically the place of sympathetic block and sympathectomy as definitive treatment for patients with causalgia.[5,14] Since then similar methods of treatment have been found effective in the management of the mimocausalgia states. Relief of pain and improvement in the other symptoms follows sympathetic ablation, whether chemical or surgical, in most cases.

The basis for proper treatment of all the various clinical entities is early recognition. If a patient begins to complain of pain that is out of proportion to that expected from the particular extremity wound, one should suspect a posttraumatic pain syndrome. Not all pain is causalgia or mimocausalgia, however, and one must rule out other complications, such as thrombophlebitis, arterial occlusion, tight cast or dressing infection, acute compression from edema, etc. If no other cause is found, the patient may be developing sympathetic dystrophy. In the early stages it may be relieved by symptomatic treatment. The use of heat with elevation of the extremity is frequently helpful as are various drugs. For pain, ordinary analgesics and tranquilizers may be employed. Anti-inflammatory agents at times will abort the syndrome. Diuretics may help by reducing edema. If vasospasm is present, vasodilators, either orally or intra-arterially, may be used. Steroids may also be of benefit.[16]

If symptoms are not relieved promptly by the measures just listed, or if they become intensified over the course of several days, one should proceed directly to sympathetic blocks, which are both diagnostic and therapeutic. In early cases relief of pain may last well beyond the duration of the block and even be curative. Repeated blocks should be performed until pain is controlled. If the results of sympathetic block are equivocal, a control block with normal saline may be performed. If relief from repeated sympathetic blocks becomes less effective or static and the initial response is dramatic but of short duration, surgical sympathectomy should be considered. Early sympathectomy will prevent the occurrence of irreversible trophic changes as well as obviate the establishment of fixed pain patterns that may become refractory even to sympathectomy if the syndrome is allowed to be prolonged without definitive therapy.

For the upper extremity, stellate ganglion blocks are employed with the use of 1 percent lidocaine or 0.25 percent bupivacaine (Marcaine), bathing the stellate ganglion, which lies at the level of C7-D1. A satisfactory technique for stellate ganglion block of the upper extremity is as follows: With the patient's head extended and turned away from the surgeon, the needle is inserted at a point 4 cm lateral to the midline and 4 cm up from the clavicle to a depth of 4 cm in the neck, with the needle directed medially and somewhat inferiorly toward the lateral bony mass of C7-D1. Ten milliliters of local anesthetic are injected. Profound Horner's syndrome with warming and drying of the hand and relief of pain follows immediately upon satisfactory block of the stellate ganglion. Recently, sympathetic block by means of intravenous guanethidine injection has also been used for relief of sympathetic dystrophy.[3]

Lumbar block is somewhat more difficult than stellate block. The preferred technique involves three needles placed 5 cm laterally to the midline opposite the transverse processes of L1, L2, and L3 or L2, L3, and L4. When the transverse processes are encountered, the needles are redirected above or below and inserted to a depth of 3.5 to 4 cm, so that their tips encounter the sympathetic trunk, lying along the anterolateral border of the lumbar vertebrae. Ten milliliters of 1 percent lidocaine are then injected into each needle. Within a few moments a sympathetic effect is apparent, with warming and drying of the foot and relief of pain.

When surgical sympathectomy is found to be necessary, for the upper extremity, ganglia D2 and D3 are all that have to be removed. When dorsal sympathectomy is necessary, several techniques may be employed. A common one is the transaxillary approach; the classic posterior approach of Smithwick through the bed of the third rib in the extrapleural plane may also be employed. With this type of operation, Horner's syndrome is not produced, but this degree of sympathectomy is completely effective in relieving pain.

For patients requiring lumbar sympathectomy, the standard lumbar approach through an abdominal incision via the retroperitoneal plane is employed, and ganglia L2 and L3 are removed.

Once pain is relieved, physical therapy is an important part of the ancillary treatment for rehabilitation.

RESULTS OF TREATMENT

A series of 147 patients with various posttraumatic syndromes will be reviewed. Of 27 patients with true causalgia, gunshot wounds were the most common cause, occurring in 11 individuals. Of 120 cases of mimocausalgia, fracture was the cause in 49, while minor trauma, such as a sprain or laceration, was a common cause in 34 patients. There were 62 males and 85 females in the series. The average duration of symptoms was 5 months, the shortest being 1 week and the longest being 60 months. In many patients, significant symptoms could be documented to be present within 7 days or less from the time of injury. The upper extremity was the site of injury in 99 patients while the lower extremity was injured in 48 patients.

One of the characteristic features important to note is the delay between trauma and diagnosis; in our series this was 5 to 5½ months. Because the cause of pain is not clear, many patients are thought to be malingering or psychoneurotic. Of these patients, 83 percent had sympathetic hyperactivity, 86.5% showed decreased function, and 68.5 percent already had trophic changes when first seen.

It is interesting to review the forms of treatment used on these patients prior to the time that we first saw them. Twenty-three had had no prior treatment; 88 had physiotherapy without relief, and 16 patients had immobilization in the absence of fractures. Eighteen patients had undergone operations such as neurolysis or carpal tunnel release. The rest of the patients in the series had various types of therapy such as the use of vasodilators, cortisone injections, and manipulations. Some patients were seen not because the diagnosis of causalgia was suspected or even known about by the referring physician but for "vascular evaluation" because of a cold, cyanotic, sweaty, painful part.

Among patients with causalgia, definitive therapy in all instances (27) was surgical sympathectomy. Among patients with mimocausalgia states, 59 patients were treated definitively with sympathetic blocks alone, while 55 patients (46 percent) required surgical sympathectomy. Six patients required only vasodilators, physical therapy, or other medical measures.

In the causalgia group, 89 percent had excellent results, and 11 percent had poor results for relief of pain, whereas 33 percent had residual symptoms. This last category is important. A patient with a serious fracture or injury to a major nerve, muscle, or joint may still have severe disability even though pain and swelling are relieved.

Among 120 patients with mimocausalgia, 80.8 percent had excellent results, 13.3 percent had good results, and 5.8 percent had poor results as far as pain relief was concerned. However, it is distressing to find that 30 percent of these patients have residual symptoms even after relief of pain. Some of these residual symptoms are due to the original injury, in which soft tissue, muscle, nerve, bone or joint loss occurred; but in many instances of mimocausalgia no major tissue loss was present, and residual symptoms resulted from stiffness of joints and limitation of motion, irreversible occurrences because of pain and trophic changes arising from the mimocausalgia itself.

Of the several reasons for treatment failures, probably the most important is delay between the onset of injury and institution of appropriate therapy, usually because the diagnosis is simply not suspected. By the time therapy is begun, the patient already has a central fixation or irreversible disability in the extremity. Another cause of failure is inadequate sympathectomy. Irreversible trophic changes are serious matters because of resulting disability and also from the standpoint of litigation and permanent compensation. Finally, it is occasionally difficult to separate dystrophy patients from true neurotics or malingerers who are trying to get compensation. Placebo sympathetic blocks with saline may be carried out in an effort to detect these individuals.

REFERENCES

1. Doupe J, Cullen CH, Chance GQ: Post-traumatic pain and causalgia syndrome. J Neurol Neurosurg Psychiatr 7:33, 1944
2. Freeman NE: Treatment of causalgia arising from gunshot wounds of peripheral nerves. Surgery 22:68, 1947

3. Hannington-Kiff JG: Relief of Sudeck's atrophy by regional intravenous guanethidine. Lancet 1:1132, 1977
4. Homans J: Minor causalgia: A hyperesthetic neurovascular syndrome. N Engl J Med 222:870, 1940
5. Kirklin JW, Chenoweth AI, Murphey F: Causalgia: A review of its characteristics, diagnosis and treatment. Surgery 21:321, 1947
6. Kleinert HE, Cook FW, Kutz JE: Neurovascular disorders of the upper extremity. Arch Surg 90:612, 1965
7. Kwan ST: The treatment of causalgia by thoracic sympathetic ganglionectomy. Ann Surg 101:222, 1935
8. Lankford LL, Thompson JE: Reflex sympathetic dystrophy, upper and lower extremity: Diagnosis and management. In Instructional Course Lectures. St. Louis, Mosby, 1977, pp 163–178
9. Livingston WK: Pain Mechanisms: A Physiological Interpretation of Causalgia and Its Related States. New York, MacMillan, 1943
10. Melzack R, Wall PD: Pain mechanisms: New theory. Science 150:971–979, 1965
11. Mitchell SW, Morehouse GR, Keen WW: Gunshot Wounds and Other Injuries of Nerves. Philadelphia, Lippincott, 1864, p 164
12. Mitchell SW: On the diseases of nerves, resulting from injuries, in contributions relating to the causation and prevention of disease and to camp diseases. In Flint A (ed): Memoirs. New York, United States Sanitary Commission, 1867, Chap. 12, pp 412–468
13. Patman RD, Thompson JE, Persson AV: Management of post-traumatic pain syndromes: Report of 113 cases. Ann Surg 177:780, 1973.
14. Shumacker HB Jr, Abramson DI: Post-traumatic vasomotor disorders. Surg Gynecol Obstet 88:417, 1949
15. Spurling RG: Causalgia of the upper extremity: Treatment by dorsal sympathetic ganglionectomy. Arch Neurol Psychiat 23:784, 1930
16. Thompson JE, Patman RD, Persson AV: Management of post-traumatic pain syndromes (causalgia). Am Surg 41:599, 1975

TWENTY-TWO
Arterial Injuries Caused by Blunt Trauma

Malcolm O. Perry

INCIDENCE AND ETIOLOGY

Most arterial injuries are the result of penetrating trauma, but some of the most difficult problems in diagnosis and management occur when blunt trauma is the cause of the injury.[11] The peripheral arteries are more susceptible to all types of vascular trauma, and this is true for blunt as well as penetrating wounds, as illustrated in the author's overall experience in 665 cases (Table 1). Most of these injuries were the result of gunshot wounds, and a smaller number were caused by stab wounds; in only 9 percent was blunt trauma the etiology. In the report by Reynolds et al.,[11] 46 of 191 arterial injuries were caused by blunt trauma, but 14 of these involved the thoracic aorta, and only 13 the popliteal, while the brachial and superficial femoral arteries were wounded 6 times each. Killeen[6] collected 1300 cases of patients who had sustained blunt trauma to the abdomen, and found only 1 patient in whom the abdominal aorta was injured, yet Dajee et al.[2] and Thal et al.[14] reported several cases of blunt trauma injuring the abdominal aorta, thought to be in association with the use of seatbelts. Plume and DeWeese[9] report a series of 20 patients who were treated for aortic rupture, and of these one patient had an injury to the abdominal aorta.

It therefore appears that, although blunt trauma is not the most common cause of injury to major arteries it does occur with sufficient frequency to be of great concern and it is especially likely to be present in the thoracic aorta, the popliteal artery, and those vessels in close proximity to the long bones.

330 Critical Problems in Vascular Surgery

Table 1. Distribution of Arterial Injuries
(in the Author's Experience)

Extremity	501
Aorta	31
Visceral	37
Cervical	96
Total	665

Connolly[1] states that the incidence of arterial injury with long bone fracture is between 0.6 and 3 percent; Ster [12] reported 10 arterial injuries in 355 patients with fractures or dislocations of the long bones. Wadell and Lencner[16] in a 10-year study of 40 arterial injuries noted 20 popliteal artery injuries, and nine of these subsequently went on to amputation. The seriousness of these injuries is underscored by Lefrak's report[8] of 152 knee dislocations, of which 42 were popliteal injuries, and 24 amputations eventually were necessary. Synder's[13] large series of 83 popliteal artery injuries included 22 cases that were caused by blunt trauma.

The abdominal aorta is relatively protected from blunt trauma, but the vessels in the root of the neck may be injured by the same forces that produce injury to the thoracic aorta, although this is not frequent. Reul,[10] reporting on a large series of injuries to the great vessels, had only a 14 percent incidence of blunt trauma, and in Flint's[4] 146 cases only 3 percent were caused by blunt trauma.

MECHANISMS AND TYPES OF INJURY

Major vessels may be injured by direct blows sustained in assaults, falls, or motor vehicle accidents. In such cases, the artery may be transected or lacerated, or there may be only mural contusions, or perhaps intimal dissection and thrombosis. Figure 1 is an example of an injury of the common carotid artery caused by a direct blow. There was a complete intimal fracture; continuity of the vessel is maintained only by the adventitia. A similar pathologic picture is found in injuries of the thoracic aorta. In other cases in which fractures or dislocations occur, the displaced bony fragments may produce direct injury, stretching, angulation, or compression.[3,7] Such mechanisms of arterial injury are thought to be involved particularly with fractures of the distal femur, fracture dislocations at the knee, and fractures of the clavicle (Fig. 2). Atherosclerotic arteries are especially susceptible to wall disruption caused by blunt trauma, and such wounds predispose to thrombosis and dissection.

The relative compressability of the chest also may permit injury of the great vessels as a result of direct trauma (Fig. 3). An almost complete

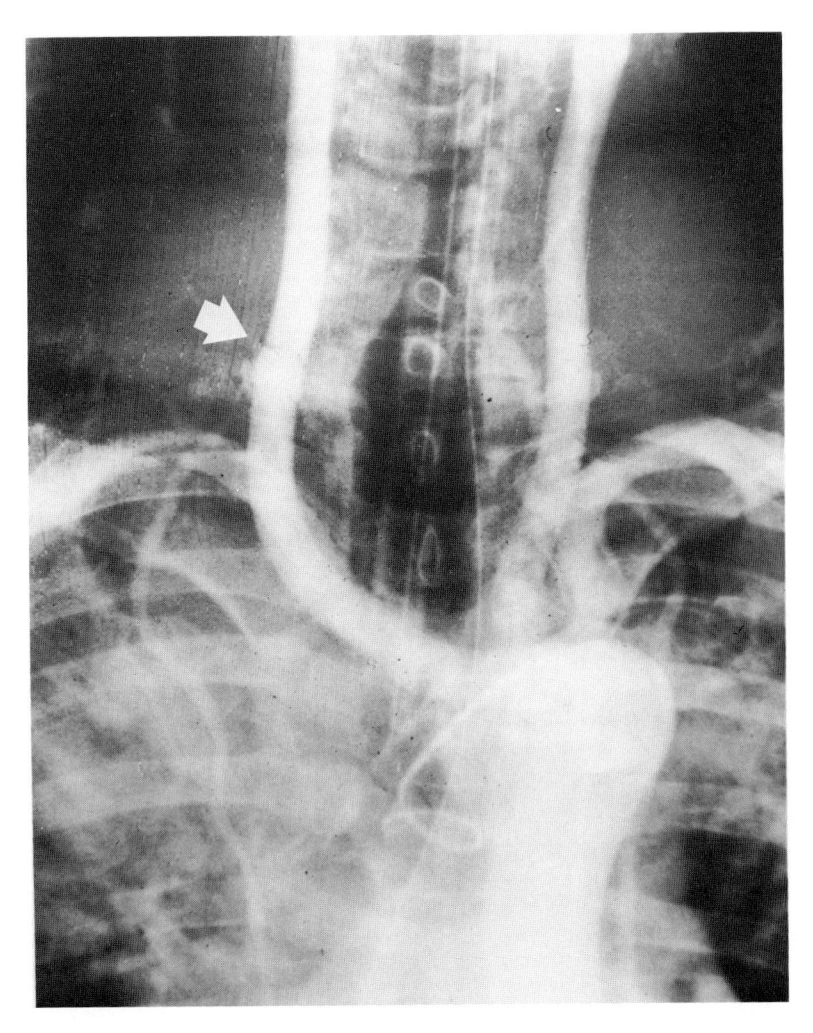

FIGURE 1. The intimal fracture seen in this arteriogram of the common carotid artery was the only indication of what proved to be extensive arterial damage.

disruption of the innominate artery was caused by a crush injury inflicted by the fall of a load of wood. As seen in this photograph, the blood is contained only by the intact adventitia.

Another mechanism of injury may follow hyperextension of the joints, fractures, and dislocations. The vessel may be severely stretched and the relatively elastic adventitia remain intact, but the media and intima may be torn in several locations, predisposing to delayed thrombosis. This is especially dangerous in vessels such as the internal carotid artery. Figure 4 illustrates the multiple intimal tears in the internal carotid

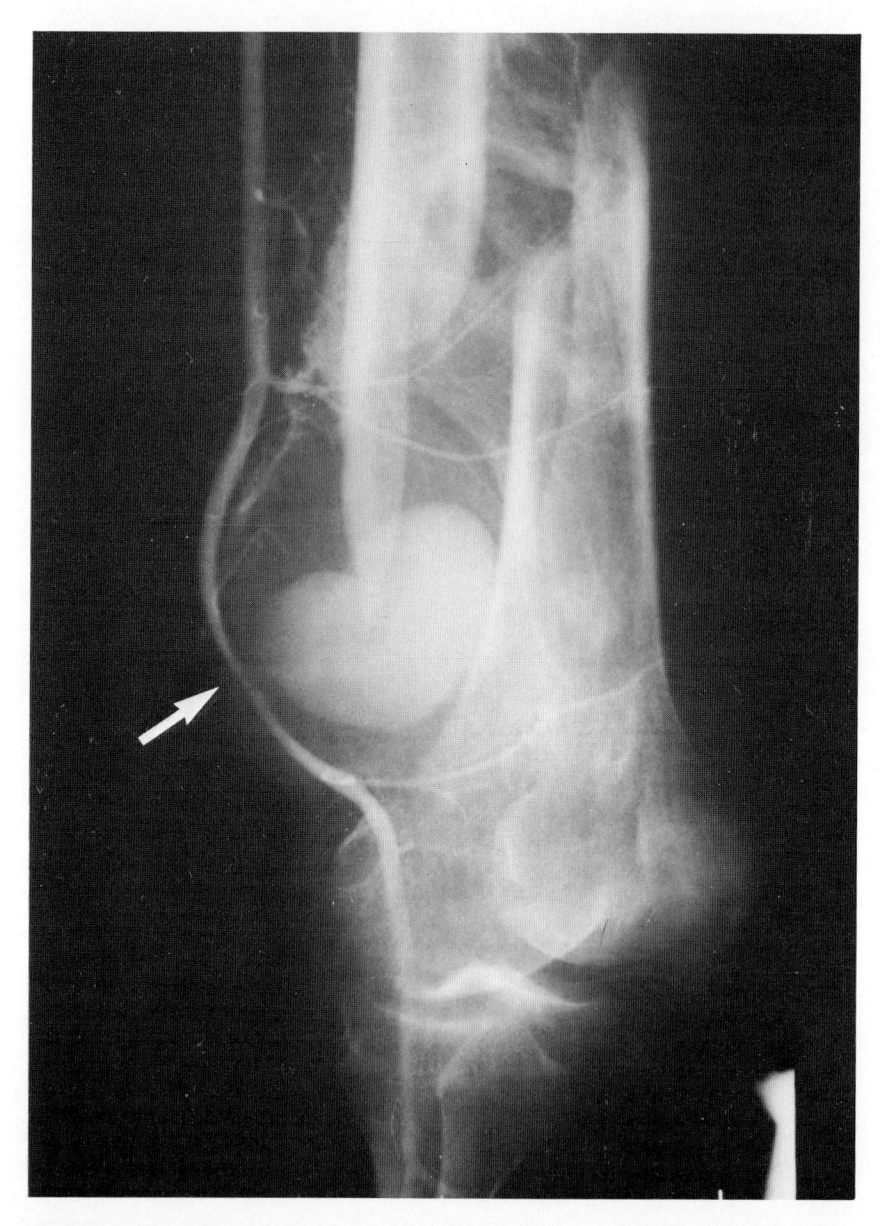

FIGURE 2. Despite the obvious arterial injury seen here, the distal pedal pulses and blood pressures were not sufficiently changed to support a diagnosis of the vascular wound.

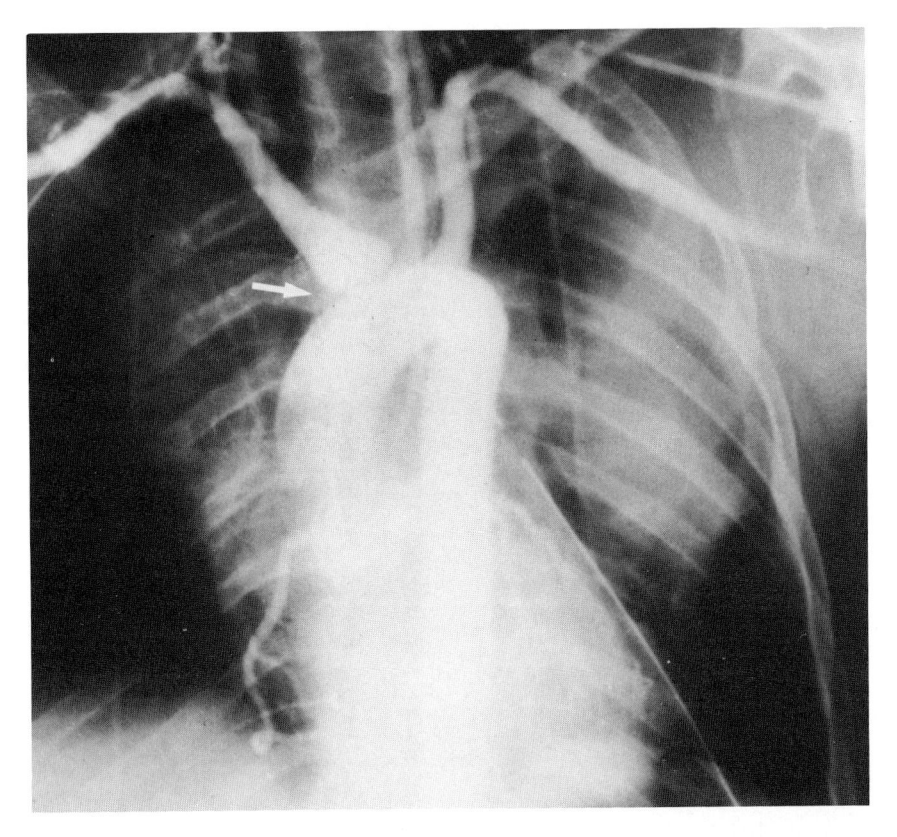

FIGURE 3. Only the adventitia was holding the innominate artery intact. A bypass graft was needed for repair.

just below its entrance into the skull; this resulted from hyperextension of the neck caused by a blow to the side of the face. Most of these lesions do not produce immediate disruption and bleeding, but lead to thromboembolic events. In certain cases, such as with fractures of the long bones and dislocations at the knee or elbow, there may be complete transection of the artery, but this often results in retraction of the vessel, thrombosis, and cessation of bleeding. Blunt trauma is not as likely to produce massive bleeding as a tangential laceration of a major vessel caused by penetrating wounds.

CLINICAL FEATURES

In most patients with arterial injuries caused by single penetrating wounds, those signs and symptoms listed below are often helpful in making the diagnosis.

334 Critical Problems in Vascular Surgery

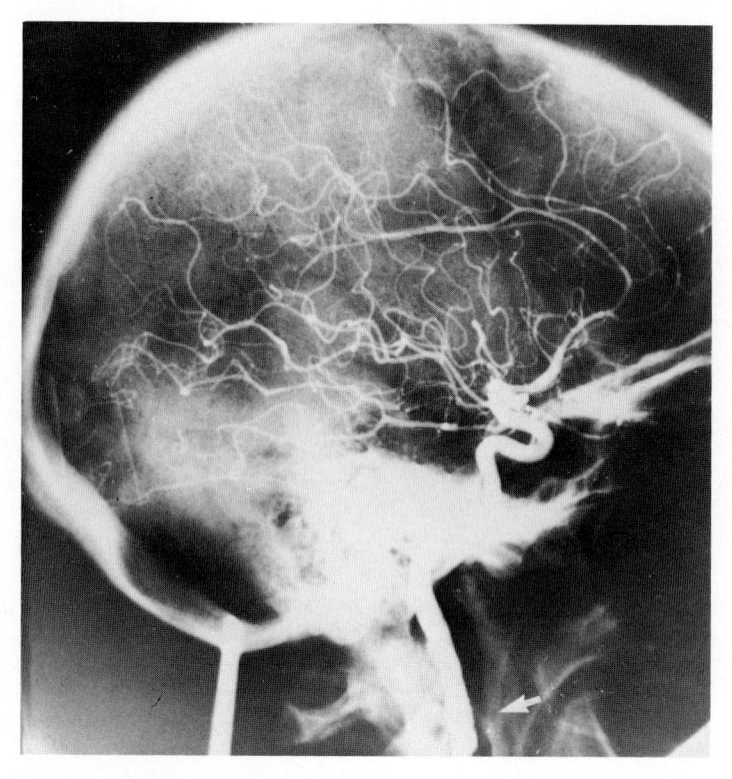

FIGURE 4. The diffuse damage and multiple intimal tears are seen in this internal carotid artery injured by hyperextension and stretching.

Diminished or absent pulse
Major hemorrhage with hypotension
Large or expanding hematoma
Bruit at or distal to injury
Anatomically related neurologic defect
Proximity of injury to major vessel

The signs and symptoms suggesting arterial wounds usually include pulse deficits and bleeding. Proximity of the wound tract to a major vessel is usually an indication for arteriography. The precise diagnosis may be more difficult to reach when the patient has had multiple wounds, as is likely when blunt trauma is the etiology. This is especially a problem in motor vehicle accidents in which the patient is likely to sustain multiple contusions, fractures, closed head trauma, and even injuries of the parenchymal organs in the abdomen.

Those patients with fractures of the long bones often have a great deal of soft tissue damage because of the tremendous forces released when a heavy bone, such as the femur or the tibia, is fractured. When the bone falls back into near-normal position, the extent of the injury may not be appreciated. In addition, the deformity associated with such injuries makes precise clinical evaluation difficult. Moreover, it is very common to have associated injuries that have a higher priority. Despite these multiple factors, in Synder's series[13] only 1 of the 22 patients with blunt trauma of the popliteal artery presented with equivocal signs; most of them had clear evidence of arterial damage with weak or absent pulses and signs of ischemia. Peroneal nerve injury is also common with these types of vascular injuries, and associated nerve injury may be a prominent finding in patients with vascular injuries caused by blunt trauma involving the neck and shoulder.

The popliteal artery is particularly vulnerable to shearing forces because it is relatively fixed proximally by the adductor muscles of the thigh, and distally by the soleus muscle. Such injuries are particularly common after posterior dislocation of the knee.[3,8] The collateral arteries of the genicular system are small and fragile, and covered only by thin tissue layers that are easily torn. In the course of evaluating and treating a patient after a motor vehicle accident, it is easy to miss an unstable knee, especially when more dramatic injuries are present. Although some distal ischemia may be noted, there is often a tendency to assign the cause to external compression or spasm of the artery. This results in untoward delays and should be avoided.

Blunt trauma involving the common or internal carotid artery produces a special sequence of events in which there is often a delay in the onset of symptoms as thromboembolism supervenes. The clinical features described by Gardner and Jernigan[5] are:

Hematoma of lateral neck
Horner's syndrome
Transient attack of ischemia
Lucid interval
Limb paresis in an alert patient

The delay in the onset of symptoms is particularly insidious and may permit the artery to progress to complete occlusion and produce irreversible neurologic deficits.[15,17] Arteriography, therefore, occupies a special role in the management of these patients, as it does in many patients who have arterial injuries caused by blunt trauma. Less than half of the patients with blunt trauma involving the head and neck have any external features that reflect the severity of the trauma, and arteriograms may be essential in the early evaluation. Indeed, even in those situations in which the diagnosis is fairly well established the arteriogram may be extremely useful in planning the operation, and preparing for adjunctive measures which may be needed during the vascular repair. The indications for arteriography that have proved to be especially useful in the author's experience are:

Blunt trauma, fractures
Penetrating injuries, chest
Cervical injuries, base of skull
Assessment multiple pellet wounds
Injuries forearm, leg

If the patient is hemodynamically unstable, however, it is best to proceed directly to the operating room and complete the resuscitation there. If arteriograms are required they can be performed during the course of the surgical procedure.

METHODS OF REPAIR

In a majority of cases, direct arterial reconstruction is satisfactory, and in large vessels lateral suture repair of tangential lacerations or puncture wounds is often possible. Many patients with arterial injuries caused by blunt trauma have a rather diffuse injury that often necessitates resection and anastomosis of the artery. If this is not possible because of the extent of the damage, reconstruction with an interposition graft of autogenous tissue is recommended. Saphenous vein, hypogastric artery, or the external iliac artery are often the autograft of choice. Failure to completely repair the vessel is likely to predispose to thromboembolic events and in the innominate, the carotid, and the popliteal arteries, these types of wounds can lead to thrombosis and serious embolic complications, and cause severe irreversible neurologic deficits or limb loss.

Initial repair of these lesions is much simpler than delayed repair. Moreover, if a false aneurysm or an arteriovenous fistula does occur, it is best to repair these at the time of identification. Spontaneous cure of false aneurysms occurs in less than 6 percent of reported cases, and less than 2 percent of the arteriovenous fistulas will spontaneously resolve. Because the lesions often enlarge and become more complex, and the technical problems presented to the surgeon become more formidable, it is advisable to repair these lesions at the outset. Very good results can be expected if the initial repair is performed without unnecessary delay.

RESULTS

Table 2 lists the results obtained in the author's experience with over 665 arterial injuries of which 9 percent were caused by blunt trauma. There is a 10 percent mortality, usually the result of multiple wounds of the major vessels in the thorax and abdomen. The amputation rate was 1.8 percent in the entire series, but injuries caused by blunt trauma were less favorable. Most series report an amputation rate greater than 35 percent in these patients, but it was 14 percent in this series.

Table 2. Results of Treatment (in the Author's Experience)

	(%)
Failure of repair	5.2
Bleeding	2.0
Infection	3.1
Amputation	1.8
Mortality	10.4

Many patients, who have complete occlusion of the internal carotid artery as a result of blunt trauma, are likely to have severe neurologic deficits that may not be improved by surgery.[17] In most of these patients, it appears that the outcome is largely the result of the initial neurologic deficit that occurs at the time that the artery becomes occluded, although in some cases distal embolization may lead to the delayed appearance of a stroke. When prograde carotid artery flow has not been interrupted, arterial repair is indicated. Conversely, if the artery is completely occluded as a result of blunt trauma, and the patient has a severe neurologic deficit associated with coma, the results of arterial repair are likely to be unfavorable. In addition, complete repair of the artery and removal of all the distal clots are necessary in order to prevent extension of the neurologic deficit.[15] If this is not technically possible, surgical repair may be contraindicated.

REFERENCES

1. Connolly J: Management of fractures associated with arterial injuries. Am J Surg 120:331, 1971
2. Dajee H, Richardson ITN, Iype MO: Seat belt aorta: Acute dissection and thrombosis of the abdominal aorta. Surg 85:263, 1979

3. Dart CH, Braitman HE: Popliteal artery injury following fracture or dislocation at the knee. Arch Surg 112:969, 1977
4. Flint LM, Synder WH, Perry MO et al.: Management of major vascular injuries in the base of the neck. An 11 year experience with 146 cases. Arch Surg 106:407, 1973
5. Jernigan WR, Gardner WC: Carotid artery injuries due to closed cervical trauma. J Trauma 11:429, 1971
6. Killeen DA: Injuries of the SMA vessels secondary to nonpenetrating abdominal trauma. Ann Surg 30:306, 1964
7. Klingersmith W, Oles P, Martinez H: Arterial injuries associated with dislocation of the knee or fracture of the lower femur. Surg Gynecol Obstet 120:961, 1965
8. Lefrak EA: Knee dislocation: An illusive cause of critical arterial occlusion. Arch Surg 111:1021, 1976
9. Plume S, DeWeese JA: Traumatic rupture of the thoracic aorta. Arch Surg 114:240, 1979
10. Reul GJ, Beall RC, Jordon GL, et al.: The early operative management of injuries to the great vessels. Surg 74:862, 1973
11. Reynolds RR, McDowell HA, Diethelm AG: The surgical treatment of arterial injuries in the civilian population. Ann Surg 189:700, 1979
12. Sher MH: Principles in the management of arterial injuries associated with fracture dislocations. Ann Surg 182:630, 1975
13. Snyder WH, Watkins WL, Whiddon LL, Bone GE: Civilian popliteal artery trauma: An eleven year experience with eighty three injuries. Surg 85:101, 1979
14. Thal ER, Perry MO, Crighton J: Traumatic abdominal aortic occlusion. Southern Med Jour 64:653, 1971
15. Thal ER, Snyder WH, Hays RJ, Perry MO: Management of carotid artery injuries. Surg 76:955, 1974
16. Waddell JP, Lencner EM: Arterial injury associated with skeletal trauma. Injury 6:28, 1974
17. Yamada S, Kindt GN, Youman TR: Carotid artery occlusion due to nonpenetrating injury. J Trauma 7:333, 1967

Part Six

Problems in Carotid Surgery

TWENTY-THREE

Role of Noninvasive Testing and Imaging in Carotid Disease

David S. Sumner

A plethora of noninvasive methods for diagnosing disease at the carotid bifurcation have been introduced over the past two decades. As a result of numerous articles, presentations, and meetings devoted to the subject, these methods are commanding ever increasing attention. Manufacturers have responded with a host of instruments designed to implement the various techniques. The result today is confusion. Some of the questions being asked are: Which method is best? Which instrument is best? But more to the point, one might ask what is the role of noninvasive testing in the diagnosis of extracranial carotid arterial disease?

Although some skeptics maintain that these studies have yet to find a use and others cautiously suggest that they may have a limited but ill-defined role, a growing body of enthusiasts feel that they have proved to be accurate and should be an integral part of every evaluation for carotid occlusive disease. In this chapter, I shall endeavor to steer a course between negativism and overenthusiasm by reviewing the accuracy and limitations of the various tests, listing the roles that have been suggested, and, when possible, providing evidence to support their value.

ACCURACY

The accuracy of a test is best defined in terms of its sensitivity (ability to detect the presence of disease) and specificity (ability to recognize the absence of disease). These terms are independent of the relative numbers of true negatives and true positives in the total population and are, therefore, more meaningful than the overall accuracy. When the test is being applied to a population with a high probability of carotid disease, a high sensitivity is desirable to avoid missing clinically important lesions. If it is being used to screen an asymptomatic population with a low incidence of carotid disease, however, the test should have a high specificity to avoid unnecessary arteriography.

Accuracy of noninvasive tests for disease at the carotid bifurcation is currently assessed by comparing the results with contrast arteriograms. What is considered to be a "positive" or "negative" arteriogram will vary depending upon the population being examined and the questions being asked. Any lesion, regardless of size, that could be responsible for emboli might be called "positive" in patients with stroke, TIAs, or amaurosis fugax. On the other hand, only those lesions that are hemodynamically significant (narrowing the arterial diameter by more than 50 percent) might be considered positive in patients with asymptomatic bruits.

Finally, it is important to know what percentage of the tests are uninterpretable and whether the test can distinguish no disease from minimal disease, minimal disease from severe disease, and severe disease from total occlusion. Unfortunately, few reports answer all of these questions.

METHODS

Noninvasive methods for examining the carotid system may be classified into those that depend upon alterations in blood flow or blood pressure (physiologic tests) and those that attempt to depict the pathologic anatomy of the carotid bifurcation (imaging techniques). Not only do the sensitivities and specificities of the tests vary widely, but also different investigators report markedly different accuracies for the same test. None of the methods can reliably detect ulceration in a nonstenotic artery; but ulceration in the absence of any degree of stenosis is rare, occurring in only 6.5 percent of patients with TIAs.

Physiologic Tests

Included in the group of physiologic tests are supraorbital Doppler sonography,[5] and photoplethysmography,[1] thermography, pulse delay oculoplethysmography (OPG—Kartchner),[20] ophthalmodynamometry, and ocular pressure plethysmography (OPG—Gee).[12] Because these methods all depend upon recognition of hemodynamic changes at sites remote from the carotid bifurcation, they cannot be expected to detect diameter stenoses less than 40 to 50 percent (64 to 75 percent reduction in cross-sectional area). All are more accurate for lesions in the 75 to 100 percent range and are rather insensitive to lesions in the 50 to 75 percent range. They cannot distinguish between total occlusion and severe disease or between minimal disease and no disease. In general, they tend to have a high specificity but only a moderately good sensitivity (Table 1). For optimal accuracy, some of these tests require carotid compression, a maneuver that may introduce a small risk.

Table 1. Reported Accuracy of Physiologic Tests for Distinguishing Hemodynamically Significant From Nonhemodynamically Significant Lesions

	Number of Reports	Stenosis Considered Positive on X-Ray (%)	Sensitivity Median % Range	Specificity Median % Range
Phonoangiography	9	40–50	58 (16–85)	93 (82–96)
Supraorbital Doppler	19	40–75	76 (17–96)	96 (69–100)
Photoplethysmography	4	33–50	67 (30–100)	87 (63–91)
Pulse delay OPG	14	40–60	62 (48–91)	91 (35–97)
Pressure OPG	10	50–75	88 (28–97)	94 (39–100)
Ophthalmodynamometry	3	50	63 (58–90)	86 (86–87)

Other physiologic tests, such as carotid phonoangiography (CPA), audio frequency analysis of carotid bruits, and Doppler flow signal analysis, assess flow patterns in close proximity to the carotid bifurcation. Although the specificity of the CPA is usually good, its sensitivity is poor (Table 1). Audio frequency analysis of the bruit may afford a more accurate determination of the severity of the lesion than is possible with simple phonoangiography.

Doppler flow signals, detected at the carotid bifurcation, can be interpreted audibly by a skilled examiner; but analogue recordings permit a more detailed analysis of changes in the contour of the flow pulse. Many of these changes have been found to correlate with the degree of stenosis. Analysis of the frequency spectrum of the Doppler signal can now be performed in real-time by multiple filter or fast-Fourier-transformation methods. Initial reports indicate that many lesions with stenosis less than 10 percent, the majority of those with stenosis between 10 and 50 percent, and over 90 percent of those with greater than 50 percent stenosis can be detected by these techniques.[3] Furthermore, they differentiate between total occlusion and severe stenosis with a

344 Critical Problems in Vascular Surgery

high degree of accuracy. They may not, however, be quite as specific as the other physiologic tests in distinguishing between minimal (< 50 percent) and severe stenosis (> 50 percent) (Table 2).

Imaging Techniques

Two methods for depicting the carotid bifurcation are currently available: B-mode scanning and Doppler flow signal mapping. The Doppler instruments, which produce an image resembling a conventional arteriogram, are popularly called "ultrasonic arteriographs." They employ either continuous wave or pulsed ultrasonic energy, the latter having the potential advantage of allowing cross-sectional images to be made (Fig. 1). Small hemodynamically insignificant lesions are frequently recognized; about 90 percent of the more severe lesions are detected; and severe stenosis can be differentiated from total occlusion with a moderate degree of accuracy.[13,23] Moreover, they provide some estimate of the degree of stenosis. None of the Doppler devices are real-time. B-mode scans, on the other hand, may be obtained in real-time, but they have the disadvantage of being unable to detect thrombi and some plaques that have an acoustic impedance similar to that of blood. When used alone, they frequently miss total occlusions. Combining B-mode scanning with Doppler flow signal analysis tends to eliminate these errors (Table 3).[3]

Table 2. Reported Accuracy of Doppler Signals from Carotid Bifurcation

	Stenosis Considered Positive on X-Ray (%)	Sensitivity (%)	Specificity (%)
Audible signal	50	95	83
	> 0	55	95
Analogue signal*	> 0	100	94
Spectral analysis			
Continous wave	70	63	85
	60	75	80
	50	90–100	34–63
	> 0	64–90	55–64
Pulsed	50	100	95
	10	84	76
	> 0	85	88

* *Retrospective analysis.*

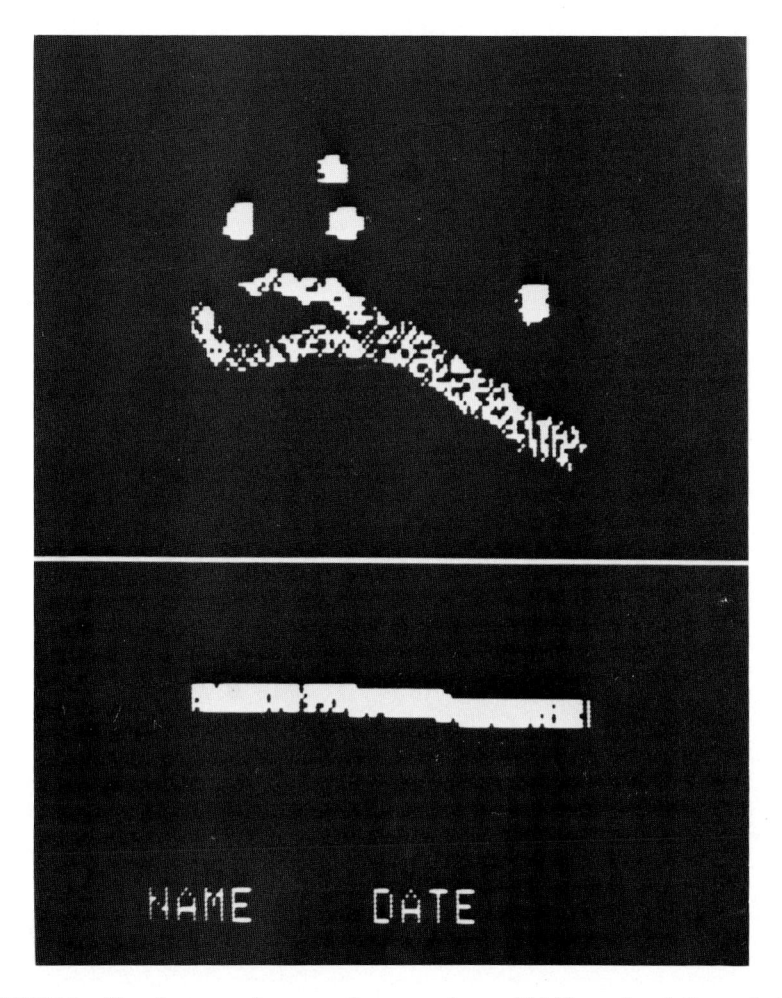

FIGURE 1. Simultaneous images of a normal carotid bifurcation in lateral view (upper panel), anteroposterior view (lower panel), and cross-sectional views (above lateral view in upper panel). In the lateral view, the internal carotid artery is shown below the external. The external carotid artery is not depicted in the anteroposterior view. Images were made with a microcomputer attachment for the Hokanson ultrasonic arteriograph. (Designed by R. D. Miles.)

Combined Approaches

Combinations of various tests will increase sensitivity and specificity when the results agree; but when they disagree, the examiner is forced to weigh one test against another and make a decision. In such cases, both sensitivity and specificity are usually decreased (Table 4).

Table 3. Reported Accuracy of Imaging Techniques

	Stenosis Considered Positive on X-Ray (%)	Sensitivity Median % Range	Specificity Median % Range
Pulsed–Doppler	40–50†	88 (48–93)	85 (55–92)
	10–25‡	80 (75–96)	75 (44–87)
	>0‡	75 (70–77)	81 (77–88)
Continuous wave–Doppler*	50‡	89 (86–92)	94 (77–99)
	>0	75	81
Continuous wave–Doppler, with color-coded velocity*	50	97	86
	25	91	90
	>0	69	94
B-mode	50	73	86
	?>0	100	81
B-mode, real time	50§	66 (57–75)	67 (36–98)
	>0§	92 (84–100)	57 (22–91)
B-mode (duplex scan)*	50	92	92
	>0	78	100

* *Doppler velocity signal analysis used in interpreting results.*
† *Six reports.*
‡ *Three reports.*
§ *Two reports.*

Table 4. Accuracy When Two Tests Agree

Tests*	Stenosis Considered Positive on X-Ray (%)	Sensitivity (%)	Specificity (%)	Concordant (%)
UA and OPG	40	95	94	67
SOD and PPG	50	100	100	47
SOD and PPG	50	95	100	89
SOD and OPG	50	86	100	85

* *UA, pulsed–Doppler imaging; SOD, supraorbital Doppler; PPG, photoplethysmography; OPG, pulse delay oculoplethysmography.*

Another approach is to call a combined study positive when any one of the tests are positive and to call it negative only when all tests are negative. This method, which yields an increased sensitivity but a decreased specificity, may be advantageous when one is dealing with a population having a high incidence of carotid disease (Table 5).

Table 5. Accuracy of Combined Studies*

Tests†	Stenosis Considered Positive on X-Ray (%)	Sensitivity Median % Range	Specificity Median % Range
OPG and CPA‡	40–60	86(65–97)	88(70–89)
OPG and SOD	50	89	95
OPG and UA	40	97	66
OPG, CPA, and UA	60	77	84
OPPG and CPA	50	91	93
OPPG, CPA, and SOD	? 50	94	78

* Study is positive if any test is positive and negative if all tests are negative.
† OPG, pulse delay oculoplethysmography; CPA, carotid phonoangiography; SOD, supraorbital Doppler sonography; UA, pulsed–Doppler imaging; OPPG, oculopneumoplethysmography.
‡ Four reports.

PURPOSE

The major purpose of noninvasive tests of the carotid system is to improve the selection of patients for arteriography. At present, none of the noninvasive tests can match the accuracy of a skillfully performed roentgenographic study; however, arteriography is expensive, time-consuming, requires hospitalization, and demands considerable technical skill. Aside from being uncomfortable, it has a modest complication rate, carries some risk of stroke, and has a low risk of mortality. Furthermore, some patients are allergic to contrast media. For these reasons, many physicians and patients are unwilling to perform arteriography, especially in situations where the incidence of disease is apt to be low.

In addition, noninvasive tests may yield important physiologic information not readily derived from the arteriogram. Occasionally, such tests will reveal surgically important anatomic features that were not perceived on the arteriogram. And finally, noninvasive methods provide a better assessment of extracranial carotid arterial disease than can be obtained by history and physical examination alone. Therefore, these tests have a role in following patients after surgery and in documenting the natural history of the disease.

TRANSIENT ISCHEMIC ATTACKS (TIAs) AND AMAUROSIS FUGAX

Because strokes, TIAs, and amaurosis fugax are often caused by stenoses or ulcerated plaques that narrow the arterial lumen by less than 50 percent, noninvasive tests (especially those that are hemodynamically based) will not indicate the presence of an appreciable number of operable lesions. As pointed out earlier in this chapter, none of the tests in use today can reliably detect an ulcer that does not impinge on the arterial lumen. For these reasons, noninvasive tests are not generally considered to have a prominent role in the evaluation of TIAs and amaurosis fugax, since patients with these manifestations should have angiography even if noninvasive tests are negative.

When the risk of arteriography is great or the symptoms are ill-defined, however, an argument can be made for using noninvasive tests to identify those patients who are most likely to have a lesion at the carotid bifurcation. In this situation, it is desirable to use a test or battery of tests with a high sensitivity. To evaluate whether it is better to obtain arteriograms on all patients with TIAs or just on those with TIAs and positive noninvasive tests would require a carefully controlled prospective study of mortality, strokes, and other morbidity in groups of patients managed by both approaches. No such study is available. Nevertheless, it is possible to make some judgments as to which approach is best based on figures available in the literature. In making such a comparison, as attempted in Tables 6 and 7, it is necessary to consider all events that happen to the patient from the time that it is decided on clinical examination alone that he has a TIA until the study is terminated several years later. This encompasses all deaths, strokes, continued symptoms, and new symptoms that occur at each stage during diagnosis and treatment. It also necessitates knowledge of the natural history of the untreated disease as well as the long-term results of surgery (Figs. 2, 3). Finally, one must consider all the avenues that can be followed after noninvasive

Table 6. Predicted Results in 100 Patients Presenting with Clinical TIAs When Arteriography Is Performed on All or Only on Those with a Positive Noninvasive Test*

	71 Patients with Operable Lesions			
	Total Number Deaths	*Total Number Strokes*	*Total Number TIAs*	*Number Operations†*
In all patients	20–25	5–12	2–6	70
In only those with positive noninvasive test	18–21	12–15	8–10	35

* *Noninvasive test: sensitivity, 90%; specificity, 84%; dividing line between positive and negative, 50% stenosis.*[23]
† *Operation performed on all operable lesions detected by arteriography.*

Noninvasive Testing and Imaging 349

Table 7. Predicted Results in Patients Having Operable Lesions when Arteriography Is Performed on All Patients Presenting with a Clinical TIA or Only on Those with a Positive Noninvasive Test*

	Deaths (%)	Strokes (%)	TIAs (%)	Operations (%)
In all patients	29–35	7–16	2–8	99
In only those with positive noninvasive test	26–29	17–22	11–14	50

* Denominator is total number of patients minus those without operable carotid lesions.

testing (Fig. 3). These tests can be positive in association with a variety of angiographic findings, from normal to total occlusion, and negative in the same groups. The computations in Tables 6 and 7 were prepared using the flow charts illustrated in Figures 2 and 3 and were derived from the following data: relative number of occlusions, stenosis greater than 50 percent, stenosis less than 50 percent, ulcers without stenosis, inaccessible lesions, and normal arteries in a group of patients with TIAs[8]; the incidence of death and stroke following arteriography[24]; the natural history of unoperated patients with TIAs and stroke[15,26]; and the incidence of death, stroke, and continued TIAs in patients following surgery.[7,25,26,29]

As shown in Tables 6 and 7, obtaining arteriography only in those patients in whom the noninvasive test is positive does not seem to affect the overall mortality rate adversely over a 3- to 5-year period; however, the number of strokes and the number of patients who continue to have TIAs would be almost doubled. Of 100 patients originally presenting with TIAs, however, restriction of angiography to only those patients with positive noninvasive studies would result in only 3 to 7 more strokes and 4 to 7 more patients who continue to have TIAs (Table 6).

This analysis is not intended to justify the use of noninvasive tests as a means of selecting patients for arteriography, in fact, it does just the opposite, but it does support the use of this approach under adverse circumstances, since the absolute risk in terms of the number of additional strokes or TIAs does not appear to be great.

STROKE

Patients with a completed stroke may continue to have TIAs or remain in jeopardy for a subsequent stroke when the responsible lesion is still present. In the event that the ipsilateral carotid is totally occluded, a

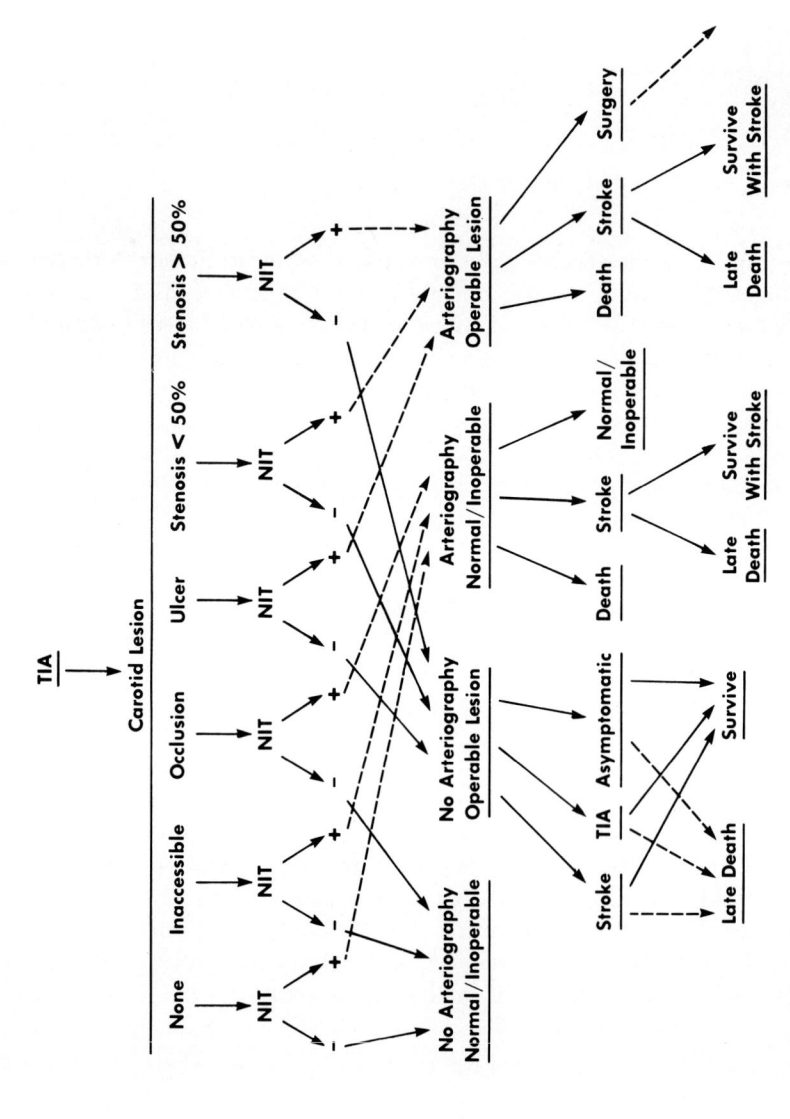

FIGURE 2. Flow chart depicting outcome of patients with transient ischemic attacks, all patients subjected to arteriography. Data derived from this chart are shown in Tables 6 and 7.

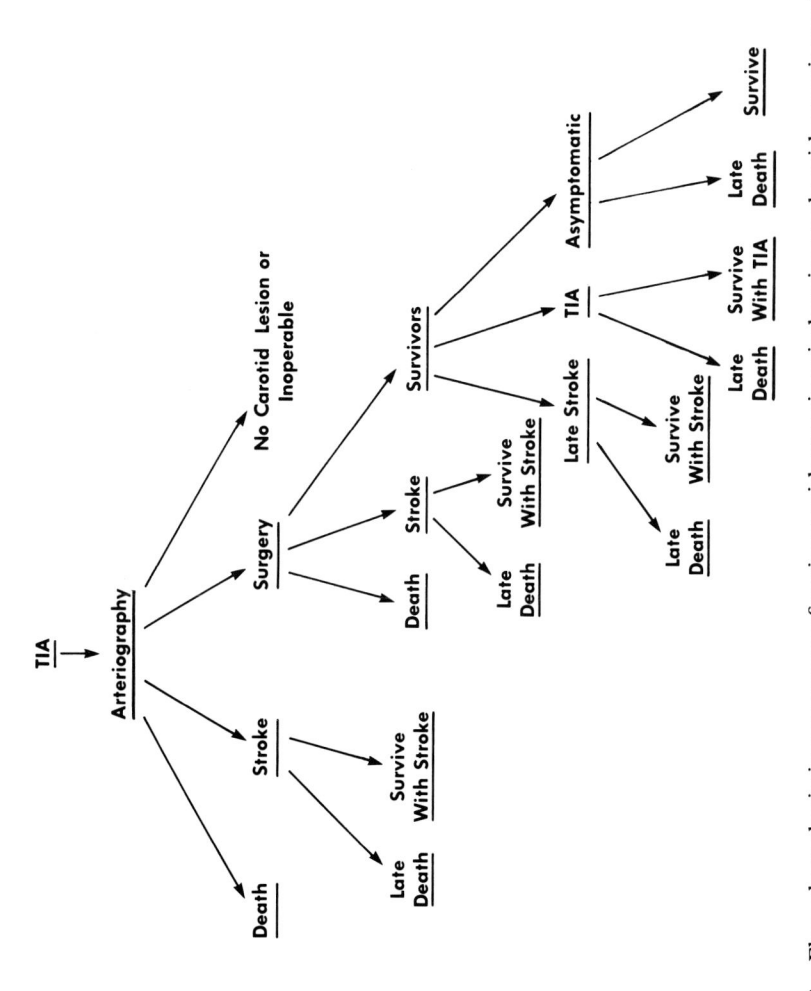

FIGURE 3. Flow chart depicting outcome of patients with transient ischemic attacks with arteriography reserved for patients with positive noninvasive tests (NIT). Data derived from this chart are shown in Tables 6 and 7.

stenotic lesion in the opposite carotid may pose a significant hazard. Some of these patients, particularly those with minimal deficits, are candidates for delayed endarterectomy. The surgical morbidity and mortality in this group are considerably higher, however, the protection against further strokes is less evident, and the functional improvement is harder to define than in patients with TIAs. Although many surgeons, including the author, advocate arteriography in many stroke patients with a mild neurologic deficit who are good surgical candidates, there is more justification for using noninvasive tests to select those patients who should have arteriography in this group than in patients with TIAs. If subjected to an analysis similar to that applied to the TIA group, the approach using noninvasive testing to select patients for angiography (3- to 5-year mortality, 36.5 percent; new strokes 27.0 percent) compares favorably with the approach using arteriography on all patients (mortality, 37.3 percent; new strokes 25.6 percent).[8,14,15,18,24,25]

NONLOCALIZING SYMPTOMS AND SIGNS

Patients with nonhemispheric symptoms, such as dizziness, lightheadedness, vertigo, ataxia, syncope, drop attacks, diplopia, bilateral visual blurring, dysarthria, confusion, bilateral paresis, or bilateral paresthesias, frequently present a difficult diagnostic problem. Although many of these patients will have carotid or vertebrobasilar lesions, the relationship of these lesions to the symptoms is seldom clear. Because it is unlikely that the symptoms are the result of emboli from the carotid bifurcation, it is hard to rationalize treatment of a hemodynamically insignificant carotid lesion. It is easier to justify an operation on a flow-reducing stenosis, since augmentation of cerebral blood pressure or flow may alleviate relative ischemia in other areas of the brain. Noninvasive tests may be used to identify those patients who are most likely to have a significant stenosis of the carotid arteries, thus, sparing the majority the need for arteriography.[20]

ASYMPTOMATIC BRUIT

Many bruits in the neck do not signify a significant stenosis of the common or internal carotid artery and, therefore, do not merit investigation. Yet, not all asymptomatic bruits are benign. The problem is to identify those patients in whom the risk of cerebrovascular symptoms is great enough to justify surgical intervention. Stenoses severe enough to be hemodynamically significant are considered to be more hazardous than those that compromise the lumen to a lesser extent. Support for this concept has been provided by Kartchner and McCrae,[20] who found that 12 percent of their patients with asymptomatic bruits who had a positive OPG and CPA suffered a stroke during the follow-up period, while only 2 percent of those with negative tests did so. Such studies provide the rationale for using noninvasive tests to select patients for arteriography and possible surgery. As a corollary, when the noninvasive tests are negative, it is safe to forego further investigation. This reasonable approach has yet to be proven correct by the results of a prospective, randomized, controlled study; because of the known propensity for lesions to progress, however, patients with bruits should be examined at yearly intervals.

PRIOR TO MAJOR VASCULAR PROCEDURES

Several studies have failed to demonstrate that the presence of an asymptomatic bruit increases the risk of stroke in patients undergoing major vascular reconstruction.[6,9,27] These studies, however, did not define the actual incidence of hemodynamically significant carotid lesions in either the patients with bruits or in the control group. That cerebral ischemia could develop during a period of hypotension in the territory supplied by a severely stenosed carotid artery (especially one that is poorly collateralized) is a reasonable assumption. McCrae and associates[20] reported a 17 percent incidence of strokes occurring in the perioperative period in patients with positive OPGs. In contrast, only 1 percent of the patients with a negative OPG suffered a perioperative stroke. It can be argued, therefore, that all patients undergoing a major vascular or cardiac operation should be screened noninvasively whether or not they have a cervical bruit. If a hemodynamically significant lesion is found, arteriography should be performed. If this reveals a stenotic lesion, a prophylactic carotid endarterectomy probably should be performed. Although this approach seems reasonable, final proof of its efficacy would require a prospective, randomized, controlled study. Such studies have been proposed but none as yet has been completed.

EVALUATION PRIOR TO EXTRACRANIAL CAROTID SURGERY

Although noninvasive testing has a limited role in the diagnostic evaluation of patients with classical TIAs, strokes, and amaurosis fugax, a preoperative baseline study is valuable if postoperative follow-up examinations are planned. Moreover, angiography is not infallible. Some angiograms are technically inadequate, others are incomplete, and some can be misinterpreted. Occasionally, an unequivocally positive noninvasive study will be obtained when the angiogram has been read as negative. In these cases, a rereading or a repeat angiogram may reveal a hitherto unsuspected lesion at the aortic arch or in the intracranial carotid or ophthalmic arteries. Imaging techniques or Doppler surveys of the carotid bifurcation may reveal patency of the extracranial external and internal carotid arteries when the common carotid is occluded up to, but not including, the bifurcation.[2] This situation, which is readily amenable to a subclavian-carotid bypass, can sometimes also be overlooked on the angiogram owing to timing factors or inadequate concentration of the contrast medium.

Measurements of ophthalmic arterial pressure with the oculopneumoplethysmograph (OPG-Gee)[12] and the direction of supraorbital blood flow as determined by Doppler sonography[5] have been shown to correlate well with the internal carotid stump pressure when these noninvasive tests are performed during common carotid compression. Such estimates have, perhaps, a limited use in predicting the need for an intraoperative shunt, but this remains unproven. For example, when the estimate of the stump pressure is high (> 60 mm Hg) or when supraorbital Doppler or photoplethysmographic studies demonstrate excellent intracranial collaterals, it is probably safe to proceed with carotid ligation in patients with inaccessible aneurysms of the internal carotid artery or intracranial arteries, subintimal carotid dissection, traumatic lesions of the carotid syphon, or carotid-cavernous sinus fistulas.

Noninvasive studies may aid in the selection of patients for extra- and intracranial (EC-IC) bypass. It is unlikely that EC-IC bypass would be of much value when supraorbital Doppler sonography indicates normally directed flow on the side of an occluded carotid artery or when the ipsilateral ophthalmic arterial pressure exceeds 60 mm Hg.[11]

When bilaterally equal carotid lesions are present, noninvasive tests may be of value in deciding which lesion to operate on first.[5,12] The initial operation should be performed on the side with the best collateral circulation as determined by noninvasive techniques, since the improved pressure head may benefit the opposite side, making subsequent operations safer.

Finally, Stanton and his colleagues have shown that the OPG can be used to determine the hemodynamic significance of kinked internal carotid arteries.[22] A delay in pulse arrival time with the neck turned implies that the lumen of the carotid artery is being functionally compromised with position change.

INTRAOPERATIVE MONITORING

Intraluminal shunts may become obstructed during the course of the operation due to kinking of the internal carotid artery or impingement of the distal end of the shunt on the arterial wall. Such occlusions are apt to go unrecognized by the surgeon. Application of a sterile Doppler probe to the common carotid artery below the shunt can be used to demonstrate continuing adequate flow. Continuous monitoring of shunt patency is also possible with the air-filled OPG or the supraorbital photoplethysmograph.

Operative arteriography will show residual defects in 2 to 4 percent of external carotid arteries, 2 to 3 percent of internal carotid arteries, and 1 to 2 percent of common carotid arteries. Because operative arteriography carries some risk, is time consuming, and the pictures are often inadequate, it is not commonly performed; consequently, some potentially correctible defects are undoubtedly missed. By using a sterile Doppler to survey the operative area, the surgeon will be able to detect most of the major defects.[10] The supraorbital photoplethysmograph may also be used to evaluate the patency of the internal and external carotid arteries following endarterectomy.[10]

POSTOPERATIVE MONITORING

When a patient awakens with a hemiparesis or awakens normal and then develops a neurologic defect, the reconstructed carotid artery may have thrombosed. Many of these defects can be reversed by immediate surgery. Seldom is there time for an arteriogram. Finding an occluded carotid artery by noninvasive testing dictates the proper course. If, however, the carotid artery is unequivocally open, then one can assume that the neurologic defect is probably related to intraoperative ischemia or to emboli and surgery can be avoided.[10] Because of its portability, the Doppler with supraorbital or direct recording over the internal carotid is particularly useful for these studies.

POSTOPERATIVE FOLLOW-UP

The mere fact that a carotid reconstruction is patent at the end of the procedure does not ensure its continued patency. While symptomatic restenosis is rare (1.5 to 3.6 percent), asymptomatic narrowing is probably much more common. In an arteriographic study of asymptomatic patients examined one or more years following carotid endarterectomy, 54 percent were found to have residual or recurrent narrowing.[19] Noninvasive methods have shown that complete obstruction can occur without symptoms in the first 4 or 5 postoperative days. Garrett and associates,[10] using the Doppler and the photoplethysmograph, found external carotid obstruction in 6.9 percent and internal carotid obstruction in 3.4 percent of patients examined in the early postoperative period. Long-term studies with the OPG-Gee, Doppler imaging, and with the Duplex-Scanner (spectral analysis) suggest that significant restenosis occurs in 9 to 49 percent of patients.[4,17,28] Because of these findings, early noninvasive examination of the endarterectomy site and follow-up studies at yearly intervals are indicated. Even if repeat surgery proves to be unnecessary, such studies will provide information regarding the natural history of the endarterectomized artery.

Some degree of narrowing is commonly found in the nonoperated contralateral carotid artery. The risk of stroke from these lesions does not appear to be high, but whether or not a minor lesion should be operated on remains controversial. It has been demonstrated angiographically that stenosis becomes more severe in 59 percent of nonoperated carotid arteries over an average period of 3 years.[16] Doppler imaging has also shown a 20 percent incidence of progression on the nonoperated side.[28] Consequently, periodic noninvasive studies of the nonoperated side have been advocated as a method for detecting the development of potentially dangerous stenoses.

NATURAL HISTORY, THERAPEUTIC TRIALS, AND SCREENING

Noninvasive testing provides a safe, relatively inexpensive, reasonably accurate alternative to angiography for detecting the presence of and determining the severity of extracranial arterial lesions in patients who are not candidates for surgery. Since the studies can be repeated as often as necessary, they can be used to define the natural history of these lesions. Lack of such information is responsible for much of the current confusion surrounding the proper therapy of patients with carotid disease and its related neurologic sequelae. Consequently, an objective evaluation of the carotid arteries should be an integral part of all therapeutic trials, whether they involve surgery, antiplatelet agents, anticoagulants, or other measures. In the past, epidemiologic studies have usually dealt only with the incidence of bruits, strokes, or TIAs in the populations surveyed. Application of noninvasive tests to these populations would serve to better characterize the extent of extracranial

Table 8. Proposed Roles for Noninvasive Testing in Carotid Disease

Condition	Function of Noninvasive Testing
TIAs, amaurosis fugax, strokes	Prior to or instead of arteriography in patients with medical contraindications to surgery, allergy to contrast media, dense strokes (arteriography indicated in all surgical candidates)
Nonlocalizing symptoms, asymptomatic bruits, major cardiovascular surgery	Arteriography reserved for those with hemodynamically significant lesions
Prior to carotid surgery	Baseline for follow-up study Detect lesions missed on arteriography Establish safety of carotid ligation Suggest need for EC-IC bypass Indicate priority in bilateral carotid lesions Document hemodynamic significance of kinking
Intraoperative	Detect shunt failure, thrombosis, technical errors
Postoperative	Detect thrombosis
Postsurgical follow-up	Detect occlusion, restenosis, disease progression on nonoperated side
Follow-up of nonoperated patients, therapeutic trials, population surveys	Objective diagnosis, detect disease progression

arterial disease and help to relate overt neurologic end points to actual physiologic and anatomic aberrations.

Screening of high-risk populations (e.g., patients with diabetes mellitus, hyperlipidemia, hypertension, coronary artery or peripheral vascular disease, or those with a family history of cardiovascular or cerebrovascular disease) has been advocated. Using the same logic that has been applied to patients with asymptomatic bruits, one could justify an evaluation of prophylactic surgery on some patients with severely stenotic ulcerated carotid arteries that were discovered as a result of such a screening process. Lesions of lesser extent could be followed periodically and active therapy instituted if potentially dangerous progression occurred.

COMMENT

Table 8 contains a summary of the proposed roles for noninvasive testing in carotid diseases. As stated in the introduction, not all investigators agree with these suggestions, and it must be admitted that there is relatively little substantiating evidence. Clearly, further prospective studies are necessary before the role of noninvasive testing in extracranial carotid arterial disease is adequately defined. Perhaps the best attitude to take is the one proposed by Sandok[21] in reference to noninvasive testing of the carotid system:

While progress is being made, some will utilize the available information in the manner they deem most appropriate for the benefit of their patients . . . and that seems reasonable. There must remain some among us who will utilize the data prospectively to try to prove that the assumptions being made are indeed correct . . . that, too, seems reasonable. There will also remain some who will be uncertain about adding these new techniques to their practice. Given the current state of the art . . . that, too, seems reasonable.

REFERENCES

1. Barnes RW, Garrett WU, Slaymaker EE, Reinertson JE: Doppler ultrasound and supraorbital photoplethysmography for noninvasive screening of carotid occlusive disease. Am J Surg 134:183, 1977
2. Blackshear WM Jr, Phillips DJ, Bodily KC, Strandness DE Jr: Ultrasonic demonstration of external and internal carotid patency with common carotid occlusion—A preliminary report. Stroke 11:249, 1980
3. Blackshear WM Jr, Phillips DJ, Thiele BL, et al: Detection of carotid occlusive disease by ultrasonic imaging and pulsed Doppler spectrum analysis. Surgery 86:698, 1979
4. Bodily KC, Zierler RE, Marinelli MR, et al: Flow disturbances following carotid endarterectomy. Surg Gynecol Obstet 151:77, 1980
5. Bone GE, Slaymaker EE, Barnes RW: Noninvasive assessment of collateral blood flow of the cerebral hemisphere by Doppler ultrasound. Surg Gynecol Obstet 145:873, 1977
6. Carney WI Jr, Stewart WB, DePinto DJ, Mucha SJ, Roberts B: Carotid bruit as a risk factor in aortoiliac reconstruction. Surgery 81:567, 1977
7. DeWeese JA, Rob CG, Satran R, et al: Results of carotid endarterectomies for transient ischemic attacks—Five years later. Ann Surg 178:258, 1973
8. Eisenberg RL, Nemzek WR, Moore WS, Mani RL: Relationship of transient ischemic attacks and angiographically demonstrable lesions of carotid artery. Stroke 8:483, 1977
9. Evans WE, Cooperman M: The significance of asymptomatic unilateral carotid bruits in preoperative patients. Surgery 83:521, 1978
10. Garrett WV, Slaymaker EE, Barnes RW: Noninvasive perioperative monitoring of carotid endarterectomy. J Surg Res 26:255, 1979
11. Gee W, McDonald KM, Kaupp HA, Celani VJ, Bast RG: Carotid stenosis plus occlusion: Endarterectomy or bypass? Arch Surg 115:183, 1980.
12. Gee W, Mehigan JT, Wylie EJ: Measurement of collateral cerebral hemi-

spheric blood pressure by ocular pneumoplethysmography. Am J Surg 130:121, 1975
13. Hobson RW II, Berry SM, Katocs AS Jr, et al: Comparison of pulsed Doppler and real-time B-mode echo arteriography for noninvasive imaging of the extracranial carotid arteries. Surg 87:286, 1980
14. Houser OW, Sundt TM Jr, Holman CB, Sandok BA, Burton RC: Atheromatous disease of the carotid artery. Correlation of angiographic, clinical, and surgical findings. J Neurosurg 41:321, 1974
15. Hutchinson EC, Acheson EJ: Strokes, Natural History, Pathology and Surgical Treatment. Philadelphia, Saunders, 1975
16. Javid H, Ostermiller WE Jr, Hengesh JW, et al: Natural history of carotid bifurcation atheroma. Surgery 67:80, 1970
17. Kremen JE, Gee W, Kaupp HA, McDonald KM: Restenosis or occlusion after carotid endarterectomy. A survey with ocular pneumoplethysmography. Arch Surg 114:608, 1979
18. L'Hermitte F, Gautier JC, Derouesné C, Guiraud B: Ischemic accidents in the middle cerebral artery territory. A study of the causes in 122 cases. Arch Neurol 19:248, 1968
19. Maddison FE: Arteriographic evaluation of carotid artery surgery. Am J Roentgenol Radium Ther Nucl Med 109:121, 1970
20. McCrae LP, Crain V, Kartchner MM: Oculoplethysmography and Carotid Phonoangiography (OPG/CPA). Tuscon, Tuscon Medical Center, 1978, pp 1–87
21. Sandok BA: Reply to letter to the editor. Stroke 10:480, 1979
22. Stanton PE, McClusky DA Jr, Lamis PA: Hemodynamic assessment and surgical correction of kinking of the internal carotid artery. Surgery 84:793, 1978
23. Sumner DS, Russell JB, Ramsey DE, Hajjar WM, Miles RD: Noninvasive diagnosis of extracranial carotid arterial disease. A prospective evaluation of pulsed-Doppler imaging and oculoplethysmography. Arch Surg 114:1222, 1979
24. Swanson PD, Calanchini PR, Dyken ML, et al: A cooperative study of hospital frequency and character of transient ischemic attacks, II. Performance of angiography among six centers. JAMA 237:2202, 1977
25. Thompson JE, Austin DJ, Patman RD: Carotid endarterectomy for cerebrovascular insufficiency: Long term results in 592 patients followed up to thirteen years. Ann Surg 172:633, 1970
26. Toole JF, Janeway R, Choi K, et al: Transient ischemic attacks due to atherosclerosis. A prospective study of 160 patients. Arch Neurol 32:5, 1975
27. Treiman RL, Foran RF, Cohen JL, Levin PM, Cossman DV: Carotid bruit. A followup report on its significance in patients undergoing an abdominal aortic operation. Arch Surg 114:1138, 1979
28. Turnipseed WD, Berkoff HA, Crummy A: Postoperative occlusion after carotid endarterectomy. Arch Surg 115:573, 1980
29. West H, Burton R, Roon AJ, et al: Comparative risk of operation and expectant management for carotid disease. Stroke 10:117, 1979

TWENTY-FOUR
Re-stenosis Following Carotid Endarterectomy

Jesse E. Thompson, R. Don Patman,
C. M. Talkington, and Wilson V. Garrett

Successful immediate anatomic restoration of blood flow by operation may be accomplished by endartectomy in almost 100 percent of properly chosen patients with partially occluded carotid arteries. An occasional patient undergoes acute thrombosis early in the postoperative period caused by technical reasons, hypotension, or unrecognized distal disease in the internal carotid artery. While endarterectomy operations in other areas of the peripheral vasculature, especially the femoropopliteal and aortoiliac systems, have exhibited a fairly high incidence of recurrent stenosis during long-term follow-up periods, a number of studies have demonstrated that carotid arteries reconstructed by endarterectomy remain patent for many years with a very low incidence of re-stenosis.

Re-stenosis in the carotid artery takes two forms. One lesion, which usually occurs within the first year after operation, is a form of myointimal proliferation. Stenoses occuring two years or more following the original endarterectomy are usually due to recurrent atherosclerotic disease in the previously endarterectomized site or in the vicinity of the previous endarterectomy.

PERSONAL EXPERIENCE

During a 20-year period beginning in 1957, we have performed 1286 carotid endarterectomies on 1022 patients with cerebrovascular insufficiency.[18,19] Postoperative arteriograms have not been performed routinely, so the total incidence of late re-stenosis or occlusion is not known. During follow-up, however, 8 patients, who originally had 13 endarterectomies, developed cerebral ischemic symptoms from re-stenosis and have required re-operation giving an incidence of 0.78 percent. Eleven stenoses were found in these 8 patients, 3 of whom had bilateral recurrence. The indication for the original operations in all patients was transient ischemic attacks (TIAs). The symptoms of recurrent stenosis were TIAs in 7 patients and a stroke in one patient. The intervals from the original operation to re-operation were 11 months in one patient, and 4, 7, 9, 12, 12, 14, and 16 years in the remaining 7 patients. Ten re-do operations were performed on 8 patients. Endarterectomy plus Dacron patch graft was performed in all 8 patients; endarterectomy alone was done in one, Dacron patch reconstruction in one. A shunt was used in all cases. No mortality or stroke was associated with these operations. Pathology included recurrent atherosclerosis in 8 patients, scarring in one, and intimal hyperplasia with diaphragm formation in one, the latter being in the patient operated upon 11 months following the original surgery. All patients were relieved of their recurrent symptoms.

Although the known rate of carotid re-stenosis with recurrent symptoms in this series is 0.78 percent for 1022 patients or 0.86 percent for 1286 operations, the actual rate of re-stenosis or occlusion is undoubtedly higher since these are known to occur without symptoms. Routine postoperative arteriograms were not done on the patients in this series. The figures cited thus represent a minimal incidence.

SURVEY OF LITERATURE

A number of studies have documented the low incidence of carotid re-stenosis following endarterectomy. Nearly all these studies suffer from the same defect; namely, that routine postoperative arteriography has not been performed in all patients and hence the exact total incidence of stenosis cannot be determined. Most patients have had arteriograms performed only when symptoms have recurred.

In 1967, Blaisdell, Lim, and Hall[1] evaluated 100 patients who had undergone endarterectomy. These investigators performed operative arteriograms at the completion of endarterectomy, 2 to 8 weeks later, and at 5 years. Twenty-five percent of the arteriograms taken at operation revealed an unsuspected defect in the repair, and immediate revision was carried out in all but one patient. Two to eight weeks later, this single patient was the only one who had an occluded artery. Follow-up examination revealed continued patency at the 5-year period in all but one instance, an asymptomatic occlusion. Thus their incidence of late recurrence in this series was 1 percent.

Edwards, Wilson, and Bennett[5] reported on 93 operations in 57 patients. Thirty patients with 43 operated carotid arteries were subjected to follow-up arteriography 5 or more years after operation. Three of these 30 patients had significant symptomatic re-stenosis that was operated upon, an incidence of 7.0 percent or a total incidence of known re-stenosis in the entire group of 3.2 percent. All 3 had fibrous thickening of the wall of the carotid bifurcation without a cleavage plane of dissection. Repair consisted of patch graft angioplasty.

DeWeese et al.[4] studied 205 patients who had 227 carotid artery reconstructions. Information concerning patency of the operated arteries was available in 98 cases. Six of these were found to be thrombosed, giving a re-stenosis rate of 6.12 percent among those studied, or a total known recurrence rate of 2.7 percent.

In 1970, Schutz, Fleming, and Awerbuck[16] studied 50 patients with endarterectomized carotid arteries by postoperative arteriograms. Thirty-nine carotid endarterectomies had been performed for stenosis and 11 for occlusion. Among the 39 arteries done for stenosis, these authors found the patency rate to be 95 percent during follow-up to 6 years.

Stoney and String[17] in 1976 reported 32 recurrent lesions in 29 patients who had undergone endarterectomy from 5 months to 13 years previously. Since these cases occurred among a total of 1654 carotid endarterectomies their known recurrence rate was 1.5 percent. Recurrent atherosclerosis was present in 19 patients, intimal fibrosis in 9 patients, and external stricture in 1. All recurrent atheromas developed more than 2 years following the original operation, with a mean of 5 years. Intimal fibrosis was seen in the first postoperative year in all but one patient, with a mean of 9 months. Reconstructive techniques included endarterectomy with or without patch grafts for atherosclerosis, and patch angioplasty or resection and anastomosis for intimal fibrosis.

In discussing Stoney and String's paper, Imparato[11] reported that he used a vein patch routinely at the first operation and the incidence of recurrence was one-tenth that reported by Stoney and String. Imparato believes that the two processes causing re-stenosis, that is, early neointimal fibrosis and late atherosclerosis, are one and the same: namely, different phases of true atherosclerosis. His work suggests that the atherosclerotic process originates as fibromuscular arterial proliferation of intima or neointima and is precipitated by specific hemodynamic events.

Also discussing Stoney and String's paper, Gaspar[9] noted 5 recurrent stenoses in a series of 650 carotid endarterectomies, an incidence of 0.77 percent. He suggested that routine use of a shunt allowed for a better endarterectomy by removing all the shreds of intima and media. He also emphasized that completion arteriography was an important feature and probably contributed to the low recurrence rate.

In 1978 Cossman et al.[3] found a 3.6 percent incidence of re-stenosis within 26 months among 360 carotid endarterectomy operations. Patients in this group tended to be younger (average age of 54 years) than the overall group. Hypertension and hyperlipidemia were also more frequent. Re-stenosis occurred within an average of 12.5 months after the first operation with a range of 5 to 24 months. Re-stenosis was attributed to a rapid exuberant myointimal proliferation. Re-operation in this group of patients was difficult and was only infrequently associated with improvements in signs and symptoms.

In 1979 Hertzer et al.[10] reported on the incidence of re-stenosis in 1250 patients undergoing carotid endarterectomy at the Cleveland Clinic. Fifteen patients underwent 16 re-operations. The incidence of known recurrent stenosis was 1.04 percent. The interval between the original procedure and re-operation was 7 months to 3 years, with a mean of 45 months. Myointimal fibroplasia was confirmed microscopically in only 2 patients, one at 7 months and one at 85 months. The remaining lesions were typical atherosclerotic lesions. Ten of the 16 re-operations consisted of carotid endarterectomy with vein patch angioplasty. One patient had angioplasty without endarterectomy. Three patients had primary closure. One patient underwent endarterectomy and replacement of the carotid bifurcation with a Dacron graft. Shunts were used in 12 of the 16 operations. Fourteen of the 15 patients have had no further neurologic symptoms. These authors state that recurrent stenoses usually are discovered because of recurrent neurologic symptoms.

In an effort to detect re-stenosis without employing arteriography, several investigators have employed noninvasive techniques during long-term follow-up after carotid endarterectomy. Kartchner and McRae[12] in 1978 reported on the use of ocular plethysmography (OPG) to follow patients after endarterectomy to determine if recurrent stenosis occurred. These investigators followed over 700 patients with this method. Postendarterectomy progression of abnormalities was noted in 34 patients with arteriographic confirmation in 28, for an incidence of 4.85 percent. In chronic postoperative cases, re-stenosis was noted in 24 patients or 3.42 percent. Twelve cases occurred within 2 to 24 months and 12 occurred after 24 months. Re-stenosis in the 2- to 24-month period was due to a fibrotic stenosis of the arterial wall, while after 24 months, re-stenosis resulted from recurrence of atheromatous plaque.

In 1979 Kremen et al.[13] reported on 141 patients having 173 carotid endarterectomies and surveyed postoperatively by OPG-Gee. Seventeen (12 percent) of the patients had positive OPG examinations. Three (1.7 percent) demonstrated symptomatic recurrent stenosis. An additional 1.1 percent of the operated arteries had asymptomatic recurrent stenosis. A total recurrence rate of 9.8% was found; however, these were not all confirmed by arteriography. A 9.8 percent recurrence rate may well be too high if the OPG alone is used for evaluation without confirmation by arteriography. A number of positive OPGs have been observed after operation when arteriograms done later did not reveal any lesions responsible for the positive test. This has occurred in our own series and has also been noted by Kartchner. Nevertheless, the OPG would appear to be an acceptable way of following patients postoperatively to screen for recurrence.

ROLE OF ANTIPLATELET AGENTS

The role of antiplatelet agents in the prevention of ischemic cerebral episodes and of carotid re-stenosis following endarterectomy remains controversial. Two recent randomized studies in patients with transient ischemic attacks have been reported. In the American study,[7] aspirin and a placebo were used. The results are shown in Table 1. There was no statistically significant reduction in the incidence of stroke in the aspirin-treated patients compared with controls. There was, however, a significant reduction in the incidence of TIAs among patients treated with aspirin. Follow-up was from 5 to 37 months with an average of 24 months. In the Canadian study,[2] aspirin, sulfinpyrazone, and a combination of the two drugs were compared with a placebo in two groups of patients with TIAs (Table 2). In women, no reduction in stroke incidence could be claimed for the treated patients. In men, no significant reduction occurred in stroke occurrence in the group treated with aspirin alone or with sulfinpyrazone alone. At this point in time, it cannot be demonstrated that aspirin is effective in stroke prevention in patients with TIAs.

In another study, Fields et al.[8] administered aspirin and a placebo

Table 1. Comparison of Aspirin and Placebo in Reducing Incidence of Stroke and TIA*

	Aspirin	Placebo
No. of subjects	88	90
Strokes	11 (12.5%)	15 (16.7%)
TIAs	8 (9.1%)	20 (22.2%)
Total	19 (21.6%)	35 (38.9%)

From Fields WS, Lemak NA, Frankowski RF, Hardy RJ: Stroke 8:301, 1977.
* Follow-up was from 5 to 37 months.

Table 2. Results of the Canadian Cooperative Study*

	Sulfinpyrazone	Aspirin	Both	Neither
Subjects (men)	115	98	102	91
Strokes	25	14	6	15
Incidence (%)	21.7	14.3	5.9	16.5
Subjects (women)	41	46	44	48
Strokes	4	8	8	5
Incidence (%)	9.8	17.4	18.2	10.4

From Canadian Cooperative Study Group: N Engl J Med 299:53, 1978.
* Follow-up was on the average 26 months.

postoperatively to 125 patients undergoing carotid endarterectomy (Table 3). Follow-up was to 24 months. A reduction in strokes and recurrent TIAs in the aspirin-treated group is apparent. However, the incidence of ischemic episodes in the control group, which is small, is higher than that reported in several other larger series with longer follow-up.

The influence of aspirin and dipyridamole on the incidence of neointimal hyperplasia at suture lines when various prosthetic materials have been sutured to host arteries has been studied in experimental animals by several investigators. Oblath et al.[15] studied the effects of aspirin and dipyridamole on the formation of neointimal fibrous hyperplasia in dogs when knitted Dacron velour and PTFE grafts were used to bypass short segments of canine femoral arteries. Although the doses of the drugs were considerably higher than comparable doses usually employed in humans, these investigators found that antiplatelet therapy prevented the development of neointimal fibrous hyperplasia at the anastomoses of prosthetic vascular grafts, presumably secondary to reduced platelet adherence to the graft.

Table 3. Effect of Aspirin in Postendarterectomy Patients Follow-up to 24 months

	Aspirin	Placebo
Subjects	65	60
Operations	70	68
Recurrent TIAs	4	8
Nonfatal strokes	1	3
Fatal stroke	0	1

From Fields WS, Lemak NA, Frankowski RF, Hardy RJ: Stroke 9:309, 1978.

Feins et al.[6] in similar experiments from the same laboratory studied the effect of aspirin and dipyridamole on human umbilical vein grafts and negatively charged bovine heterografts placed as bypasses in the femoral arteries of dogs. Autogenous vein grafts were placed as controls. Platelet aggregation inhibition significantly improved the patency of human umbilical vein grafts (from 10 to 60 percent) but had no effect on patency of autogenous veins (100 percent) or on negatively charged bovine heterografts (0 percent patency). Neointimal fibrous hyperplasia at both proximal and distal anastomoses was shown to be intimately associated with late graft occlusions.

In 1980, McCann, Hagen, and Fuchs[14] reported the effects of aspirin and dipyridamole in monkeys who had bilateral vein bypass grafts placed in the iliac arteries followed by injury to the intima of the vessels. All vessels with intimal injury in the placebo group, except one, exhibited intimal hyperplasia compared to the drug-treated group, in which over half were normal. Their data suggest that vascular intimal hyperplasia can be reduced by treatment with antiplatelet agents.

Further studies in humans are necessary before final conclusions can be drawn regarding the effect of the various antiplatelet agents on the formation of neointimal fibrous hyperplasia and the rate of long-term stenosis or occlusion in vessels treated by endarterectomy and bypass operations.

SUMMARY

Carotid endarterectomy carries a low but definite incidence of late known re-stenosis of from less than 1 percent to 7 percent. Re-stenosis within the first year is due to myointimal proliferation while atherosclerosis is the cause of later occurrence. Patch graft angioplasty is the most common method of repair. Antiplatelet agents have not resulted in any reduction in the incidence of stroke in patients with TIAs. However, aspirin appears to reduce the incidence of recurrent TIAs in unoperated patients and to lower the frequency of such attacks in postendarterectomized patients. Experimental studies in animals suggest that antiplatelet agents reduce the incidence of neointimal fibrous hyperplasia at suture lines constructed with various prosthetic grafts.

REFERENCES

1. Blaisdell WF, Lim R Jr, Hall AD: Technical result of endarterectomy. Arteriographic assessment. Am J Surg 114:239, 1967

2. Canadian Cooperative Study Group: A randomized trial of aspirin and sulfinpyrazone in threatened stroke. N Engl J Med 299:53, 1978
3. Cossman D, Callow AD, Stein A, Matsumoto G: Early re-stenosis after carotid endarterectomy. Arch Surg 113:275, 1978
4. DeWeese JA, Rob CG, Satran R, et al.: Surgical treatment for occlusive disease of the carotid artery. Ann Surg 168:85, 1968
5. Edwards WS, Wilson TAS, Bennett A: The long-term effectiveness of carotid endarterectomy in prevention of strokes. Ann Surg 168:765, 1968
6. Feins RH, Roederscheimer LR, Green RM, DeWeese JA: Platelet aggregation inhibition in human umbilical vein grafts and negatively charged bovine heterografts. Surgery 85:395, 1979
7. Fields WS, Lemak NA, Frankowski RF, Hardy RJ: Controlled trial of aspirin in cerebral ischemia. Stroke 8:301, 1977
8. Fields WS, Lemak NA, Frankowski RF, Hardy RJ: Controlled trial of aspirin in cerebral ischemia, Part II: Surgical group. Stroke 9:309, 1978
9. Gaspar MR: In discussion of Stoney and String. Surgery 80:705, 1976
10. Hertzer NR, Martinez BD, Benjamin SP, Beven EG: Recurrent stenosis after carotid endarterectomy. Surg Gynecol Obstet 149:360, 1979
11. Imparato AM: In discussion of Stoney and String. Surgery 80:705, 1976
12. Kartchner MM, McRae LR: Noninvasive assessment of the progression of extracranial carotid disease. In Diethrich EB (ed): Noninvasive Cardiovascular Diagnosis, Current Concepts. Baltimore, University Park Press, 1978, p 13
13. Kremen JE, Gee W, Kaupp HA, McDonald KM: Re-stenosis or occlusion after carotid endarterectomy. A survey with ocular pneumoplethysmography. Arch Surg 114:608, 1979
14. McCann RL, Hagen P-O, Fuchs JCA: Aspirin and dipyridamole decrease intimal hyperplasia in experimental vein grafts. Ann Surg 191:238, 1980
15. Oblath RW, Buckley FO Jr, Green RM, Schwartz SI, DeWeese JA: Prevention of platelet aggregation and adherence to prosthetic vascular grafts by aspirin and dipyridamole. Surgery 84:37, 1978
16. Schutz H, Fleming JFR, Awerbuck B: Arteriographic assessment of carotid endarterectomy. Ann Surg 171:509, 1970
17. Stoney RJ, String ST: Recurrent carotid stenosis. Surgery 80:705, 1976
18. Thompson JE, Austin DJ, Patman RD: Carotid endarterectomy for cerebrovascular insufficiency: Long-term results in 592 patients followed up to thirteen years. Ann Surg 172:663, 1970
19. Thompson JE, Patman RD, Talkington CM: Asymptomatic carotid bruit: Long-term outcome of patients having endarterectomy compared with unoperated controls. Ann Surg 188:308, 1978

Part Seven

Problems in Aortic Surgery

TWENTY-FIVE
Management of Infected Aortic Grafts

Frank J. Veith and Sushil K. Gupta

An infection involving a vascular reconstructive operation on the aorta is one of the most catastrophic complications in surgery. Full knowledge of the natural history of this complication and appropriate principles of treatment, however, make it possible to salvage the life and limbs of some patients that have such infections. This chapter will consider infections that involve prosthetic grafts that have at least one anastomosis with the infrarenal abdominal aorta, although the principles of management can also generally be applied to the rare infections that complicate aortic thrombendarterectomy or operations elsewhere on the aorta.

INCIDENCE AND PREVENTION

The incidence of infection involving aortic prosthetic grafts is fortunately low, even though it will vary somewhat in different population groups and different institutions. Szilagyi and his colleagues[21] provide a reasonably representative appraisal of incidence in their important analysis of infections in arterial reconstructions with synthetic grafts. They found the incidence of serious infection in aortic reconstructive operations performed solely through an abdominal incision to be 0.7 percent, while there was a 1.6 percent incidence of infection in aortofemoral operations. These authors were also the first to point out that superficial wound

---

This work was supported in part by a grant from the John Hilton Manning and Emma Austin Manning Foundation.

infections that did not involve the prosthesis were of little consequence after arterial reconstructions.[21] It must be recognized, however, that even a superficial infection in a groin wound of an arterial reconstruction must be a serious concern because of the possibility that the superficial infection will spread to involve the nearby vascular prosthetic graft and the arterial suture line.

Although the incidence of infection should be higher after operations for ruptured aortic aneurysm than after elective procedures because of the requirement for haste, the probability of shock, and the inevitable hematoma, this is difficult to prove conclusively. The frequency of positive intraoperative cultures, however, has been significantly greater from ruptured than from nonruptured aneurysms.[9] Furthermore, even in elective aortic procedures, poor surgical technique, the presence of wound hematoma, and the need for re-exploration probably increase the hazard of graft contamination and septic complications. To minimize the incidence of aortic graft sepsis, therefore, the surgeon should, if possible, avoid these errors.

Because infections involving operations on the arterial tree have serious consequences, many vascular surgeons have long advocated the use of so-called prophylactic antibiotics in conjunction with aortic surgery. Despite experimental evidence that supported their use,[1,4,16] the value of prophylactic antibiotics in human arterial surgery remained unproven until the prospective, randomized, double-blind controlled study of Kaiser and colleagues[13] clearly demonstrated a diminished incidence of infection in reconstructive arterial surgery if appropriate doses of cefazolin were given immediately before and for 24 hours after operation. Although this study had the defect of only including a small number of graft infections, all of these were in the placebo group. Moreover, a second randomized, controlled study has recently confirmed the value of appropriately administered prophylactic cephalosporin antibiotics in arterial surgery.[18] Accordingly, the appropriate use of prophylactic antibiotics *is* presently indicated to minimize the incidence of infections involving aortic prosthetic grafts.

ETIOLOGY

Staphylococci have been the predominant organism responsible for infections of aortofemoral prostheses while gram-negative coliform bacteria have predominated in aortoiliac infections.[21] The organisms responsible for most infections involving aortic prosthetic grafts are probably introduced from the operating room environment or the patient's skin at the time of operation, as is the case with most infections that involve clean surgical procedures. There are other possible sources for bacterial infection that involve aortic prostheses, however. These include any transient bacteremia that can inoculate a vascular prosthetic, particularly before it is well healed.[3,14,15,17] Furthermore, bacteria that transgress the intestinal wall can sometimes be cultured from the fluid that exudes from the eviscerated bowel during aortic operations, and some positive bacterial cultures have been obtained from the clot that is contained within the lumen of many aortic aneurysms.[9,10] The frequency of positive bacterial cultures from these sources makes it somewhat surprising that the incidence of true infection in aortic procedures is as low as it is and provides further justification for the use of prophylactic antibiotics.

In addition to these sources of bacterial contamination that are generally present, there are three other specific sources that may be present in some instances; first are patients in whom the jejunoileum or the duodenum may be injured in gaining aortic exposure. If this is detected, serious consideration must be given to postponing the aortic operation or avoiding the insertion of any prosthetic graft material in the contaminated area. The latter requirement may necessitate the performance of an extra-anatomic axillofemoral procedure to revascularize the lower extremities. Second, if the presence of localized or generalized cloudy peritoneal fluid raises the question of pre-existing bacterial contamination of the operative field, the surgeon can obtain an immediate smear and Gram stain examination for bacteria. The absence of organisms helps to justify cautious continuation of the operation whereas the presence of bacteria mandates termination of the operation, or if this is not possible, the performance of an axillofemoral bypass with elimination of the need for placing any foreign vascular prosthetic material in the known contaminated field. The third specific source of contamination, a preoperatively infected abdominal aortic aneurysm,[12,19] can be suspected from a septic course; a sharply circumscribed, saccular aneurysm with relatively normal aorta proximally and distally on angiography; or the presence of retroperitoneal pus. If suspected, this entity can often be confirmed by Gram stain examination of smears and is best managed by control of the aneurysm by proximal and distal ligation, excision of all infected tissue usually with drainage, and performance of an axillofemoral bypass.

NATURAL HISTORY AND DIAGNOSIS

Serious infection involving an aortic prosthesis may be a simple matter to detect in some cases; in others, it may be extremely difficult to diagnose, particularly in the early stages. To understand this apparent contradiction, one must have insight into the variable natural history of infections involving aortic prosthetic grafts. This variable natural history is represented by the many different ways that such infections can be classified as shown in Table 1.

Infections may present at any time during the first postoperative month, or they may be extremely delayed in their presentation with their first signs or symptoms not appearing until several years after the initial operation. Whether this means that the infecting organisms have been lying dormant since their introduction at operation or whether it means they have been newly introduced is not known. It is known, however, that some infections have a rapid course with serious local and systemic manifestations and rapid progression to catastrophic end points, whereas others can have an indolent course with minimal consequences being manifest for a long time before the lethal end phases of the infection occur.

Groin Infection

One reason for this variability in course is the intrinsic virulence of the infecting organism in a given patient; another more important reason is the localization of the infection. Whether or not the infection is present in a groin incision is important in determining its presentation and behav-

Table 1. Classifications of Infections Involving Aortic Prosthetic Grafts

By time of onset	Early: 0–30 days after operation
	Late: 1 month to 5 years after operation
By localization	Groin involvement
	Intra-abdominal involvement
	Total involvement
By severity	Superficial wound: grades I and II of Szilagyi[21]
	Deep wound—perigraft*
	Bacteria in graft interstices*
	Breakdown of anastomosis*
By manifestation	Systemic: fever, leukocytosis, bacteremia, septicemia
	Back pain, ureteral obstruction
	Abscess, sinus
	Thrombosis
	False aneurysm, enteric fistula (especially aortoduodenal), hemorrhage

* *Grade III of Szilagyi.*[21]

ior. Many infected aortofemoral prosthetic grafts present only with an abscess or persistent draining sinus in the groin incision.

This alone must be regarded as an ominous sign, irrespective of the time after the original operation that it occurs and whether or not it is accompanied by fever or leukocytosis. The graft itself may or may not be involved, and other parts of the graft may or may not be infected. If the abscess cavity or the sinus communicates with the prosthetic graft, and if the treatment is expectant or conservative, one of two serious consequences will occur even if the infection is initially restricted to the groin incision. One consequence is that the involved limb of the graft will thrombose with possible spread of the infection to involve the entirety of the thrombosed portion of the graft. Persistent local evidence of infection will continue until all of the infected foreign material is removed. The second and even more serious consequence of unaggressive management of infection in the distal end of an aortofemoral prosthesis is disruption of the graft to artery suture line with formation of an anastomotic false aneurysm or bleeding to the exterior via the previously noted sinus tract. This bleeding is often small in amount at first and may appear to be of little consequence. If the nature and origin of this "sentinel bleeding," however, is not recognized and managed aggressively, it can lead to exsanguination and death.

Once an arterial prosthetic infection has progressed to the point where bleeding occurs, it means that the artery at the level of the anastomosis is also infected and no attempt to preserve the continuity of that vessel will succeed. The prosthetic graft must be removed and the involved vessel ligated or oversewn with or without a prior or subsequent extraanatomic bypass in a clean field to maintain arterial continuity and extremity viability.

It has been thought that infection in a wound surrounding a functioning prosthetic graft (perigraft infection), even without anastomotic disruption or bleeding, also required similar treatment. This is still true if the aortic end of a prosthetic graft is involved in the septic process. Recently, however, we have observed five patients with purulent wound infections at the site of prosthetic graft anastomosis to the external iliac, common femoral, or popliteal artery. In two patients, the grafts were of woven Dacron; in three, the graft material was expanded polytetrafluoroethylene. In all five, one graft to artery suture line was visible in the infected wound and obviously bathed in pus. In these five patients, surgical debridement or excision of the wound in the operating room, daily packing with povidone-iodine, and appropriate systemic antibiotics resulted in healing of the wound and preservation of graft and artery patency that have persisted 1 to 5 years. In two similarly managed cases, graft-to-artery anastomotic disruption occurred and required the radical treatment already outlined. Nevertheless, our recent experience supported by the previous observations of Carter, Cohen, and Whalen[5] would appear to justify cautious use of aggressive surgical management *without* graft removal in selected prosthetic infections that are restricted to the groin and in which the graft to artery suture line remains intact. If the latter approach is attempted, it must be recognized that massive bleeding can occur and the patient should, therefore, never be left unattended.

Intra-abdominal Infection

In patients whose aortic operation does not have a groin incision and in those whose aortofemoral prosthesis is primarily infected at the proximal end, the infection usually presents differently and may be more difficult to diagnose. The occurrence of otherwise unexplained fever or leukocytosis with or without back pain at any time after an aortic procedure should be enough to arouse suspicion. Gas bubbles in the retroperitoneal area surrounding the graft and absence of the left psoas shadow may also be noted. Performance of an intravenous pyelogram may show hydronephrosis.[20] In fact, this finding may be the first evidence of an infected aortic graft. Other diagnostic modalities that may be helpful include abdominal sonography, which can reveal an echolucent mass surrounding the aortic graft (Fig. 1), and computed axial tomography, which can reveal an abnormal water density mass in the retroperitoneal area surrounding the graft or radiolucent areas posterior to the graft (see Chap. 2). If the patient has a septic course, positive blood cultures obtained by arterial puncture downstream to the graft are persuasive evidence that there is bacterial involvement of the luminal aspect of the prosthesis and that radical treatment is required. In the early phases of such an infection, angiography may not be helpful and will probably show intact anastomotic lines and absence of luminal irregularities.

If the proximal end of an aortofemoral prosthesis or either end of a totally intra-abdominal prosthesis become infected and radical surgical treatment with removal of the graft is not undertaken, disruption of the involved suture line will occur. This may lead to prompt exsanguination, although more commonly it presents as a pulsatile abdominal mass that represents a false aneurysm. If untreated, this can produce pressure effects on adjacent viscera and ultimately exsanguination. If time permits, angiography is the most helpful diagnostic procedure and localizes the involved anastomosis if two or more are at risk. Another possible presentation of an infected aortic or iliac artery anastomosis is by communication with the gastrointestinal tract. Aortoduodenal fistulas are most common in this regard and are best diagnosed by fiberoptic endoscopy.

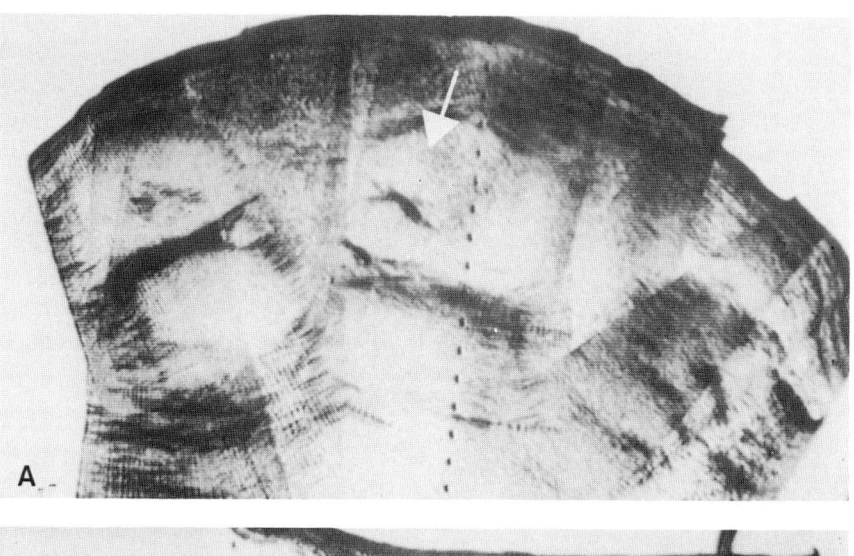

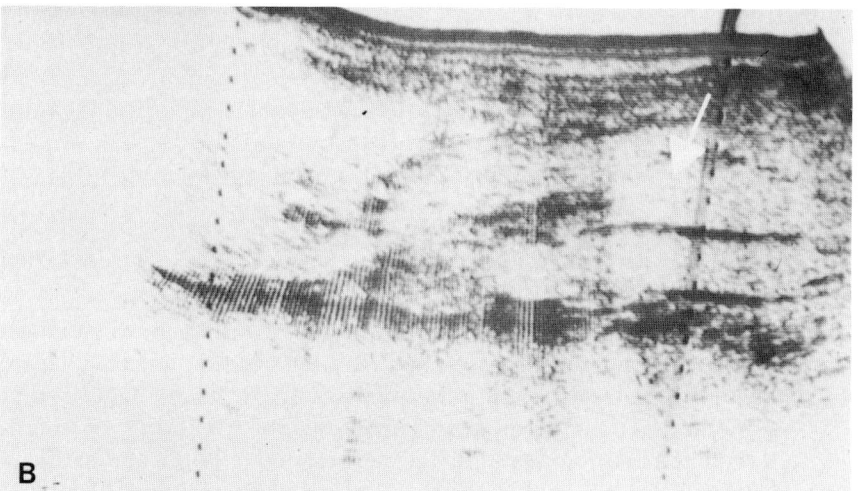

FIGURE 1. Transverse (A) and sagittal (B) sonographic cuts demonstrating an echolucent area (arrows) anterior and lateral to an infected aortic prosthesis following operation for ruptured abdominal aortic aneurysm. (From Veith FJ: Surgery of the infected aortic graft. In Bergan JJ, Yao JST (eds): Surgery of the Aorta and its Body Branches. New York, Grune & Stratton, 1979.)

It should be noted that other causes of disruption of the proximal aortic suture line and other graft-to-artery anastomoses exist. False aneurysms unassociated with sepsis may occur from a variety of other causes including a weakened artery wall, loss of suture tensile strength, excessive graft tension, or improper surgical technique with inadequate suture bites. Fistulas between the proximal aortic suture line and the adherent duodenum can occur without initiating sepsis and can be prevented by the interposition of vascularized, viable soft tissue or the onlay of a patch of graft material between the anastomosis and the duodenum. Absence of systemic or local evidence of infection and negative smears for bacteria, cultures, and histologic examination should permit the surgeon to differentiate these noninfectious complications from those due to infection so that treatment may be appropriate. It should be pointed out, however, that the absence of bacteria on a gram-stained smear *does not* reliably rule out infection. Graft-to-artery anastomotic problems truly unassociated with the presence of infection do not require extraanatomic bypass in a clean field.

TREATMENT

Effective management of infected aortic reconstructions must be based on a clear knowledge and understanding of their variable natural history and the classifications by localization, severity, and manifestation listed in Table 1. Infections that are established as being superficial require only good local treatment and appropriate antibiotics to prevent spread. They are not of serious import and will not be considered further in this discussion.

Infections Restricted to the Groin Wound

When these do not involve the interstices of the prosthesis or the femoral artery at the distal anastomosis, they may be treated by radical local debridement or excision of all infected tissue from the involved wound in the operating room followed by povidone-iodine packing and high-dose intravenous antibiotics as dictated by wound cultures and sensitivity. It must be recognized that this is a relatively new and unproven approach to such infections based largely on our own limited experience and that it is associated with a substantial risk that the infection may progress in extent with disruption of the anastomosis and serious arterial hemorrhage. If this approach is chosen, appropriate precautions to permit immediate control of bleeding by direct pressure and rapid operation must be taken until the wound is fully healed. Furthermore, if there is any evidence of even minor "sentinel" bleeding, the management should parallel the following classic treatment for infection restricted to the groin incision of an aortofemoral prosthesis. The principles of this treatment were first enunciated by Shaw and Baue[20] and mandate removal of the prosthetic graft to the extent that it is involved in the infectious process, ligation of the involved artery proximal and distal to the infected anastomosis, and, if necessary and possible, salvage of the involved limb by an extra-anatomic bypass in a totally separate, clean operative field. This method of treatment is still clearly the one of choice when an infection localized to the groin is or becomes associated with hemorrhage, false aneurysm, graft thrombosis, or persistent septicemia.

In such circumstances, the operation consists of two stages. One stage removes the infected limb of the graft and controls bleeding by ligature or oversewing of the artery or arteries proximal and distal to the infected anastomosis. The other stage provides extra-anatomic revascularization of the involved limb. Both stages can be performed at one operation through totally separate surgical fields, or either stage can be performed first at a separate operation depending on the preference of the surgeon and the urgency of the situation with regard to bleeding or limb ischemia.

One approach is to perform first, through an abdominal and distal thigh incision, an obturator bypass from the uninfected aortic graft or its opposite iliac limb to the uninvolved distal superficial femoral, deep femoral, or popliteal artery. The technique of obturator bypass has been well described and illustrated elsewhere.[11,20] Then, through the abdominal incision, the involved limb of the graft can be ligated and divided in an area proximal to any evident infection, and the external iliac artery can be ligated as far distally as possible. After all the wounds are closed and sealed, or possibly at a second operation, the second phase is performed. This consists of removal of the previously divided graft and proximal and distal oversewing or preferably ligation of the common femoral artery and sometimes its branches in the region of the infected anastomosis. Dissection of the arteries in this infected, scarred wound can be extremely difficult and dangerous. It is facilitated by the previous distal external iliac artery ligation but may require further temporary intraluminal control by balloon catheters.

Another simpler approach is the one that we favor. The first phase of this consists of gaining access to the retroperitoneum through an oblique or transverse abdominal incision well above the infected groin. Through this clean field, the limb of the graft is ligated and divided and the external iliac artery is ligated as far distally as possible. An axillary-to-superficial femoral artery or axillopopliteal bypass is performed using an expanded polytetrafluoroethylene graft that is tunneled lateral to the infected groin wound and diagonally across the anterior surface of the thigh below the infection to join the superficial femoral artery or to enter the popliteal fossa.[24] After closing and sealing all these clean incisions, the infected graft and groin wound is managed as already described.

A third albeit somewhat different approach to the infected prosthetic graft has been recommended by Wylie and by Ehrenfeld, Stoney and their associates.[8,26] This approach, which will be detailed by Stoney in the following chapter, uses autogenous tissue to permit removal of all infected material. It is limited by the requirement that an arterial anastomosis be performed in an infected field, but autologous arterial suture lines can heal in this circumstance, and the approach can be used successfully.[8,26] We have not used it as often as other methods.

Infections of an Entire Aortoiliac Graft or Infections Restricted to the Aortic End of an Aortofemoral Bypass

Once diagnosed, such infections must be treated radically and aggressively with removal of the infected prosthetic graft, wide drainage, appropriate systemic antibiotics, and usually restoration of distal flow by extraanatomic bypass through separate clean operative fields. Although restoration of distal flow may not always be required, to our knowledge there are no reported instances when failure to remove the infected prosthesis was effective treatment for this problem. These infections require, therefore, a radical approach to achieve salvage of the patient and his or her limbs even though many aspects of it may be difficult.

Again, the approach comprises two phases: 1) removal of the infected graft with proximal and distal control of the artery or arteries at the anastomotic sites; and 2) restoration of distal arterial flow through a separate operative field. The latter phase, which is not difficult since the groins are uninvolved by sepsis, should be performed first if the patient is not exsanguinating. It can be accomplished best by an axillobifemoral bypass or bilateral axillofemoral bypasses. In the rare instance when neither axillary artery is suitable to provide inflow, the thoracic or supraceliac aorta may be used.[2,23]

Removal of the infected graft and control of bleeding can be far more difficult, particularly if the proximal anastomosis is immediately below the renal arteries. It is helpful and usually possible to determine by angiography how much aorta remains between the renal arteries and the proximal anastomosis. This determination is important because it indicates whether there is enough aortic length to permit ligation of the infrarenal aortic stump or whether it will be necessary to oversew it. The former procedure, if feasible, is safer and more secure than the latter since subsequent infection and aortic rupture is less likely. Wide drainage of this area and excision of all infected tissue also help to minimize the ever-present risk of hemorrhage from infection remaining in the aortic stump.[21,25]

Gaining control of the aorta distal to the renal arteries to permit ligation or oversewing may be difficult at best in a field obscured by previous operative scarring and infection. If the remaining infrarenal aortic segment is short and the anastomosis is disrupted, it may be impossible to gain this control without exsanguination. In such circumstances, we and others have found it beneficial to gain proximal control of the supraceliac aorta through the abdomen.[6,23]

This can safely be accomplished as shown in Figure 2.[22] The aorta may be occluded in this location as long as it is necessary to gain effective control below the renal arteries so that debridement and oversewing or ligation can be performed. In our hands the supraceliac aorta has sometimes been occluded for more than an hour without causing serious impairment of hepatic, enteric, or renal function.[22]

Another method has been advocated by Diethrich and his co-workers[7] to facilitate management of the infrarenal aortic segment in instances in which the proximal anastomosis is infected but intact. According to this method, removal of the proximal graft is preceded by ligation of the graft limbs and several days delay to allow the infrarenal aorta to thrombose solidly. If feasible, this approach facilitates gaining aortic control but whether it decreases the incidence of aortic stump infection as claimed remains to be shown.

After managing the proximal aortic anastomosis, the iliac arteries are controlled, debrided, and ligated or oversewn, and the entire aortoiliac prosthesis removed. The aortic and iliac stumps are covered with any viable adjacent soft tissue, and wide retroperitoneal drainage through the left flank is established. The main abdominal incision is then closed with a single layer of closely spaced, retention-type monofilament sutures. If only the upper end of an aortofemoral graft is involved in the septic process, the distal uninfected graft will have previously been ligated and divided at the time of the axillofemoral bypass. The remaining graft can then be extracted at the time of the abdominal procedure.

Infection of an Entire Aortofemoral Graft

Treatment in this situation is identical to that already outlined with two exceptions. First, graft removal usually would be preceded by bilateral axillary to superficial femoral artery or axillopopliteal bypasses if limb viability is to be maintained. The course of these bypasses is lateral to the infected groin wounds. Second, the abdominal approach to remove the infected graft must also be accompanied by groin incisions and proximal and distal ligation of the femoral arteries involved in the distal anastomosis. Management and techniques in this area are similar to those already presented for infections restricted to the groin wounds.

Although removal of the infected graft and securing of the involved

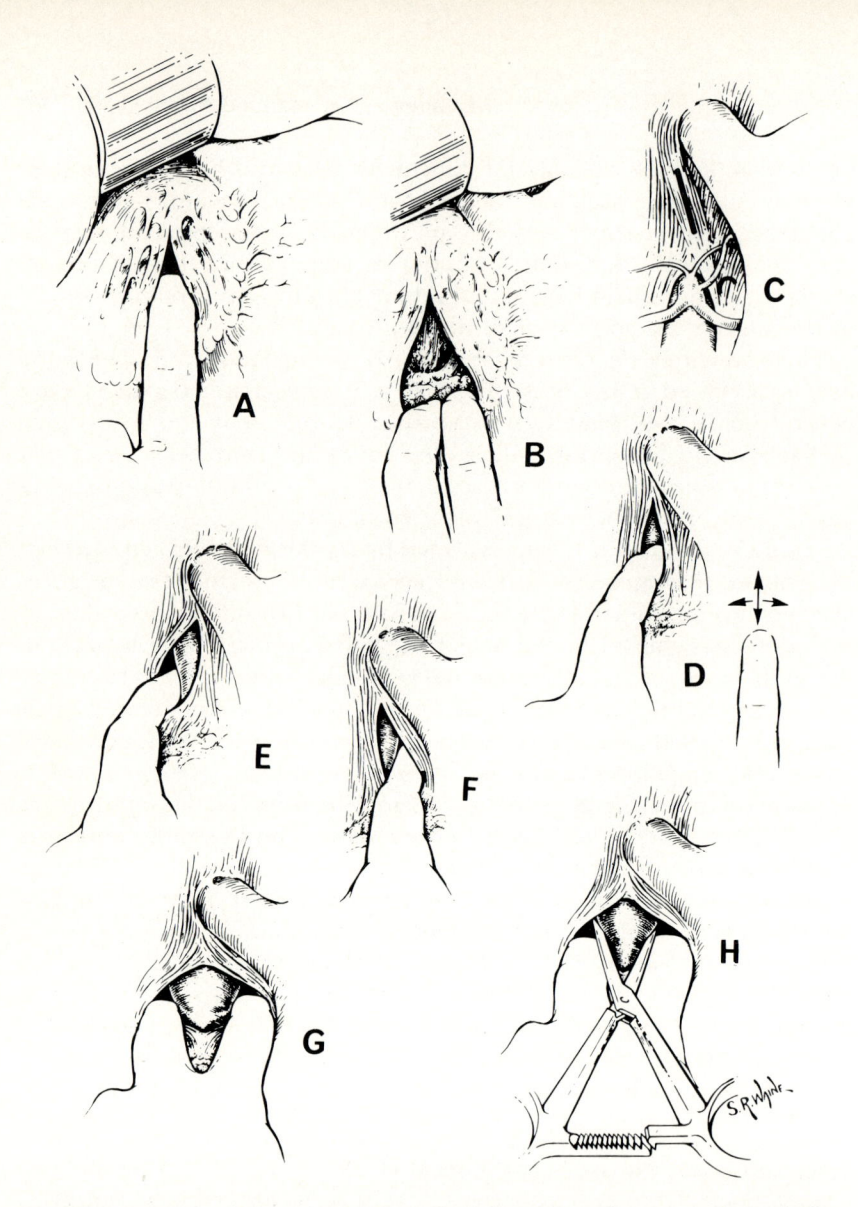

FIGURE 2. Method for gaining control of the supraceliac aorta through the abdomen. The abdomen is opened with a long midline incision extending to the xiphoid, and the liver is retracted upward and to the right with a Deaver retractor. **A.** The index finger is shown bluntly tearing the lesser omentum between the liver and the stomach. The caudate lobe of the liver is visualized through the upper portion of the lesser omentum. **B.** The opening in the lesser omentum is shown through which can be seen the peritoneum overlying the crura of the diaphragm superiorly and the upper border of the pancreas inferiorly. The celiac axis and its branches are intimately associated with the upper border of the pancreas and cannot be clearly distinguished from it without dissection. **C.** The position of these vessels is shown diagramatically with the pancreas and other nonvascular structures omitted. The heavy line indicates

remaining arteries in any of the above circumstances is best preceded by extra-anatomic bypass in a clean field, this is not always possible. Exsanguinating hemorrhage from a disrupted anastomosis may require control and graft removal before any attempt is made to restore the distal circulation. In an occasional instance, a patient's precarious condition following the graft removal and control of bleeding may force the surgeon to accept limb loss rather than perform the extra-anatomic bypass. This should be an extremely rare occurrence, however, particularly if treatment is not inadvisably delayed.

CONCLUSIONS

Infection involving a vascular reconstruction of the aorta if untreated or inadequately treated will have a fatal outcome. By knowing the natural history of such infections, it is possible to suspect and diagnose them with relative certainty so that appropriate treatment can often be carried out deliberately before the patient is critically ill or moribund. Even though this treatment may involve complex and radical surgery, it is justified by the lethal nature of this complication and can lead to a successful outcome with salvage of the patient and his or her extremities. This chapter emphasizes those aspects of the natural history of the infections that occur in aortic reconstructions so that a proper diagnosis can be made and appropriate principles of management can be applied.

REFERENCES

1. Baker WH, Bodensteiner JA: The administration of antibiotics in vascular reconstructive surgery. A comparison of the effectiveness of systemic cephaloridine versus cephaloridine-soaked grafts in preventing graft infections in dogs. J Thorac Cardiovasc Surg 64:301, 1972

---

the location of the incision in the posterior peritoneum overlying the diaphragmatic crura. This incision is made with the fingernail of the left index or middle finger. **D.** The method for digitally splitting and, with posteriorly directed pressure, transgressing the muscle fibers of the diaphragmatic crura to gain access to the periadventitial plane of the aorta is illustrated. **E, F.** This plane is widened medial and lateral to the aorta. No attempt is made to dissect the aorta circumferentially since this can be difficult because of limited exposure and access. **G, H.** Inferior traction, illustrated with the fingers, creates a space on either side of the aorta so that a totally occluding large clamp with slightly curved blades can be applied. (From Veith FJ, Gupta S, Daly V: Technique for occluding the supraceliac aorta through the abdomen. Surg Gynecol Obstet 151:427, 1980; by permission of Surgery, Gynecology & Obstetrics.)

2. Blaisdell FW, DeMattei GA, Gauder PJ: Extraperitoneal thoracic aorta to femoral bypass graft as replacement for an infected aortic bifurcation prosthesis. Am J Surg 102:583, 1961
3. Bradham RR, Cordle F, McIver FA: Effect of bacteria on vascular prostheses. Ann Surg 154:187, 1966
4. Burke JF: The effective period of preventive antibiotic action in experimental incisions and dermal lesions. Surgery 50:161, 1961
5. Carter SC, Cohen A, Whelan TJ: Clinical experience with management of the infected Dacron graft. Ann Surg 158:249, 1963
6. Crawford ES, Manning LG, Kelly TF: "Redo" surgery after operations for aneurysm and occlusion of the abdominal aorta. Surgery 81:41, 1977
7. Diethrich EB, Noon GP, Liddicoat JE, DeBakey ME: Treatment of infected aortofemoral arterial prosthesis. Surgery 68:1044, 1970
8. Ehrenfeld WK, Wilbur BG, Olcott CN, Stoney RJ: Autogenous tissue reconstruction in the management of infected prosthetic grafts. Surgery 85:82, 1979
9. Ernst CB, Campbell HC, Daugherty ME, et al: Incidence and significance of intra-operative bacterial cultures during abdominal aortic aneurysmectomy. Ann Surg 185:626, 1977
10. Fry WJ: Vascular prosthesis infections. Surg Clin North Am 52:1419, 1972
11. Guida PM, Moore SW: Obturator bypass technique. Surg Gynecol Obstet 128:1307, 1969
12. Jarrett F, Darling RC, Mundth ED, Austen WG: Experience with infected aneurysms of the abdominal aorta. Arch Surg 110:1281, 1975
13. Kaiser AB, Clayson KR, Mulherin JL, et al: Antibiotic prophylaxis in vascular surgery. Ann Surg 188:283, 1978
14. Lindenauer SM, Fry WJ, Schaub G, Wild D: The use of antibiotics in the prevention of vascular graft infections. Surgery 62:487, 1967
15. Malone JM, Moore WS, Campagna G, Bean B: Bacteremic infectability of vascular grafts: The influence of pseudointimal integrity and duration of graft function. Surgery 78:211, 1975
16. Moore WS, Rosson CT, Hall AD: Effect of prophylactic antibiotics in preventing bacteremic infection of vascular prostheses. Surgery 69:825, 1971
17. Moore WS, Rosson CT, Hall AD, Thomas AN: Transient bacteremia: A cause of infection in prosthetic vascular grafts. Am J Surg 117:342, 1969
18. Pitt H, Postier R, Frank L, et al: Prophylactic antibiotics in vascular surgery: Topical, systemic or both? Ann Surg 192:356, 1980
19. Scher LA, Brenner BJ, Goldenkranz RJ, et al: Infected aneurysm of the abdominal aorta. Arch Surg 115:975, 1980
20. Shaw RS, Baue AE: Management of sepsis complicating arterial reconstructive surgery. Surgery 53:75, 1963
21. Szilagyi DE, Smith RF, Elliott JP, Vrandecic MP: Infection in arterial reconstruction with synthetic grafts. Ann Surg 176:321, 1972
22. Veith FJ, Gupta S, Daly V: Technique for occluding the supraceliac aorta through the abdomen. Surg Gynecol Obstet 151:427, 1980
23. Veith FJ, Hartsuck JM, Crane C: Management of aortoiliac reconstruction complicated by sepsis and hemorrhage. N Engl J Med 270:1389, 1964

24. Veith FJ, Moss CM, Fell SC, et al: New approaches to limb salvage by extended extra-anatomic bypasses and prosthetic reconstructions to foot arteries. Surgery 84:764, 1978
25. Vellar IDA, Doyle JC: Axillofemoral bypass in the management of infected aortic bifurcation Dacron graft. Aust NZ J Surg 40:58, 1970
26. Wylie EJ: Discussion in RS Shaw and AE Baue. Management of sepsis complicating arterial reconstructive surgery. Surgery 53:75, 1963

TWENTY-SIX

The Use of Autogenous Tissues in the Management of Infected Aortic Prosthetic Grafts

Ronald J. Stoney

Chronic infection involving a prosthetic graft used for aortic reconstruction is the gravest complication in vascular surgery. Fatal aortic hemorrhage or ischemia of the lower limbs requiring high thigh amputation are frequently reported following surgical management by experienced vascular surgeons.[3,8] Resolution of chronic perigraft sepsis demands removal of the involved prosthesis; however, the viability of pelvic viscera and the lower extremities usually depend upon the blood supplied by the graft. Alternate methods for revascularization of these critical vascular beds are essential in order to achieve a successful outcome for the threatened patient.

This chapter will describe the clinical manifestations of chronic aortic perigraft sepsis, discuss the techniques useful in defining the presence and extent of perigraft involvement, and review the principles of autogenous revascularization and the results achieved in managing 22 consecutive such patients (Table 1).

Chronic perigraft infection results from the successful bacterial colonization of the tissues that incorporate the prosthetic graft itself. The graft provides a permeable latticework or scaffold to promote the ingrowth of host fibroblast tissue. When this tissue becomes colonized in close proximity to the foreign material (graft), the resulting infection progressively involves all the tissue that is in intimate juxtaposition to the prosthetic fibers. The infected soft tissue cannot be effectively sepa-

---

Portions of this work reproduced from Wylie EJ, Stoney RJ, Ehrenfeld WK: Manual of Vascular Surgery, Vol. II. New York, Springer-Verlag, 1980.

Table 1. Chronic Perigraft Infection

Graft Size	No. of Pts.	Repair Technique Prosthetic	Repair Technique Autogenous	Results Deaths	Results Amputations	Results Stroke
Carotid	2	0	2	—	—	0
Innominate	2	0	2	—	—	0
Femoropopliteal	4	0	4	—	—	—
Aortofemoral	21	11	10	2 (10%)	2 (5%)	—
Aortoiliac	1	1	0	—	—	—
Total	30	12	18	2 (6.6%)	2	0

rated in situ from the foreign body, so the involved graft together with this infected perigraft tissue must be removed in order for the infection to be resolved. Clinical experience with more than 50 patients with perigraft infection in various anatomic sites suggests that the infection most commonly begins outside the graft rather than by a bacteremic colonization of the pseudointima from the bloodstream.[2,6] Aortic prostheses within the abdominal cavity are infected by enteric organisms usually originating from an adjacent viscus that has been eroded by the prosthesis (i.e., small intestine, colon, or ureter). Aortic prostheses that extend beyond the abdominal cavity are attached to the arteries within the groin, and are infected by skin staphylococci present in the groin or peroneal areas. This may originate from a groin or extremity wound infection or infected groin lymphatics draining a distal ischemic and infected lesion of the limb.

Chronic perigraft infection is usually diffuse and often involves the entire implanted prosthesis and perigraft tissue. This results when the infection begins in the perigraft tissue before the graft is completely enveloped in the host tissue (incorporated). The time of incorporation varies but is probably complete within a year following graft implantation unless healing complications or impairment of the healing response are present (e.g., steroids, immunosuppression, diabetes mellitus).

Localized perigraft infection occurs when a portion of a chronically implanted graft is exposed and then subsequently infected. This classically occurs following local operations on a portion of a graft limb to manage late graft complications such as occlusion or a false aneurysm. The techniques of thrombectomy and revision of the outflow arteries or local excision and regrafting necessarily remove a portion of the host tissue that envelopes the original prosthesis. The ensuing infection involves the new graft and its perigraft tissue. The infection's progression is impeded by the host–graft incorporation of the proximal graft limb. This adjacent, adherent, undisturbed perigraft tissue resists septic dissolution and the underlying graft remains free of infection. This observation allows one occasionally to simplify surgical management by removal of the portion of an aortofemoral prosthesis that is involved with infection. Provisions for providing blood supply to the involved extremity may then be simpler than if removal of the entire prosthesis together with the aortic portion of the graft were required. The contralateral graft limb then remains undisturbed by the revascularization method employed to manage the localized perigraft infection.

DIAGNOSIS

Chronic perigraft infections involving an aortic prosthesis contained within the abdomen may be difficult to detect on clinical grounds alone. Occasionally back pain, low-grade fever with a disproportionately high white blood cell count, and elevated erythrocyte sedimentation rate are present. More often, this infection is undetected unless graft limb thrombosis, hemorrhage from an eroded adjacent viscus, or septic embolization to the limbs are detected. Chronic perigraft infection involving an aortic prosthesis in which one or both limbs are extended to the femoral area may be more obvious clinically. Signs of infection occasionally involve the wound or scar in the groin where the graft limbs have been attached. Sinus formation, purulent drainage, intermittent bleeding or pain, erythema, swelling, and tenderness are the findings of chronic perigraft infection in a subcutaneous location in the groin.

Diagnostic aids may be required in suspected chronic perigraft infection and are listed and discussed below.

1. *Contrast radiography of the wound sinus tract* may define the proximal extent of the graft infection which involves the perigraft space. Graft corrugations may be identified in the proximal portion of the sinogram, and this may, in fact, track proximally to an eroded adjacent viscus (Fig. 1A,B).
2. *Needle aspiration of perigraft space* can be performed over the course of subcutaneous grafts in the femoral (groin) region, or in the retroperitoneal space. Sterile technique is employed. The needle is introduced into the region adjacent to the pulsatile graft and aspirations are attempted. It may be necessary to inject a small amount of saline and then withdraw this saline to recover organisms and fluid if the perigraft space is small. Subsequent smear and culture of recovered fluid will confirm the diagnosis of chronic perigraft sepsis.
3. *Computed axial tomographic (CAT) scans* may be helpful using contrast enhancement to show the perigraft space, gas, or fluid accumulations, particularly in inaccessible portions of aortofemoral grafts in the pelvis or retroperitoneum (Fig. 2).[5]

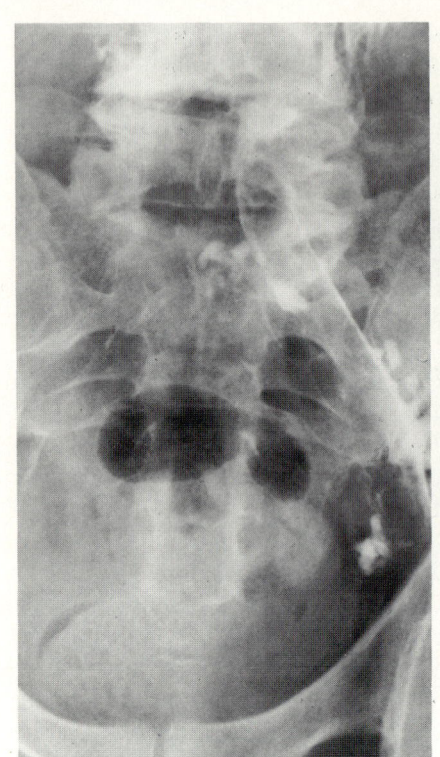

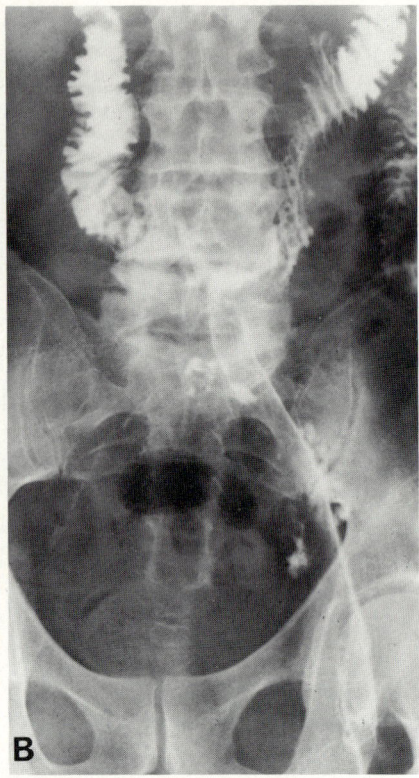

FIGURE 1.A. Sinogram from the left groin showing left perigraft space surrounding an infected aortofemoral graft limb. B. Sinogram from the left groin showing proximal extension of contrast from perigraft space into the duodenum.

4. *Ultrasonography* has been useful to assess the status of healing of grafts and complications of healing which include false aneurysm and perigraft fluid accumulations.[4] Longitudinal sonography may be helpful to assess the status of the iliac and femoral portions of aortofemoral graft limbs (Fig. 3).
5. *Gastrointestinal endoscopy* may be helpful when an aortic prosthesis is suspected of eroding the gastrointestinal tract. This may be associated with occult chronic perigraft sepsis or occasionally with insidious or massive gastrointestinal hemorrhage.[1] The most common site of gastrointestinal erosion is the duodenum overlying the aortic portion of the graft. Occasionally fistulas have occurred by erosion of the graft into the colon. The cecum or sigmoid colon are the most likely sites for this. Colonoscopy may be of use if this type of enteric-prosthetic communication is suspected.

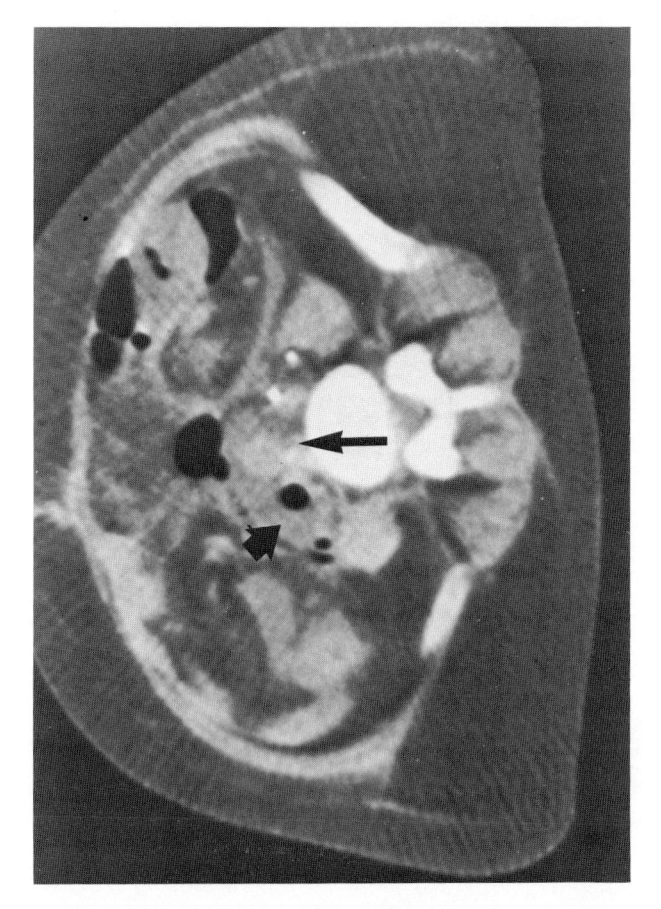

FIGURE 2. CAT scan in a patient with an infected aortic prosthetic graft. Thin arrow indicates calcification in native bypassed aorta. Large arrow shows a paragraft mass containing gas.

6. *Direct surgical exploration* of the graft is necessary on occasion to confirm or exclude the possibility of chronic perigraft sepsis. The findings of a failure of graft incorporation, the presence of perigraft fluid, or suture line disruption with false aneurysm formation may be present even when other methods of defining perigraft infection have been inconclusive.

SURGICAL MANAGEMENT

An accurate definition of the location of the involved graft, its route, and the anastomotic sites are useful before planning surgical manage-

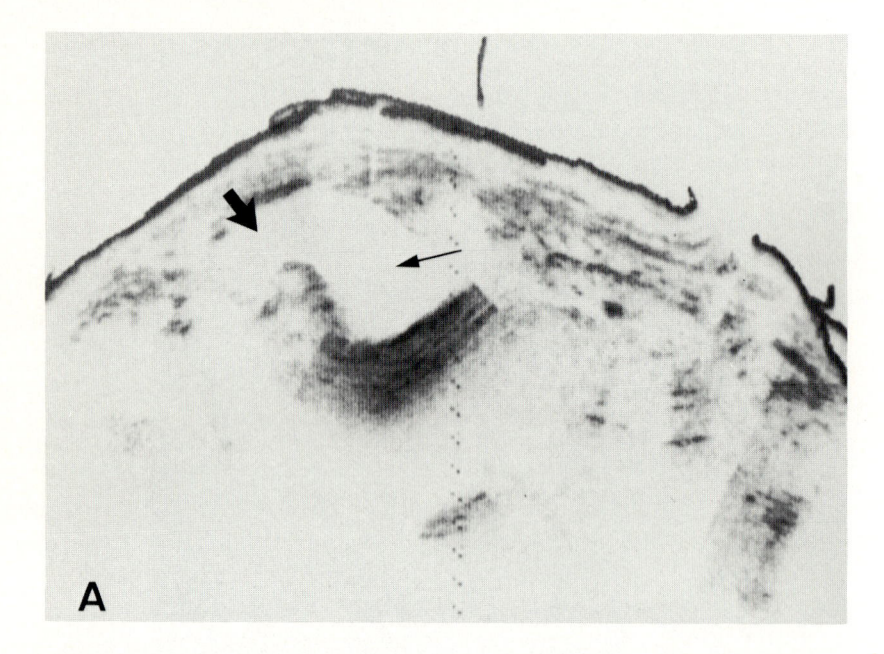

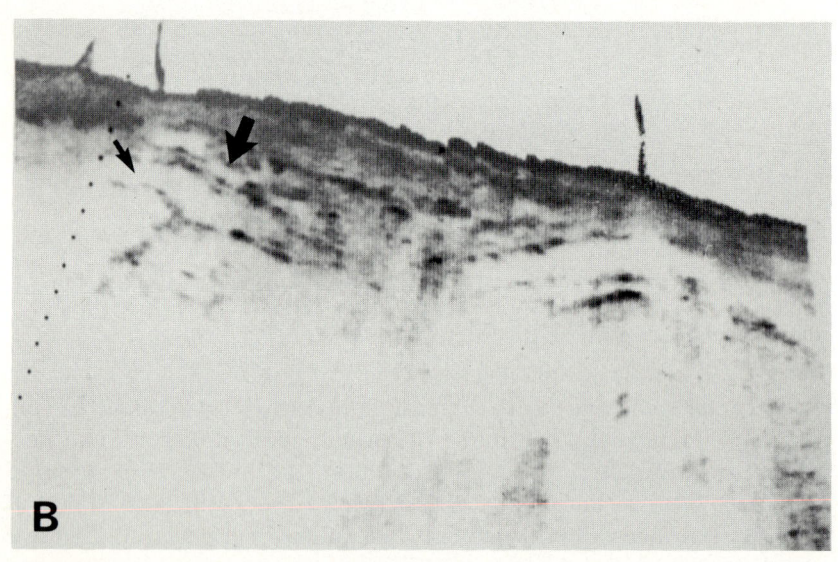

FIGURE 3.A. Transverse sonogram in patient with an infected aortofemoral prosthetic graft. Thin arrow points to graft limb and lumen. Thick arrow indicates paragraft space, which contained purulent fluid. **B.** Longitudinal sonogram showing course of iliac-femoral limb of an infected aortofemoral prosthetic graft. Graft lumen in groin indicated by small arrow. Paragraft fluid space shown by large arrow.

ment. Review of details of the original graft operation with particular attention to the type of graft and arterial pathology treated may be of particular value. In addition, knowing the method and type of anastomoses and suture material employed may be helpful when available. A current arteriogram is obtained to define the related arterial status as well as the patency of the graft itself. This will provide information necessary to plan and execute a safe, durable procedure, which usually includes removal of the infected graft material and simultaneous autogenous arterial repair to provide or maintain critical flow to the involved extremity or organ supplied by the graft.

Autogenous Tissue Techniques

1. *Patch angioplasty* is applicable to cover any partially circumferential arterial defect that is in continuity with the arterial tree, for example, arteriotomy sites which remain infected when a previous bypass graft has been removed (Fig. 4).
2. *Endarterectomy* is a useful and fundamental technique for restoring flow through obstructed or stenosed arterial segments that had previously been bypassed by the infected prosthetic graft. For example, aortoiliac and aortofemoral endarterectomy may be used to restore lower limb perfusion when an infected aortofemoral bypass graft has been removed.

Patch Graft
(open endarterectonmy)

Conduit Graft
(eversion endarterectomy)

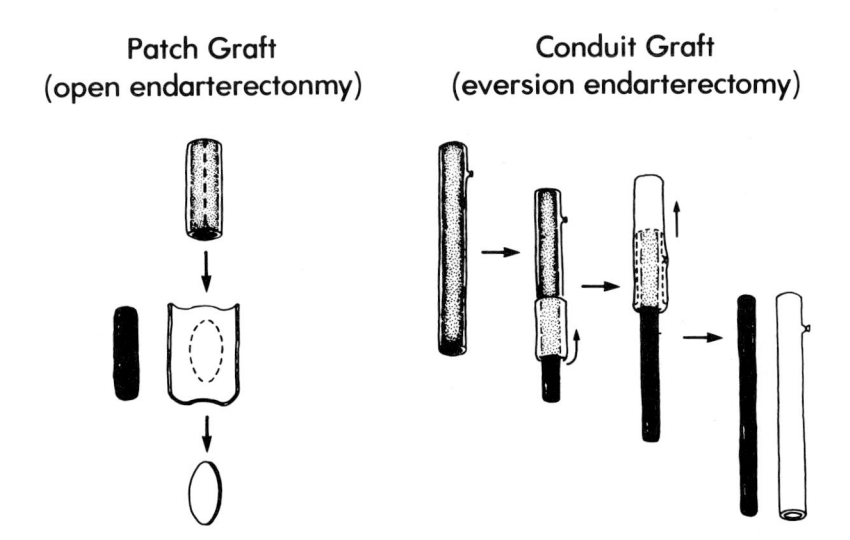

FIGURE 4. Diagram showing the use of the occluded superficial femoral artery as an autogenous graft.

3. *Autogenous graft replacement* is necessary to bridge circumferential defects in the arterial tree usually caused by the removal of infected grafts employed for aneurysmal or occlusive atherosclerosis (Fig. 4).[7,8]

Autografts are used to replace the aortoiliac or femoral segments when aneurysmal atherosclerosis of the native arteries makes endarterectomy impossible. The autograft may frequently be obtained by excising the occluded superficial femoral arterial segments in the thigh and disobliterating them using the eversion endarterectomy technique.

The most common and lethal chronic perigraft infection occurs in aortofemoral bypass grafts. The mortality rate for diffuse aortofemoral graft infection as reported by Szilagyi and Fry was 100 percent and 70 percent, respectively. If no provisions for lower extremity perfusion are made, the amputation rate exceeds 80 percent (bilateral midthigh level). The details of two surgical management variations employing autogenous revascularizations will be discussed in order to provide the reader with various technical considerations that have evolved in managing these problems.

Abdominal and Groin Prosthetic Graft Infection

Prosthetic grafts attached to the abdominal aorta (usually by the end-to-side technique) and extended to the anterior and medial surface of the common femoral arteries unilaterally or bilaterally are the most common configuration of prosthetic grafting in use for occlusive atherosclerosis of the aortoiliac arteries (Fig. 5A). Infection usually originates from skin bacteria native to the groin or peroneal area. Since the groin areas are immediately adjacent to the infected graft itself, the exposure of the femoral limbs of such a graft to facilitate removal necessarily contaminates the groin wound and precludes placing another prosthetic graft in this location. Therefore, the successful surgical management of an aortofemoral perigraft infection may at times be impossible to manage using conventional techniques of ex situ remote bypass to preserve extremity blood flow. Surgical management of such complicated graft infections requires a thorough knowledge of the related arterial anatomy, as well as the region traversed by the graft and the technique of graft insertion. Finally, the surgeon must be familiar with autogenous techniques of endarterectomy and other autogenous graft materials in order to restore lower extremity perfusion following removal of this type of infected graft. Diffuse involvement of the entire graft is usual. When the graft is removed, restoration of limb blood flow is usually crucial for extremity salvage.

Use of Autogenous Tissues 395

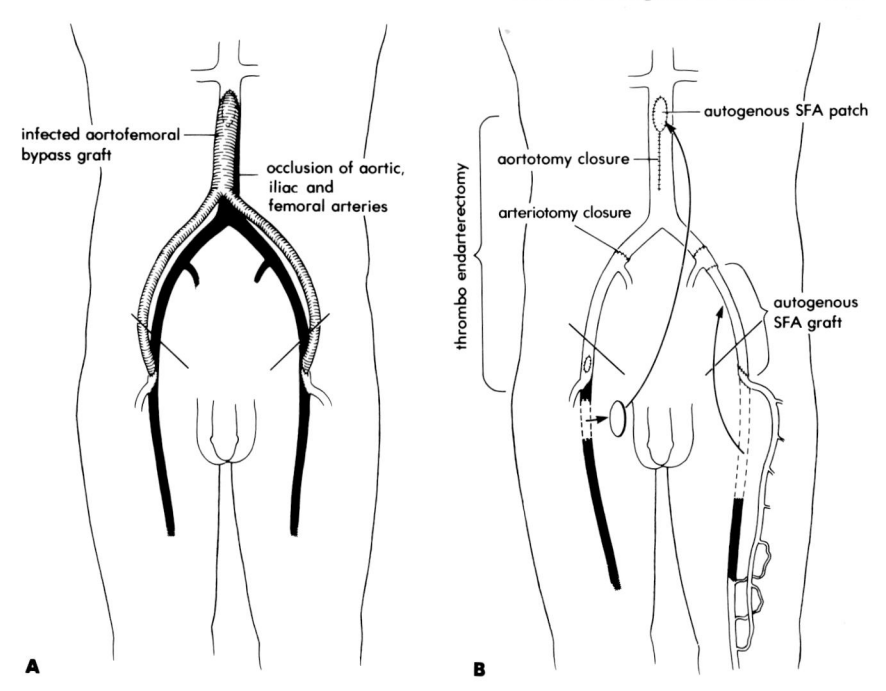

FIGURE 5.A. Diagram of an infected aortofemoral prosthetic bypass graft in its usual configuration. End-to-side anastomosis proximally as well as distally with runoff through the profunda femoris arteries. The superficial femoral arteries are chronically occluded. **B.** Diagram of various autogenous techniques useful in managing chronic infection of an aortofemoral prosthetic bypass. In situ thromboendarterectomy; autogenous arterial patch angioplasty, and conduit grafting are shown.

The extent of the aortoiliac atherosclerotic occlusive disease that is bypassed by an aortofemoral graft varies, but diffuse lesions of the aortoiliac as well as the femoropopliteal artery are usually present. Because the superficial femoral artery is occluded, the outflow of the femoral graft limbs is usually restricted to the profunda femoris artery. The profunda femoris is the important artery that provides abundant collateral flow to the lower leg and must be reperfused when the aortofemoral graft is removed in order to preserve the limb. Because there are no patent arterial segments present in the thigh, a remote bypass (axillofemoral bypass) cannot be employed. Autogenous reconstruction may be accomplished by either autograft reconstruction or in situ endarterectomy (Fig. 5B). Autogenous grafts may be obtained by removing the occluded superficial femoral arteries and restoring luminal patency using the eversion endarterectomy technique. The two arterial conduits thereby obtained can be anastomosed to substitute for the aortofemoral graft that must be removed. If portions or all of the original bypassed abdominal aorta and iliac arteries are suitable and can be disobliterated by in situ endarterectomy, use of the extremity autografts may not be necessary. Aortoiliofemoral thromboendarterectomy is facilitated by introducing loop strippers through the arteriotomies that were originally used to attach the bypass graft. These arteriotomies are closed using autogenous patches of saphenous vein or endarterectomized superficial femoral artery wall as necessary. Figure 6 shows pre- and postoperative aortograms. An aortoiliofemoral endarterectomy was performed after removal of an infected aortofemoral and crossfemoral bypass graft.

If adequate lengths of the native iliac arteries or the autograft of superficial femoral artery are not adequate to bridge defects in arterial continuity, a composite autogenous graft, including segments of available saphenous or other veins, is useful in revascularizing the limbs within the infected field. Figure 7 shows a composite aortofemoral autograft used to restore aortofemoral flow, with a reversed saphenous vein as a femorofemoral crossover graft.

The use of autogenous tissue technique permits the surgeon to restore or maintain aortic continuity in managing the septic aortic graft. Deliber-

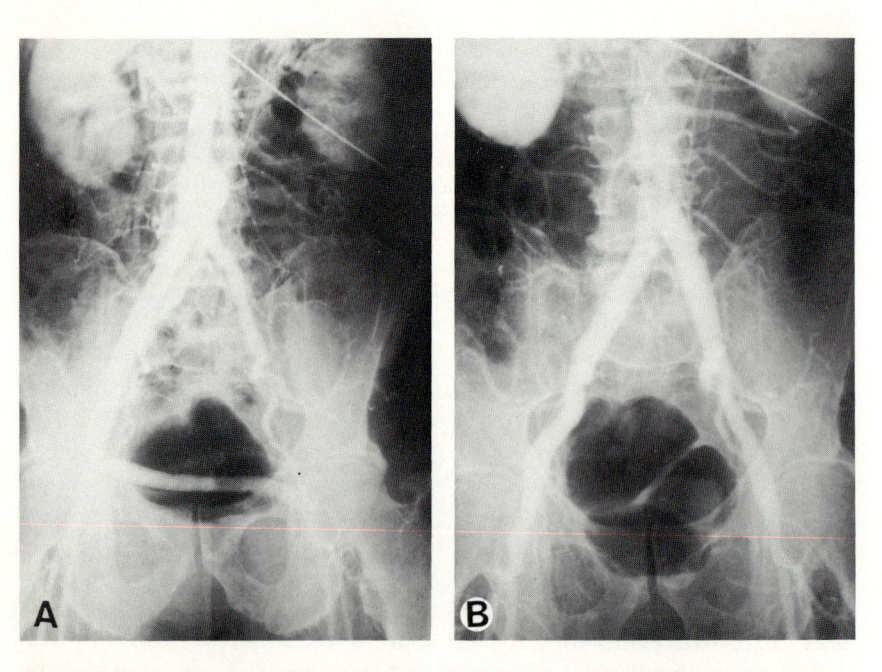

FIGURE 6.A. Preoperative aortogram showing patent aortofemoral cross femoral infected prosthetic graft. B. Postoperative aortogram showing patent aortoileofemoral segments following in situ thromboendarterectomy.

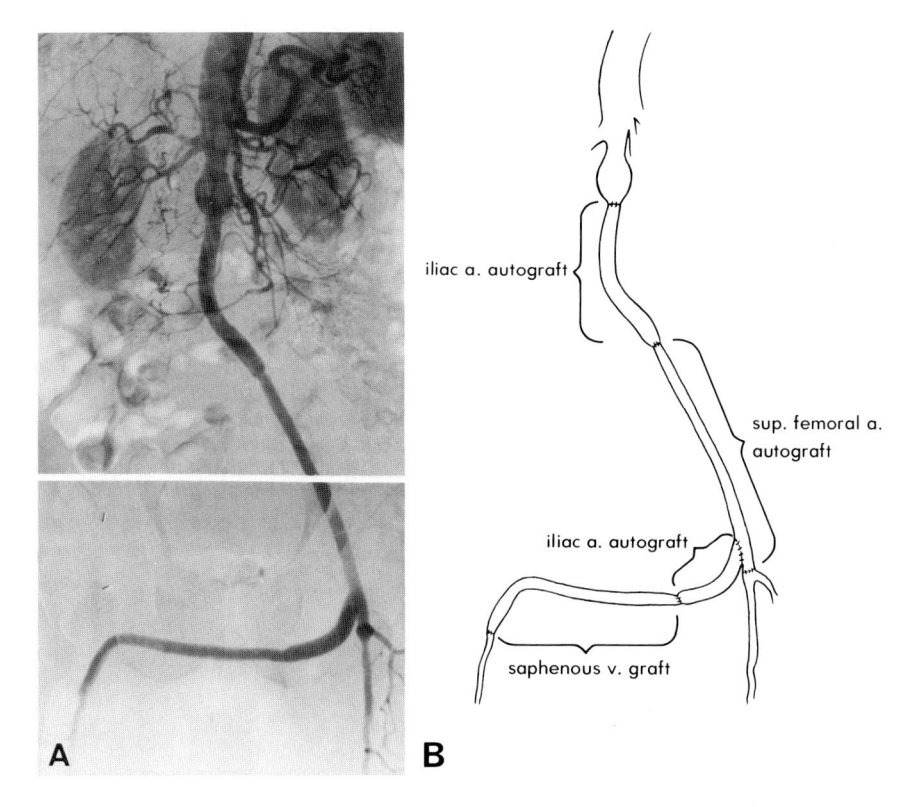

FIGURE 7.**A.** Postoperative aortogram. **B.** Diagram showing autograft aortofemoral reconstruction following removal of an infected aortofemoral replacement graft.

ate subrenal aortic division and ligation are unnecessary and its two focal sequellae, stump dehiscence and proximal aortorenal thrombosis, are avoided. No instances of early or late hemorrhage or thrombotic complications have occurred among the entire group of patients in whom autograft revascularization methods within the infected field were used.

SUMMARY

This chapter has attempted to outline problems of chronic perigraft infection complicating aortic prosthetic arterial repair. The clinical presentations and diagnostic methods useful in identifying these problems are reviewed. The successful management corollaries include these principles:

1. Removal of all involved prosthetic material
2. Restoration or maintenance of critical blood flow (originally provided by the graft) using autogenous tissues within the infected field

Familiarity with endarterectomy and the techniques of redo arterial surgery will allow the surgeon to achieve a satisfactory outcome for the threatened patient with the dreaded complication of chronic aortic perigraft infection.

REFERENCES

1. Baker BH, Baker MS, van der Reis L, Fisher JH: Endoscopy in the diagnosis of aortoduodenal fistula. Gastrointes Endos 24:35, 1977
2. Ehrenfeld WK, Wilbur BG, Olcott CN IV, Stoney RJ: Autogenous tissue reconstruction in the management of infected prosthetic grafts. Surgery 85:82, 1979
3. Fry WJ, Lindenauer SM: Infection complicating the use of plastic arterial implants. Arch Surg 94:600, 1967
4. Gooding GAW, Effeney DJ, Goldstone J: The aorto-femoral graft: Detection and identification of healing. Complications by ultrasonography. Arch Surg (in press)
5. Haaga JR, Baldwin GN, Reich NE, et al: CT detection of infected synthetic grafts: Preliminary report of a new sign. Am J Roentgenol 131:317, 1978
6. Moore WS, Rosson CT, Hall AD, Thomas AN: Transient bacteremia: A cause of infection in prosthetic vascular grafts. Am J Surg 117:342, 1969
7. Stoney RJ, Wylie EJ: Arterial autograft. Surgery 67:18, 1970
8. Szilagyi DE, Smith RF, Elliott JP, Vrandecic MD: Infection in arterial reconstruction with synthetic grafts. Ann Surg 176:321, 1972

TWENTY-SEVEN

Aortoduodenal and Other Aortoenteric Fistulas

Victor M. Bernhard

Communication between the aorta and the intestine may be a primary event complicating an aortic aneurysm or secondary to a prior aortic reconstruction. In either case, inflammatory and/or mechanical factors promote erosion of the vascular structure into an adjacent loop of bowel.

Primary aortoenteric fistula was first recorded in 1817 by Sir Astley Cooper who described the classic picture of recurring and ultimately fatal gastrointestinal hemorrhage in a young man with a pulsatile abdominal mass. Although the underlying aneurysm was almost certainly of luetic origin in this instance, the majority are due to atherosclerotic degeneration.[2] Other degenerative processes of the aortic wall, such as mycotic aneurysm, tumor erosion, and tuberculosis, have been implicated occasionally as the primary etiologic factor.[2] In this era of aggressive surgical management of abdominal aortic aneurysm and aortoiliac occlusive disease spontaneous aortoenteric fistula is a rare occurrence.[21] Only four patients with this problem have been identified in the combined experience of the affiliated hospitals of the Medical College of Wisconsin during the past 20 years.[2]

Secondary fistula is a complication of previous aortic surgery and has become the most common form of this disease.[10] It was first described in 1953 by Brock[5] in a report of his early experiences with the replacement of abdominal aortic aneurysms by homografts. The pathophysiology of this process is similar to that of primary fistulas in that it is due to aneurysmal degeneration of the homograft wall with progressive erosion into the overlying duodenum. This specific etiology is now of historical interest only since prosthetic aortic replacements have replaced homografts. The term *secondary aortoenteric fistula* generally implies development of this problem in patients following aortic reconstruction with Dacron or other plastic materials because it is only rarely a complication of endarterectomy.

PATHOGENESIS

Several factors have been identified as important contributors to this pathologic process by inference, direct observation, or evaluation of experimental models. The location of most fistulas between the infrarenal abdominal aorta and the duodenojejunal flexure is obviously related to the anatomic propinquity of these structures, the frequency of spontaneous aneurysm in the infrarenal aorta, and the usual location of grafts and suture lines at this level for the repair of aneurysm or occlusive disease. In the experience presented from the Medical College of Wisconsin, 75 percent of fistulas involved these structures.[18] Although the colon, stomach, and esophagus are rarely involved, any segment of the gastrointestinal tract may become directly adherent to a diseased or operated segment of the aorta and consequently become the site for fistula formation.

Direct erosion of an aortic aneurysm or a graft into an adjacent loop of bowel may be the result of the mechanical trauma from recurrent arterial pulsation. This appears to be the obvious explanation for the formation of all primary and secondary fistulas due to homografts or anastomotic aneurysms (Fig. 1). Direct erosion of a prosthesis or prosthetic-aortic anastomosis into an overlying adherent loop of bowel (Fig. 1) may occur when a healthy layer of viable tissue has not been interposed between these structures at the original procedure.[10] This was the apparent cause in three of our cases in which this mechanical setting was clearly described in the initial operative report.

Reoperation on the aorta and consequent infection may have been the etiologic factor in five of our patients in whom exogenous contamination or bacterial seeding of the operative repair from inadvertent bowel injury occurred. Although graft infection per se was not clearly identified as the basis for secondary fistula formation in our series, it has been demonstrated to be an important causative factor in a carefully controlled animal study by Bussittil and co-workers[7] and clearly is a factor in some patients. Graft redundancy and kinking in two of our patients probably contributed to mechanical erosion by protruding into an adjacent loop of bowel. Although no apparent etiologic factor could be identified in a few patients, one or more factors were demonstrated in 14 of 17 determinate cases occurring secondary to a previous aortic operation.[18]

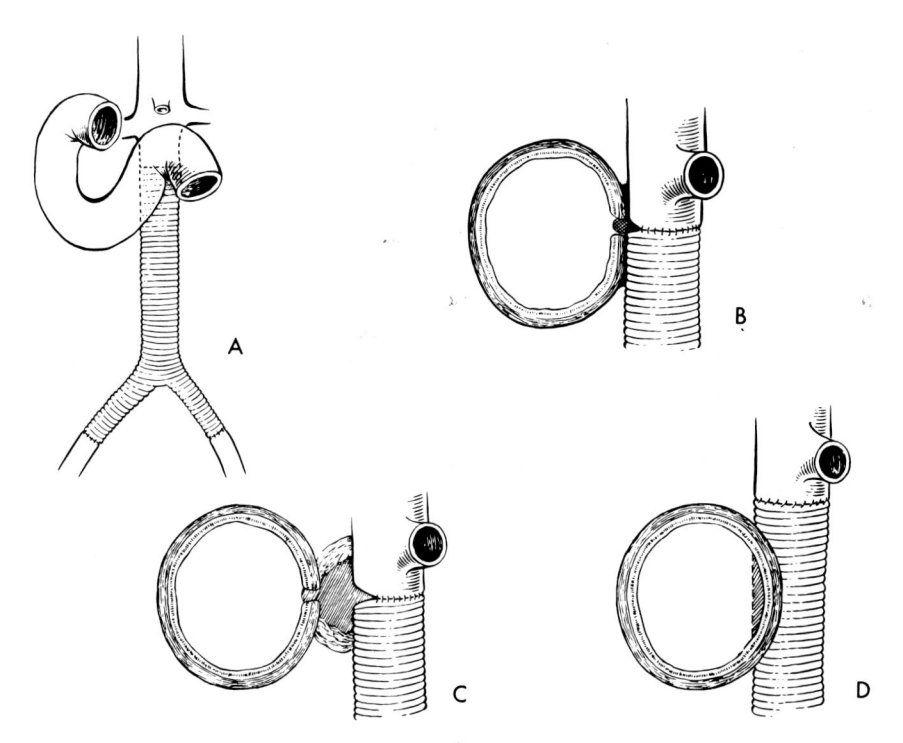

FIGURE 1. Pathogenesis of aortoduodenal fistula. **A.** Anatomic relationship of duodenojejunal flexure to the proximal graft anastomosis. **B.** Temporary thrombus occluding small direct fistula. **C.** Fistula due to erosion of anastomotic false aneurysm into the bowel wall. **D.** Graft erosion directly into bowel without direct involvement of the anastomosis (paraprosthetic enteric fistula). (From Bernhard VM: Aortoenteric fistulas. In Bergan JJ, Yao JST (eds): Operative Techniques in Vascular Surgery. New York, Grune & Stratton, 1980)

Logic dictates that technical perfection during the initial surgical procedure is the most important prophylaxis against fistula formation. This includes careful graft placement under adequate tension to avoid kinking, separation of the entire prosthesis and all anastomoses from direct contact with loops of bowel by interposition of a layer of healthy viable tissue, and prevention of perigraft infection by meticulous technique and the use of prophylactic antibiotics. During aneurysm resection, the intima of the aneurysm sac as well as the laminated thrombus should be removed in accordance with the suggestion of Ernst and colleagues[14] who identified a significant number of positive bacterial cultures from this material. Only the viable muscularis and adventitia of the sac should be left in place and used to wrap around the prosthesis.

CLINICAL PRESENTATION

Gastrointestinal bleeding in some form occurs in all patients with aortoenteric fistulas, and the characteristics of this bleeding are indistinguishable from that due to the more common primary gastrointestinal lesions. Regardless of the initial presentation, all patients will eventually succumb from massive gastrointestinal hemorrhage unless the pathologic process is interrupted by surgery. The type of gastrointestinal bleeding and its duration depend upon the location and the nature of the communication between the vascular and intestinal structures. The classic picture is one of recurrent "herald" bleeding with spontaneous remission. When a vascular anastomosis, false aneurysm, or true aneurysm is the basis for direct erosion into the duodenum, hematemesis, melena, or both occur and are indistinguishable from the bleeding caused by peptic ulceration, varices, or tumor. Hematochezia occurs when the distal small intestine or colon are involved and is similar in nature to bleeding due to diverticular disease or tumor. The initial bleeding episodes are usually mild to moderate and will stop spontaneously as long as the fistula is small enough to be temporarily plugged by thrombus formation. Thrombolysis leads to recurring hemorrhage and eventually the fistula enlarges to the point where thrombus formation is inadequate and exsanguination ensues. Less than 10 percent of patients will present with continuing massive hemorrhage as the initial event with no prior history of bleeding. Only two of 24 patients in our experience had no antecedent episode of gastrointestinal blood loss.

Graft erosion into the intestinal lumen at a point remote from an anastomosis does not present initially with gross evidence of gastrointestinal bleeding (Fig. 1). Fibrous tissue incorporating the prosthesis is digested by intestinal juices and infection thus permitting a slow, continuous ooze of blood through the interstices of the graft into the bowel lumen.[10,13,18,20] This variant is referred to as paraprosthetic enteric fistula and is characterized by a clinical picture of anemia, guiac positive stools, and fever. Blood cultures are frequently positive. Graft infection will eventually extend along the prosthesis to involve the aortic wall at an anastomosis. Thereafter, recurring episodes of "herald" bleeding develop as blood issues forth from the degenerating anastomosis and travels along the tract of the infected graft into the bowel lumen.

A pulsatile mass may be present if the fistula arises from an aortic aneurysm or aneurysmal degeneration of a graft. In most instances, false aneurysms located in the retroperitoneal space are too small to be palpated. Of the eight patients in our series who had palpable masses associated with aortoenteric fistula, four were due to primary aortic aneurysm, three to degenerated homografts, and only one was due to a large anastomotic false aneurysm.

DIAGNOSIS

Gastrointestinal bleeding of any type in a patient with a history of prior surgery on the aorta or its major branches or in a patient who has a pulsatile, abdominal mass must be assumed to be due to an aortoenteric fistula until proven otherwise. Because the initial bleeding episode is rarely exsanguinating, a period of at least a few hours after onset of symptoms is available to carry out diagnostic tests if the patient is hemodynamically stable. Upper gastrointestinal endoscopy may identify other actively bleeding lesions in the esophagus, stomach, or proximal duodenum.[18] Nonbleeding lesions, however, should not be considered the source of hemorrhage. Occasionally, a skilled endoscopist can visualize a fistula directly by passing a scope into the distal portion of duodenum.[1,19] In our experience, endoscopy was helpful in eight of nine patients by demonstrating the absence of other gastrointestinal lesions in six and actually visualizing fistula erosion into the third portion of the duodenum in two.

An aortogram may rarely identify a false aneurysm or the intraintestinal leakage of contrast media. A normal study is of no value, however, as it does not rule out fistula formation.[18]

A gallium scan may demonstrate a midabdominal perigraft inflammatory process. This study is of particular value in patients with paraprosthetic fistulas. Because of the time required to complete this test, however, it is applicable only in patients who have chronic anemia and guaiac positive stools but have not had gross hemorrhage and in whom exsanguination does not appear to be imminent. Computerized tomographic scanning may identify a false aneurysm or a perigraft inflammatory mass that may contain gas. Because this procedure can be accomplished quickly, it should be considered for any patient who is hemodynamically stable.

The barium meal is highly unreliable. It rarely identifies the fistula but frequently demonstrates extraneous lesions that are not the immediate cause of bleeding. These findings confuse the issue and cause delay in surgical intervention based on the forlorn hope that nonoperative therapy will be effective. The positive findings when present include a compression deformity of the fourth portion of the duodenum, extraluminal extravasation of barium, and contrast outlining the corrugations of a vascular graft.

Barium enema and colonoscopy are useful to rule out colonic neoplasia and diverticular disease in patients with chronic anemia and guaiac positive stools or hematochezia because colon or distal small bowel erosion by a graft is extremely rare and intrinsic bowel pathology is far more common. Although positive findings do not absolutely rule out an aortoenteric fistula, identification of a primary colon lesion directs the surgeon to prepare the bowel in anticipation of colon resection if the patient is stable.

In any patient with a suspected aortoenteric fistula, diagnostic maneuvers should be performed within a few hours of admission while the operating room is being prepared. A more leisurely approach may be used in a patient with anemia and guaiac positive stools who has not sustained massive hemorrhage or recurrent "herald" bleeding. Since major hemorrhage will eventually occur in all of these patients, however, workup under these circumstances should be expeditious and completed within a few days. It must be recognized that in most patients, preoperative investigation is primarily helpful by ruling out other causes of bleeding and infrequently directly establishes the diagnosis of a fistula directly.

In some patients in whom the diagnosis remains in doubt, the ultimate diagnostic test, surgical exploration, must be considered.

PRINCIPLES OF SURGICAL MANAGEMENT

The goals of surgical intervention in this disease are to verify the diagnosis, control hemorrhage, and restore bowel and vascular continuity. Full cardiovascular monitoring should be established prior to the induction of anesthesia. This should include insertion of a Swan-Ganz catheter if time and facilities permit. A blood culture should be obtained preoperatively and broad spectrum antibiotics administered before laparotomy to treat the mixed infection associated with the gastrointestinal flora that is invariably present around the fistula.[18] This therapy is modified as necessary depending upon the culture findings and is continued for at least 10 days postoperatively or until all evidence of infection has subsided.

The visual first step in surgical management is to stop hemorrhage or to remove the threat of exsanguination by immediate laparotomy. When preoperative diagnostic maneuvers have firmly established the presence of paraprosthetic fistula without immediate threat of massive hemorrhage, however, it is appropriate to establish an alternate route for lower extremity revascularization as the preliminary step.

Abdominal exploration is performed through a long midline incision from the xiphoid down to a point a few centimeters above the pubis. This provides the most effective exposure for intra-abdominal maneuvers and avoids contamination of the flank and suprapubic routes required for subsequent axillobifemoral bypass.

Active hemorrhage can be temporarily controlled by application of direct tamponade to the aorta at the level of the celiac artery by a mechanical compressor or the surgeon's hand. Rapid exposure of the supraceliac aorta can be achieved by incising the diaphragm at the aortic hiatus for direct application of a clamp as described in Chapter 25.[8] The infrarenal aorta just above the fistula can then be safely identified and freed from the scar of the previous surgery and the inflammatory process associated with the fistula without danger of exsanguination[3] (Fig. 2). Thereafter, the clamp is transferred from the supraceliac to the infrarenal position. If the patient is not actively hemorrhaging and the aortic wall is not obscured by scar or a false aneurysm, the infrarenal aorta can be approached directly. The fistula can be divided and the aortic opening controlled by finger tamponade (Fig. 2) until the infrarenal aorta has

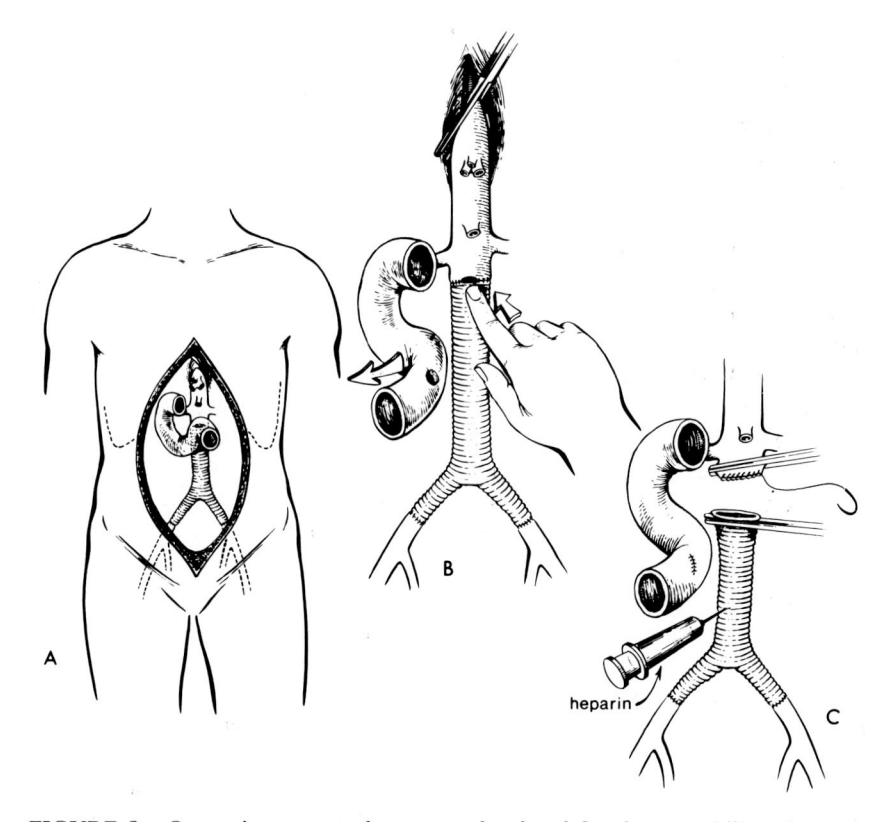

FIGURE 2. Operative approach to aortoduodenal fistula. **A.** Midline incision. **B.** Aortic control with supraceliac clamp after division of diaphragmatic crura. Finger tamponade of a small vascular defect after takedown of the fistula. **C.** Closure of enteric defect and resection of graft with oversewing of the aortic stump. Distal installation of heparin through the graft to avoid peripheral thrombosis. (From Bernhard VM: Aortoenteric fistulas. In Bergan JJ, Yao JST (eds): Operative Techniques in Vascular Surgery. New York, Grune & Stratton, 1980)

been adequately exposed and clamped. The enteric defect is closed using standard gastrointestinal suture techniques. If the bowel defect is extensive, resection and reanastomosis are preferred.

In most secondary fistulas, the entire graft should be removed because it is infected, and a new graft should not be replaced in the contaminated retroperitoneal space. Although successful results have been reported following direct repair of the fistula without graft excision,[4,11,13,16] in our experience and that reported by others,[12,15,18] sepsis, hemorrhage, and recurrent fistula formation have frequently occurred whenever old or new graft material has been left in the retroperitoneal area.

Closure of the infrarenal aortic stump is hazardous due to a high incidence of septic necrosis with hemorrhage or late aneurysm formation and refistulization.[6] Insofar as possible, all necrotic tissue, including infected aortic wall, should be excised. Stump closure should be performed at a level where the aortic wall is grossly healthy using multiple layers of 2–0 monofilament polypropylene suture[3] (Fig. 2C). A flap of anterior spinous ligament can sometimes be raised and placed over the aortic closure as a reinforcing layer.[15] Alternatively, a tongue of omentum may be placed over the aortic closure.[3] There measures have not consistently prevented stump breakdown, however. Recently, Buchbinder and coworkers[6] presented experimental evidence that a pedicle of vascularized muscle, obtained by stripping the mucosa from an isolated segment of small bowel, when sutured over the stump will prevent dehiscence of the oversewn aorta. This technique has been successfully applied in two patients.[17]

After the aortic stump is secured, all infected and necrotic tissue is debrided from the retroperitoneum and a suction drain is brought out through a flank stab wound on the side opposite to the planned axillofemoral bypass.

Lower extremity revascularization should be carried out immediately unless the limbs have been previously amputated or the excised graft has been thrombosed for a sufficient length of time to permit development of adequate collaterals. Abrupt interruption of lower extremity circulation by graft excision may produce ischemic necrosis of the colon and buttocks as well as the legs.[18] Unfortunately, the appearance of the feet immediately after graft excision is not a reliable guide. By the time the need for postponed revascularization had become apparent in two of our patients, lethal and irreversible changes had taken place in the pelvic viscera and the extremities.

Limb revascularization should not be performed until the abdominal wound has been closed and sealed. The patient should be reprepped and draped, fresh instruments obtained, and the operating team newly gowned and gloved. The simplest and most effective technique for lower extremity revascularization is axillobifemoral bypass (Fig. 3). Distal anastomoses to the common femoral arteries can be employed when the infected aortic graft is entirely confined to the abdomen. If the fistula is associated with an aortofemoral graft, however, the inguinal areas are potentially infected or may become contaminated during graft excision and will be unsuitable as anastomotic sites for the extra-anatomic prosthesis. Considerable ingenuity is required to avoid contamination from groin wounds and to carry out anastomoses to the distal patent vessels of the limbs. The axillofemoral graft can be routed laterally through a notch in the iliac crest or just medial to the anterosuperior iliac spine. The distal superficial femoral or the midprofunda artery can be approached through an intermuscular plane lateral and deep to the rectus femoris. A crossover femorofemoral graft of autogenous tissue (saphenous vein or endarterectomized superficial femoral artery) can

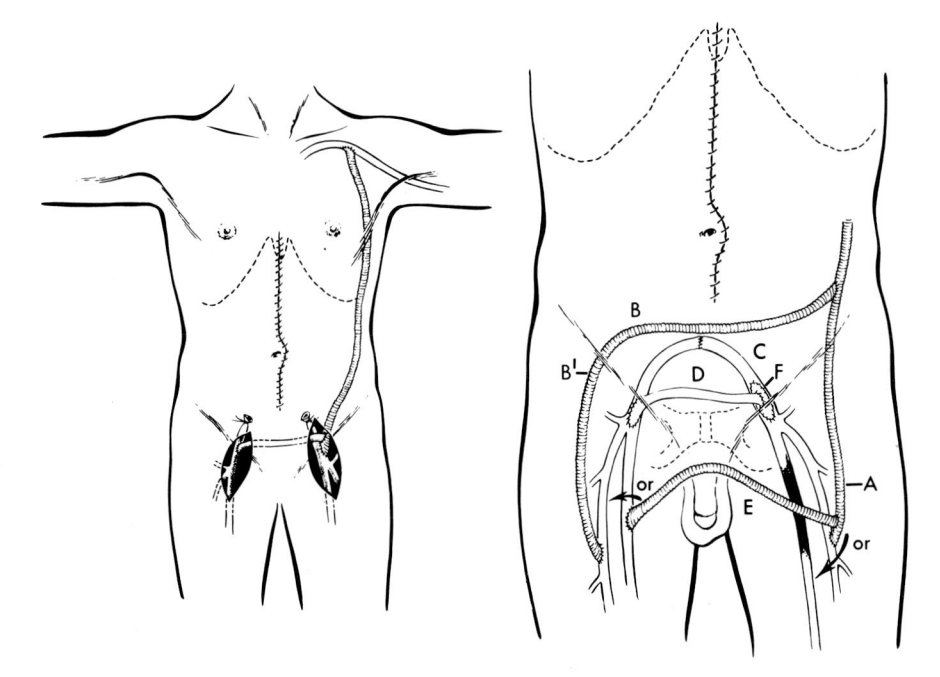

FIGURE 3. Extra-anatomic bypass for extremity revascularization. **Left.** Simple axillobifemoral bypass when the infected graft is confined to the abdomen. **Right.** Various techniques for lower extremity revascularization after excision of an aortofemoral graft to avoid secondary contamination from groin wounds. (From Bernhard VM: Aortoenteric fistulas. In Bergan JJ, Yao JST (eds): Operative Techniques in Vascular Surgery. New York, Grune & Stratton, 1980)

then be placed through the reopened groin incisions. Alternatively, a subcutaneous route inferior to the pubic symphysis can be developed on the medial aspect of the thigh to crossover to the opposite limb (Fig. 3).

The primary aortoenteric fistula should be managed somewhat differently from the secondary fistula if the initiating degenerative process in the aorta is atherosclerosis and not a mycotic aneurysm. Infection is of minor consequence because there is no foreign body to promote the process and erosion is almost invariably into the duodenum that has a low concentration of gastrointestinal flora. Daugherty and his associates[9] have clearly demonstrated that simple closure of the duodenal defect and standard resection of the aneurysm and graft replacement will resolve the problem with standard morbidity and a minimal risk of graft sepsis. The portion of aneurysm wall directly involved with the fistula should be liberally excised and the prosthetic replacement wrapped in a tongue of omentum to insure a well vascularized perigraft bed. If the primary fistula is due to a mycotic aneurysm or is accompanied by extensive infection, however, resection and extra-anatomic limb revascularization should be considered.

RESULTS

Twenty-five aortoenteric fistulas have been managed in the affiliated hospitals of the Medical College of Wisconsin in Milwaukee. Four patients had primary fistulas, three of which were not recognized and the patients died from exsanguination. The diagnosis was suspected preoperatively in the fourth patient on the basis of recurrent upper gastrointestinal bleeding and a known abdominal aortic aneurysm. The diagnosis was confirmed by endoscopy. Aneurysm resection and axillofemoral bypass were performed and the patient was recovering well until the eighth postoperative day when he suddenly died from a massive pulmonary embolism. The collected series reported by Daugherty and colleagues[9] indicated that extra-anatomic bypass is unnecessary for primary fistulas. Excision of the aneurysm, bowel closure, and standard retroperitoneal graft placement produced recovery and long-term survival in 13 of 14 patients.

Our experience with 21 secondary fistulas support the principles of excision and extra-anatomic bypass for this entity.[18] The overall mortality was 62 percent. Failure to recognize the diagnosis preoperatively or at the time of surgery was invariably associated with a fatal outcome from exsanguination. Recurrent sepsis, hemorrhage, or recurrent fistula formation and death occurred in all patients in whom the old graft was left in the retroperitoneum or was replaced by a new prosthesis. Failure to revascularize previously well perfused limbs resulted in death from extremity, buttock, and colon necrosis in two patients.[17]

Eight of ten patients (80 percent) survived when managed according to the principles previously outlined for diagnosis and surgical management of secondary fistulas. The two deaths were a result of renal failure secondary to perioperative hemorrhage in one patient and a myocardial infarct in the other. One of the survivors died from rupture of an aortic stump aneurysm eight months after successful repair of his fistula.[18]

SUMMARY

Aortoenteric fistula invariably produces some form of gastrointestinal bleeding and should be considered the primary diagnosis in any patient who has had previous aortic surgery or in whom an aneurysm has been identified. Prompt surgical intervention is mandatory to confirm the diagnosis and prevent exsanguination. Endoscopy, aortography, and other investigative maneuvers may be helpful to rule out other causes of gastrointestinal bleeding, but infrequently establish the diagnosis. Furthermore, preoperative investigation is frequently confusing, and negative findings do not rule out the diagnosis. Primary fistulas can usually be managed by closure of the bowel, excision of the aneurysm, and standard retroperitoneal graft placement. Secondary fistulas, which are much more common, require excision of the previous aortic graft and limb revascularization by extra-anatomic bypass.

REFERENCES

1. Baker BH, Baker MS, van der Reis L, Fisher JH: Endoscopy in the diagnosis of aortoduodenal fistula. Gastrointest Endosc 24:35, 1977
2. Bernhard VM, Kleinman LH: Aorto-enteric fistulas. In Bergan JJ, Yao JST: Surgery of the Aorta and Its Branches. New York, Grune & Stratton, 1979, pp 591–603
3. Bernhard VM: Aortoenteric fistulas. In Bergan JJ, Yao JST: Operative Techniques in Vascular Surgery. New York, Grune & Stratton, 1980, pp 193–202
4. Brenner WI, Richman H, Reed GE: Roof patch repair of an aortoduodenal fistula resulting from suture line failure in an aortic prosthesis. Am J Surg 127:762, 1974
5. Brock RC: Aortic homografting: A report of six successful cases. Guy's Hosp Rep 102:204, 1953
6. Buchbinder D, Leather R, Shah D, Karmody A: Pathological interactions

between prosthetic aortic grafts and the gastrointestinal tract. Clinical problems and a new experimental approach. Am J Surg, 140:192, 1980
7. Busuttil RW, Rees W, Baker JD, Wilson SE: Pathogenesis of aortoduodenal fistula: Experimental and clinical correlates. Surgery 85:1, 1979
8. Crawford ES, Manning LG, Kelly TF: "Redo" surgery after operations for aneurysms and occlusion of the abdominal aorta. Surgery 81:41, 1977
9. Daugherty M, Shearer GR, Ernst CG: Primary aortoduodenal fistula: Extraanatomic vascular reconstruction not required for successful management. Surgery, 86:399, 1979
10. DeWeese MS, Fry WJ: Small-bowel erosion following aortic resection. JAMA 179:882, 1962
11. Eastcott HHG: Discussion of Kleinman LH, Towne JB, Bernhard VM: A diagnostic and therapeutic approach to aortoenteric fistulas: Clinical experience with twenty patients. Surgery 86:868, 1979
12. Ehrenfeld WK, Lord RSA, Stoney RJ, Wylie EJ: Subcutaneous arterial bypass grafts in the management of fistulae between the bowel and plastic arterial prostheses. Ann Surg 168:29, 1968
13. Elliott JP Jr, Smith RF, Szilagyi DE: Aortoenteric and paraprosthetic-enteric fistulas: Problems of diagnosis and management. Arch Surg 108:479, 1974
14. Ernst CB, Campbell HC, Daugherty J, et al: Incidence and significance of intraoperative bacterial cultures during abdominal aortic aneurysmectomy. Ann Surg 185:626, 1977
15. Fry WJ, Lindenauer SM: Infection complicating the use of plastic arterial implants. Arch Surg 94:600, 1967
16. Garrett HE, Beall AC Jr, Jordan GL Jr, DeBakey ME: Surgical considerations of massive gastrointestinal tract hemorrhage caused by aortoduodenal fistula. Am J Surg 105:6, 1963
17. Karmody A: Personal communication
18. Kleinman LH, Towne JB, Bernhard VM: A diagnostic and therapeutic approach to aortoenteric fistulas: Clinical experience with twenty patients. Surgery 86(6):868, 1979
19. Mir-Madjlessi SH, Sullivan BH Jr, Farmer RG, Beven EG: Endoscopic diagnosis of aortoduodenal fistula. Gastrointest Endosc 19:187, 1973
20. O'Mara C, Imbembo AL: Paraprosthetic enteric fistula. Surgery 81:556, 1977
21. Reckless JPD, McColl I, Taylor GW: Aorto-enteric fistulae: An uncommon complication of abdominal aortic aneurysms. Br J Surg 59:458, 1972

TWENTY-EIGHT
The Hypoplastic Aortoiliac Syndrome

Dominic A. DeLaurentis

A fascinating variety of atherosclerotic occlusive disease is the type associated with hypoplasia of the distal abdominal aorta. Although this occlusive process can be considered a variant of the Leriche syndrome, there seem to be sufficient identifying features to warrant separate consideration. It is not unusual to find reference to patients with small aortas.[12,21] Informal discussions with vascular surgeons on this topic usually elicit some experience with "the young woman with a small aorta." This may not be considered a subgroup. The problems and hazards encountered during surgical reconstruction provided the original reason for reporting this group of patients.[5] This chapter will describe the clinical features and principles of surgical management of patients with hypoplastic distal aortas associated with atherosclerotic occlusive disease. In addition, the current etiologic theories of hypoplasia of this segment of the aorta will be reviewed. In this regard it should be noted that there are important differences and no obvious relationship between this lesion and coarctation of the abdominal aorta, which is rare.

MATERIALS AND METHODS

Between January 1965 and December 1979, 398 patients underwent surgery for aortoiliac occlusive disease. This group was made up of 262 men (66 percent) and 136 women (34 percent). The operative procedures consisted of aortofemoral or aortoiliac bypass or endarterectomy in 319 patients (80 percent) and extra-anatomic bypass in 79 patients

(20 percent). Operations for aneurysms or trauma are not included. Twenty-seven of these 398 patients (7 percent) had small or hypoplastic distal aorta and iliac arteries as defined in the section on measurements. None were treated by an extra-anatomic procedure. Of the 319 aortoiliac or aortofemoral reconstructions, therefore, 27 were done for atherosclerosis associated with a hypoplastic aortoiliac system (9 percent). An analysis of these patients constitutes the basis of this report.

Analysis of 27 Patients with Hypoplastic Distal Aortoiliac Systems

The patients included 25 women (93 percent) and 2 men (7 percent). The 25 women with hypoplastic aortas comprised 23 percent of the total number (107) of women who underwent aortoiliac or aortofemoral reconstruction for atherosclerotic occlusive disease in this area. This lesion, then, was present in an important number of women requiring aortoiliac reconstruction.

The ages of the patients with hypoplastic aortas at the time of surgery ranged from 28 to 71 years and averaged 47 years. This is considerably younger than the average age for all of the patients who underwent surgery for aortoiliac occlusive disease (60 years). If we consider the age when symptoms were first noted by the 27 patients, we find a range of 28 to 57 years and an average age of 41 years. The duration of claudication in the four oldest patients at the time of surgery was 20 years (age 71), 20 years (age 60), 12 years (age 58), and 10 years (age 50).

Clinical History

All 27 patients were heavy cigarette smokers (1–3 pack/day), which is somewhat at variance with a previous report.[13] A strong family history of serious cardiovascular disease in the mother, father, or siblings was present in 17 of 21 patients (80 percent) in which this information was recorded. Four patients (aged 50, 51, 60, and 71) had a history of angina at the time of surgery and two of these four had suffered previous mild myocardial infarctions. No other obvious clinical heart disease was detected in the remainder of this group. Thigh and leg claudication, often bilateral, was elicited in all 27 patients. Rest pain involving the toes was present in four patients. Effort anesthesia and paresthesia of the feet were present in three other patients. Eight patients had symptoms either of transient ischemic attacks or left upper extremity claudication. Five of these eight patients underwent surgical correction of the brachiocephalic atherosclerotic occlusive process before aortoiliac reconstruction (Table 1).

Table 1. Statistical Analysis of 27 Patients with Hypoplastic Distal Aortoiliac Syndrome

	No.
History and Symptoms	
Claudication	27
Cigarette smoking	27
Strong family history of cardiovascular disease	17/21
Rest pain	4
Previous brachiocephalic arterial surgery	5
TIAs	4
Upper extremity claudication	4
Coronary artery disease	4
Hormonal and Reproductive Factors	
Surgically induced menopause	9
Normal menses and pregnancies	11
Normal menses and no pregnancies	3
Still births	1
Pre-eclampsia	1
Impotence	2
Diabetes mellitus	0
Oral contraceptives	3
Height in Inches	
56	1
59	1
60	5
61	1
62	2
63	1
64	6
65	2
66	4
67	1 (man)
68	1 (man)
Physical Examination	
Weak or absent femoral pulses	27
Abdominal bruits	16
Carotid bruits and/or upper extremity pulses↓	16
Hypertension	2
Obesity	8

Surgically induced menopause preceded claudication symptoms in nine women. Another woman, aged 39, had been taking oral contraceptives for 8 years prior to operation. Another patient had been pregnant six times but had never delivered a live child. Of the remaining 14 women, 11 had normal menstrual cycles with uncomplicated pregnancies, and three had normal cycles with no pregnancies. Both men had been impotent for 3 and 6 months before surgery (Table 1).

Physical Examination

Eight patients were overweight by an average of 36 pounds (range 20–50 pounds). Although this syndrome may seem to represent merely small aortas in small women, this was not the case in our series. The height was recorded in 25 of 27 patients. The distribution is shown in Table 1. The two male patients were 67 inches and 68 inches tall. The women ranged from 56 inches to 66 inches with an average of 63 inches. Blood pressure consistently above 140/90 was found in only two patients (ages 58 and 59), one of whom had known hypertensive disease (190/120) for 28 years and had been treated for 23 years. This patient was obese and had a type IV hyperlipidemia. Her blood pressure returned to normal, and has been normal for 7 years after she lost 50 pounds. The other patient had mild hypertension (150/90) that was easily controlled with diuretics. *The absence of hypertension in this group is an important clinical difference between this pathologic process and that of coarctation of the abdominal aorta.*[2,15]

Abdominal bruits, thrills, and weak femoral pulses were found in all patients, except for those with complete aortic occlusion. Pulses distal to the femoral area were rare. Venous filling times were increased, and ankle blood pressures showed definite gradients. Thigh and buttock atrophy was not marked. Foot pallor on elevation was common. Carotid bruits or absent or very weak left upper extremity pulses were found in 16 patients (60 percent). *Brachiocephalic occlusive disease was the most frequent coexistent vascular process encountered in our group of patients with hypoplastic aortoiliac segments (Table 1).*

Laboratory Data

There was no evidence of diabetes mellitus in any of the patients. Hyperlipidema was found in 9 of 13 patients tested: 7 had a type IV pattern and 2 patients had a type II. Serum cholesterol was as low as 175 mg% (normal 120–290) with an average of 266 mg% (25 patients). Eight patients had levels above the normal range. Serum triglyceride levels ranged from 90 mg% to 420 mg% (normal 30–135) with an average of 207 mg% (14 patients). Nine patients had triglyceride levels above the normal range. These findings do not conform with those reported by Greenhalgh[9] who found that 78 percent of "little women with blocked aortas" had cholesterol levels above 270 mg% and that the incidence of elevated triglyceride levels was much lower than in our patients. Three patients demonstrated serum fibrinogen levels above 500 mg%. All other laboratory studies were within normal limits.

Angiographic Studies

Angiography was performed in all patients, usually by the translumbar method, although retrograde femoral and transaxillary techniques were also used. Bleeding and acute occlusion following retrograde femoral catheterization occurred in one patient. This complication was corrected by immediate thrombectomy and angioplasty of an extremely small femoral artery.

The area of aortic hypoplasia occurred below the renal arteries and was most pronounced in the segment between the origin of the inferior mesenteric artery and the aortic bifurcation (Fig. 1). Five patients had occlusion of this segment with prominent collaterals (Fig. 2). Half of the remaining patients had a characteristic "hourglass" constrictive lesion immediately above the bifurcation (Fig. 3). Unilateral renal artery stenosis was found in one patient. Again, this lack of renal artery involvement is markedly different from coarctation of the abdominal aorta. There was no poststenotic dilatation of the aorta. The aorta bifurcated high, and there was a marked lack of elongation and tortuosity of the iliac system. The iliac-femoral system was uniformly quite narrow and appeared to be involved in the hypoplastic process. Superficial femoral artery occlusion with reconstitution of the popliteal artery was present in seven patients.

TREATMENT

I attempted endarterectomy on several occasions, but had to abandon it because of the small size of the arteries. This is in marked contrast to a recent report in which endarterectomy was the procedure of choice.[18] In this report by Roaf and Shannon, however, the lesion was a very localized, solitary, diaphragmatic process much like that described by Staple.[21] In my series of patients, the most common method of revascularization was a bypass technique using a bifurcated knitted Dacron graft. An end-to-side anastomosis was usually performed at both the aortic site and at the distal external iliac or common femoral areas. Excision

416   Critical Problems in Vascular Surgery

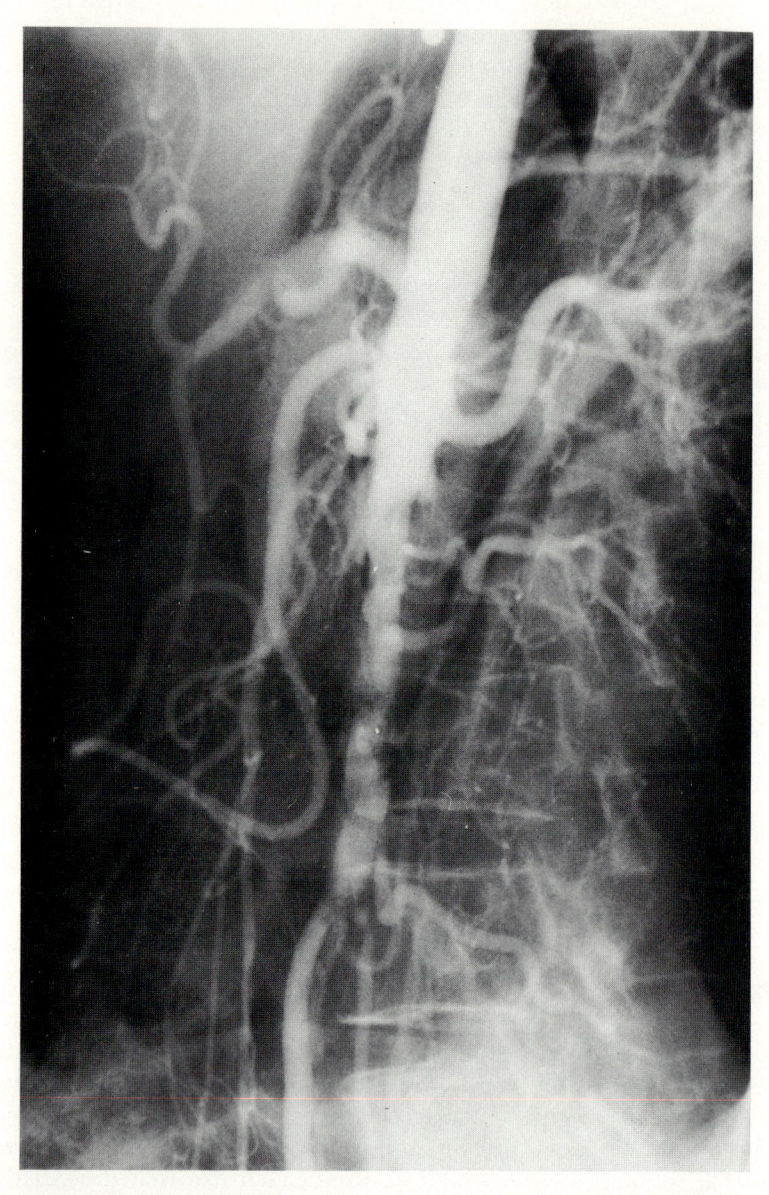

FIGURE 1. Infrarenal aortic hypoplasia and atherosclerotic narrowing in a 46-year-old woman.

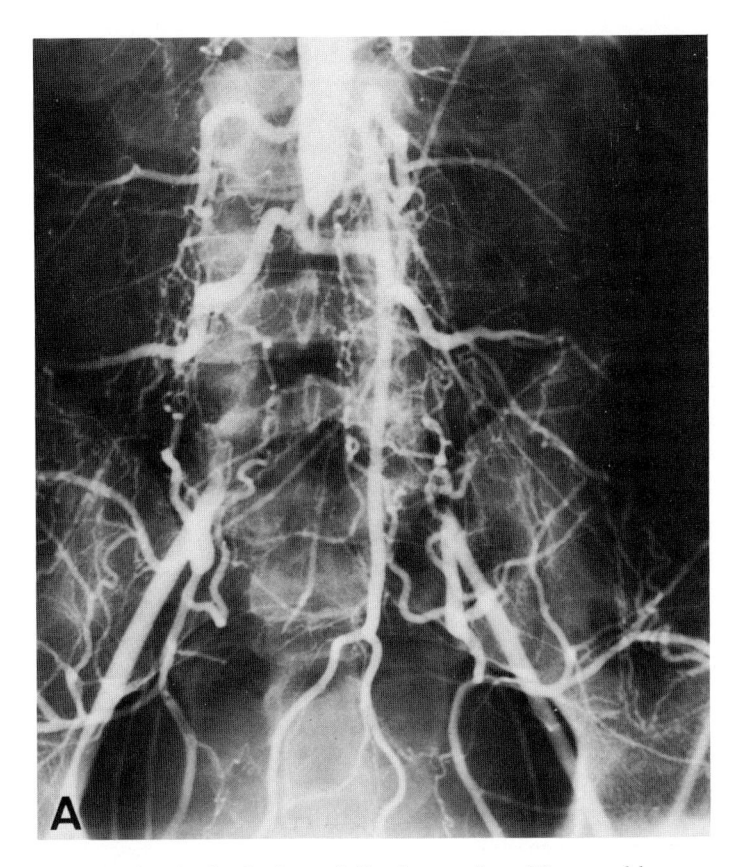

FIGURE 2. **A.** Occlusion of distal aorta in a 28-year-old man. *(Continued.)*

of the involved segment of aorta and proximal common iliac arteries was carried out in five instances. The proximal aortic anastomosis more recently has been of the end-to-end variety (11 patients). This proximal end-to-end anastomosis can be difficult and often requires a small bifurcated graft with proximal diameters of 12 or 13 mm and an oblique aortoplasty. Because of the narrow iliac and femoral arteries in these patients (diameter 2.5–3 mm), it was important to execute a meticulous and *long* end-to-side anastomosis distally, and not to attempt an end-to-end technique (Fig. 4). Systemic heparinization was instituted before aortic clamping and was not usually reversed.

The anastomosis to the aorta was performed first. It was necessary to construct the proximal anastomosis high up on the infrarenal aorta in order to avoid aortic disease and maximize aortic diameter. For proper

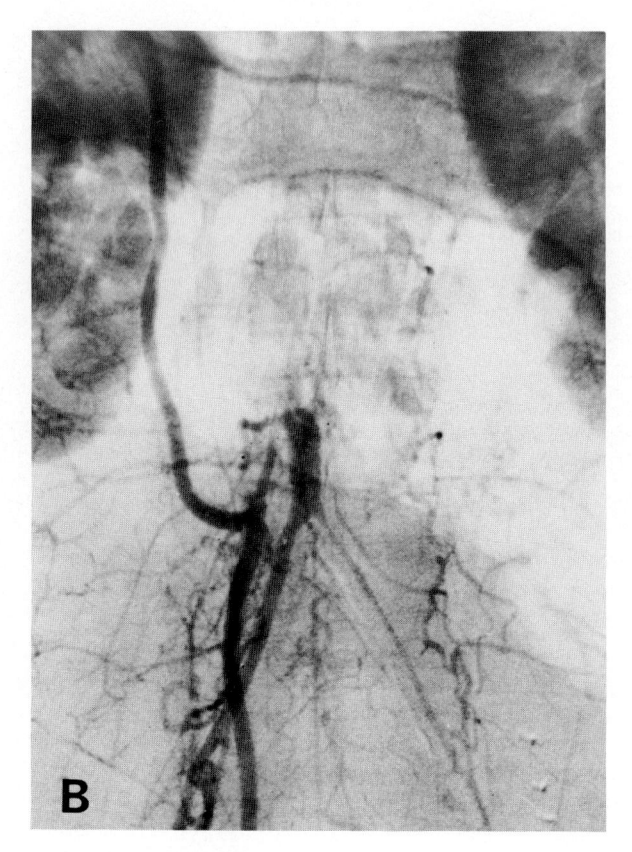

FIGURE 2. **B.** 38-year-old woman with occlusion of the aorta and reconstitution of an infantile distal aorta and iliac system.

aortic exposure, the left renal vein had to be divided in two patients, and no untoward effects resulted. The limbs of the bifurcated grafts were always brought down to the common femoral artery when there was superficial femoral artery occlusion or severe external iliac artery disease; otherwise anastomosis was to the external iliac just above the inguinal ligament. Bilateral lumbar sympathectomy was performed on the last 17 patients. There does not seem to be any marked difference between the early group of patients and the more recent ones who have had the sympathectomy. A patent inferior mesenteric artery or accessory renal arteries were never knowingly interrupted. Dacron sutures were used. Preoperative and postoperative antistaphylococcal antibiotics were given prophylactically to all patients. Anticoagulants and antiplatelet drugs were not administered postoperatively.

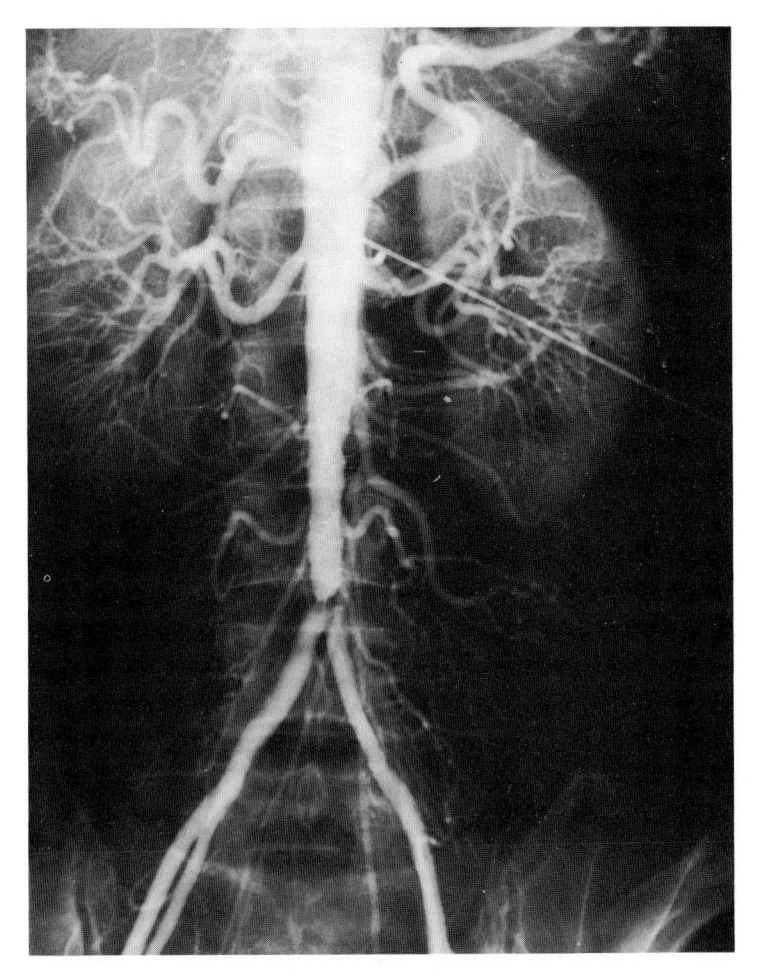

FIGURE 3. "Hourglass" stenosis at the distal aorta in a 37-year-old woman. Note the high bifurcation of the aorta, the marked narrowing between the inferior mesenteric artery origin and the bifurcation of the aorta, and the lack of tortuosity of the iliac system.

MEASUREMENTS

Although aortic, iliac, and femoral measurements in situ were made during most operations, the measuring method often varied. External diameters of the distal unclamped hypoplastic aortas ranged from 6 to 15 mm and averaged 11.25 mm. External diameters of the common iliac arteries ranged from 4 to 8 mm and averaged 5.25 mm. The external

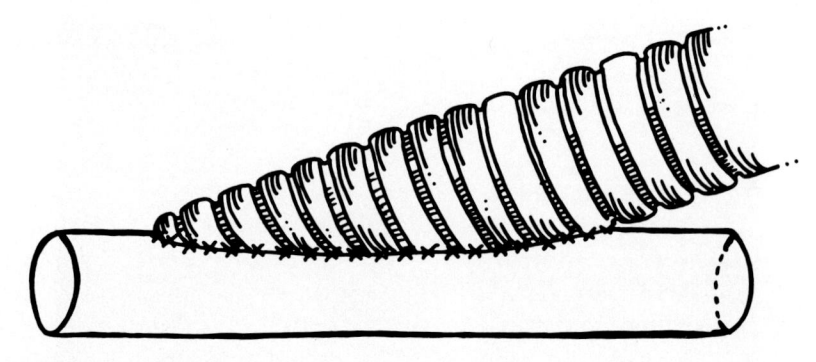

FIGURE 4. Technique of long end-to-side anastomosis between graft and hypoplastic femoral or iliac arteries.

iliac arteries ranged from 2 to 4 mm in diameter. More precise measurements were made of three resected specimens. The specimens were opened longitudinally and the circumferences at the proximal and distal aortic lines of resection were measured. The diameters of the proximal resected aortas (circumference/π) were 9 mm, 8 mm, and 2.5 mm. The diameters of the distal resected aortas were 3 mm, 2.5 mm, and 2.5 mm. In situ measurements of the same specimens àt surgery were 16 mm, 13 mm, 8 mm, and 10 mm, 8 mm, 8 mm, respectively (Table 2). What size is considered "hypoplastic" is difficult to state. A critical angiographic review of 20 normal aortoiliac systems was carried out by Wilson[5] during the preparation of our report in 1978. These angiograms were in renal donors and were only in one projection. The diameters of the aortas just below the renal arteries and just above the aortic bifurcation, however, were the same and averaged 18 mm (range 15–22 mm). The diameters of the common iliac artery averaged 11.25 mm and ranged from 8 to 22 mm. From these data, it appears that a practical guide

Table 2. Diameters of Resected Aortas in 3 Patients (mm)

Patient	Level	In Situ	Specimen
T.P.	IM	16	9
	AB	10	3
J.K.	IM	13	8
	AB	8	2.5
B.P.	IM	8	2.5
	AB	8	2.5

IM, Inferior mesenteric artery level; AB, Aortic bifurcation level.

to classify an aortoiliac system as hypoplastic would be an infrarenal diameter less than 15 mm, a common iliac diameter less than 8 mm, and an external iliac diameter less than 4 mm (Fig. 5).

RESULTS OF SURGERY

There were no operative deaths, and all of the patients were discharged improved. Graft thrombosis occurred on the fourth postoperative day in the first patient and was managed successfully by thrombectomy of the graft. This patient continues to have viable lower extremities with good peripheral pulses 15 years postoperatively. Severe back pain and postsympathectomy neuralgia occurred in three patients, but was resolved without sequelae. One patient with persistent postoperative back and thigh pain eventually was found to have herpes zoster. There were no cardiac complications postoperatively, and despite the universal smoking history, serious postoperative atelectasis did not occur. Mild and easily controlled leg edema was common. One patient who required temporary left renal artery occlusion during aortic anastomosis developed left flank pain postoperatively, which lasted for several days. An intravenous pyelogram obtained during the postoperative period revealed delayed function on that side.

FOLLOW-UP

Complete follow-up to June 1980 was achieved in 23 of the 27 patients (85 percent). Follow-up periods ranged from 1 year to 15 years and averaged 6.1 years. One death from myocardial infarction occurred in a patient 9 years after aortobifemoral and femoropopliteal bypass (at age 45 years). She had never stopped smoking. All grafts were patent.

Thus far, there has been one instance of graft occlusion at 6 months that was treated successfully by thrombectomy of the graft and construction of a femoropopliteal bypass using a reversed saphenous vein. This patient had bilateral superficial femoral artery occlusion at the time of the aortobifemoral bypass. The acute graft occlusion seemed to be caused by excessive pseudointima formation at the femoral anastomosis leading to thrombosis of the profunda femoris orifice. Thrombectomy of the profunda femoris artery and femoropopliteal bypass re-established good runoff. Because a similar situation was anticipated in the other extremity, a femoropopliteal bypass was also performed. This patient was kept on anticoagulant agents for 6 months. She had no ischemic symptoms and had excellent pulses at all levels in both lower extremities.

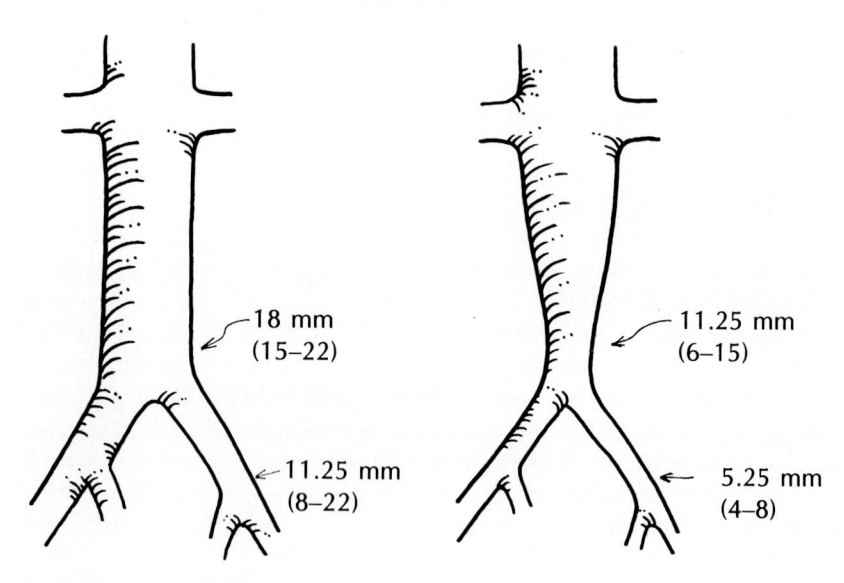

FIGURE 5. External diameters measured at surgery with arteries not clamped compared to 20 normals.

One year later she was readmitted because of infection in her aortic graft that presented in the left groin area. The aortic graft was removed following a successful right axillary-femoral bypass. An amputation below the knee was required on the left side. Three other patients with known superficial femoral artery occlusion required femoropopliteal bypass at 2 months, 3 months, and 9 months following aortofemoral bypass because of persistent claudication.

Two patients suffered strokes. One occurred 6 years postoperatively, was mild, and probably due to a carotid artery lesion. Ocular plethysmography and Doppler studies were abnormal. The patient refused carotid angiography and surgery, has taken aspirin for 6 years, and has had no further strokes or transient ischemic attacks. The other patient required surgery for an intracranial aneurysm that was treated successfully. One patient developed left subclavian stenosis that is asymptomatic. Another patient who had a subclavian occlusion at the time of her aortic surgery underwent carotid subclavian bypass 9 years later because of ischemic symptoms in the upper extremity.

New mild hypertension developed in one patient 6 years postoperatively and another developed angina 10 years postoperatively. No patients developed diabetes mellitus. Both men had restored potency. About 50 percent of patients stopped smoking.

DISCUSSION

Although the etiology of hypoplasia of the distal aorta has not been established, factors such as trauma,[16] oral contraceptives,[11] congenital rubella,[20] therapeutic radiation,[4] hormonal imbalance,[6] and inflammatory factors[19] have all been implicated. The association of this syndrome with eclampsia and recurrent intrauterine fetal death has also been described.[3] The abnormality of the aorta might also be an end result of "shrinkage" secondary to atherosclerosis.

Quain formally described hypoplasia of the distal aorta in 1847.[17] As cited by Arnot and Louw,[1] Morgagni, in 1733, described the lesion in a 33-year-old monk found to have generalized aortic hypoplasia on postmortem examination. An excellent anatomic argument for a congenital theory was presented by Arnot and Louw in 1973. These workers studied the anatomy of the posterior abdominal aorta in 100 cadavers and correlated the aortic diameter at four levels. They found that eight cadavers had a single common origin of the lowest pair of lumbar arteries and that the same specimens had a significantly smaller diameter of the aorta between the origin of the inferior mesenteric artery and the aortic bifurcation. These authors concluded that the anomaly is a congenital defect in which there is excessive fusion of the embryonic dorsal aortas around the 25th day of intrauterine life (Fig. 6). This explanation, however, does not account for the apparent difference in incidence between the sexes.

The pathologic findings in our three resected specimens demonstrated no specific histologic abnormality. Aside from marked narrowing of the aorta and iliac arteries, often associated with recent and old thrombosis, the pathologic findings were characteristic of atherosclerosis with calcification. One specimen revealed diffuse subintimal fibrosis with fragmentation of the elastic membrane. This finding gave the appearance of a vascular "jet lesion."

Atherosclerosis in humans is known to develop first and most markedly in the abdominal aorta (with no sex differentiation).[7,10,22] Lallemand[12,13] and Gosling[8] reported that premature atheromatous disease of the aortic bifurcation may be due to reflected arterial pulse waves. This hemodynamic stress is thought to be caused by abnormal vessel dimensions, and is expressed as a ratio of the sum of the cross-sectional areas of the common iliac arteries to the cross-sectional areas of the aortic bifurcation (Fig. 7). The average area ratio in our patients with hypoplastic aortoiliac segments when external diameters were used is 0.43. This is considerably lower than the average ratio of 0.78 derived from 20 normal aortograms (renal transplant donors) (Fig. 8). Glagov[7] has postulated

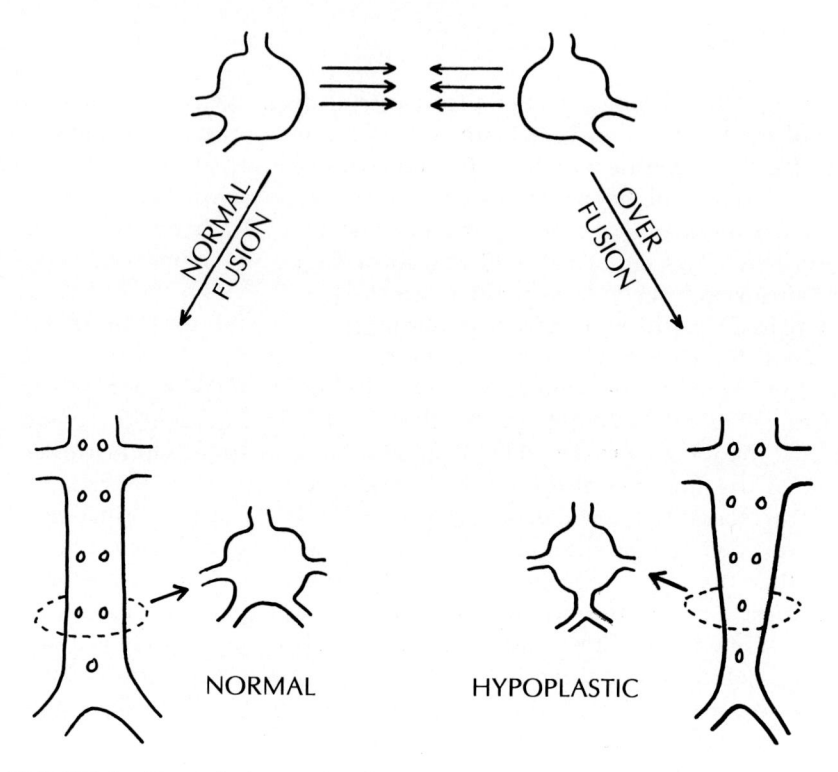

FIGURE 6. Hypoplasia may be due to overfusion of primitive dorsal aortas.

that the abdominal aortic segment of man is exceptional when compared to aortas of other mammals. The total number of lamellar structural units in the human thoracic aorta and in medias of most mammalian aortas correspond precisely to aortic diameter. The human abdominal aortic media, however, has too few layers for its diameter, thickness, and total tension. In its midportion, it has only 29 layers and is avascular. Each layer sustains a relatively elevated average tension without the nutritive support of medial vasorum. These discrepancies may place the abdominal aortic segment at a disadvantage with regard to its nutrition and its adaptive and reparative responses and lead to early atherosclerotic changes. Haimovici[10] believes that the abdominal aorta is more susceptible to atherosclerosis because of a biologic difference in this segment of the aorta. He transplanted abdominal aortic segments into various areas of the thoracic aorta in dogs who were put on an atherogenic regimen. These implants always developed marked atherosclerosis regardless of position when compared to the rest of the thoracic aorta.

$$A.R. = \frac{B+C}{A}$$

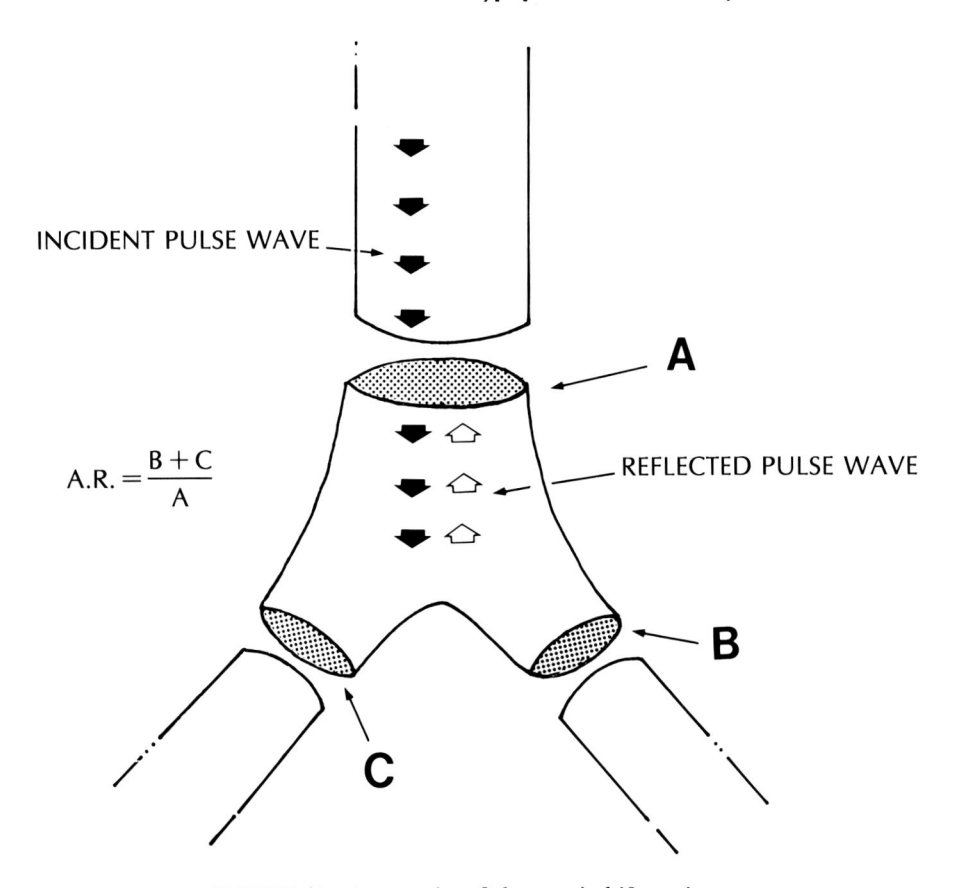

FIGURE 7. Area ratio of the aortic bifurcation.

CONCLUSIONS

On the basis of these findings, the combination of congenital hypoplasia and the normal early development of atherosclerosis in this segment appears to account for the premature occlusive symptoms in patients with the hypoplastic aortoiliac syndrome (Fig. 9). The high incidence of brachiocephalic arterial involvement and the low incidence of coronary artery disease in this group along with female predominance remains difficult to explain.

The best method of treating this entity seems to be via the bypass procedure. Endarterectomy is difficult because of the fibrotic type of

426   Critical Problems in Vascular Surgery

$$\text{Area Ratio} = \frac{B + C}{A}$$

Hypoplastic Aortae (ratio = 0.43)

20 Normal Angiograms (ratio = 0.78)

REFLECTION COEFFICIENT (%)

AREA RATIO

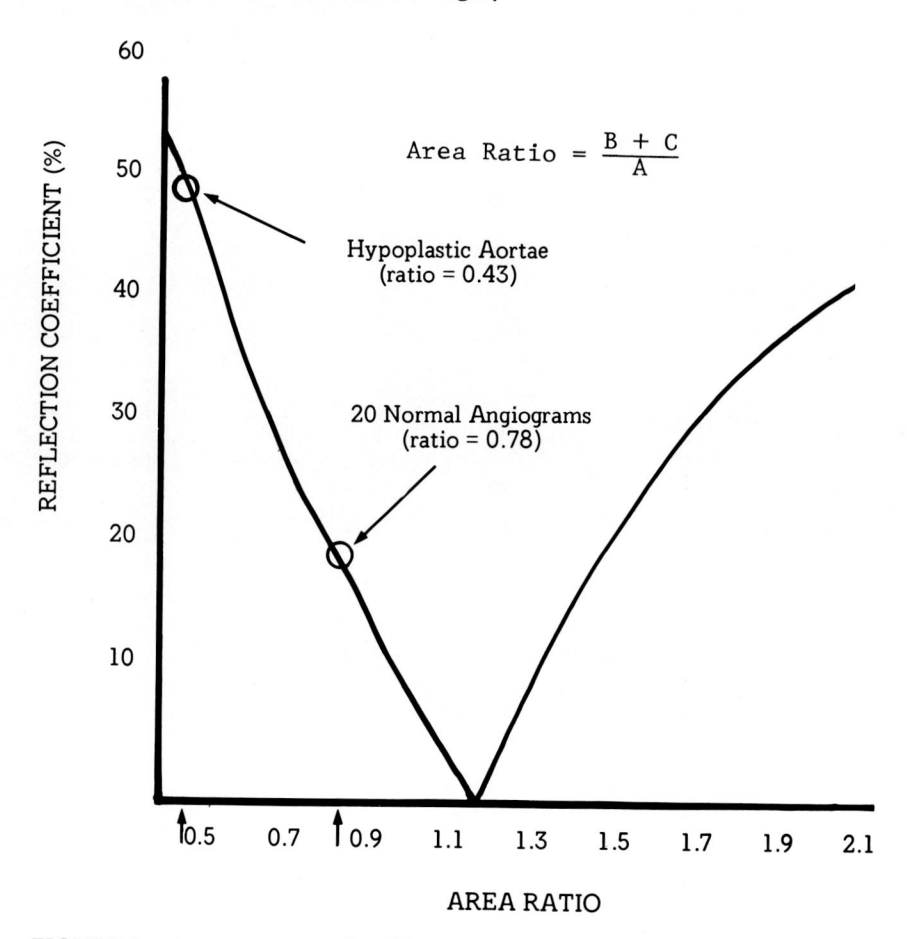

FIGURE 8. Average area ratio of hypoplastic aortas showing a reflection coefficient of almost 50 percent as contrasted to average area ratio of 20 normal aortograms with a reflection coefficient of less than 20 percent.

atherosclerosis and because of the very small diameters involved. Although I have added bilateral lumbar sympathectomy to the procedure, I cannot determine at this time how the long-term results will be affected by this maneuver. When superficial femoral artery occlusion is encountered, synchronous femoropopliteal bypass should be considered because the run-off into a small deep femoral artery in some of these patients may not be enough to prevent graft thrombosis.

Although original prognostic estimates were pessimistic, follow-up thus far warrants a more optimistic posture. Cessation of smoking, weight control, and proper treatment of existing hyperlipidemia are recom-

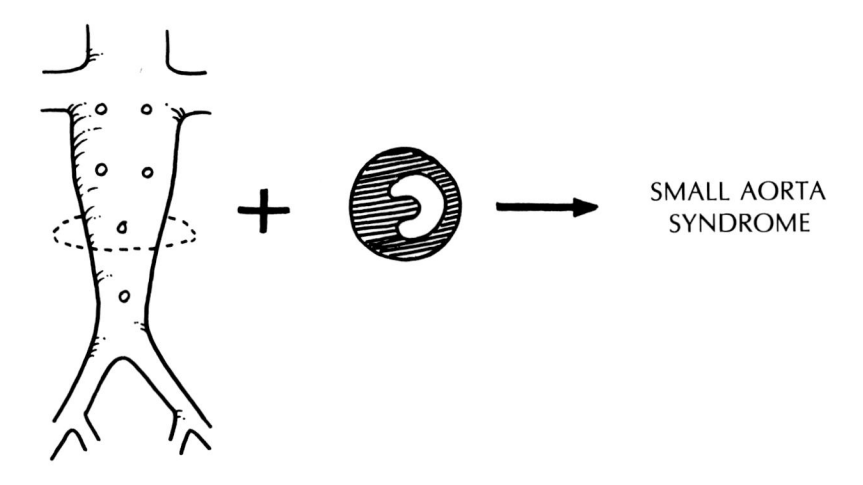

FIGURE 9. Etiology of small aorta syndrome.

mended strongly. The absence of diabetes mellitus, along with infrequency of coronary artery disease, hypertension, and renal artery involvement, probably accounts for my more optimistic view. This subgroup, therefore, may be somewhat similar to the group of men reported by Malone, Moore, and Goldstone.[14] These authors demonstrated that males undergoing aortoiliac reconstruction who did not have diabetes mellitus or coronary artery disease had "normal" life expectancy.

REFERENCES

1. Arnot RS, Louw JH: The anatomy of the posterior wall of the aorta. S Afr Med J 47:899, 1973
2. Ben-Shoshan M, Rossi NP, Korns ME: Coarctation of the abdominal aorta. Arch Pathol 95:221, 1973
3. Clemetson CAB: Aortic hypoplasia and its significance in the etiology of pre-eclamptic toxemia. Br J Obstet Gynaecol 67:90, 1960
4. Colquhoun J: Hypoplasia of the abdominal aorta following irradiation in infancy. Radiology 86:454, 1966
5. DeLaurentis DA, Friedmann P, Wolferth CC Jr, et al: Atherosclerosis and the hypoplastic aortoiliac system. Surgery 83:22, 1978
6. Friedman SA, Holling EH, Roberts B: Etiologic factors in aortoiliac and femoropopliteal vascular disease. N Engl J Med 271:1382, 1964
7. Glagov S: The role of medial structure, mechanical stress and vasa vasorum in the pathogenesis of arterial lesions. In Bergan JJ, Yao JST (eds): Gan-

grene and Severe Ischemia of the Lower Extremities. New York, Grune & Stratton, 1978, pp 3–18
8. Gosling RG, Newman DL, Bowden NLR, Twinn KN: The area ratio of normal aortic junctions. Br J Radiol 44:850, 1971
9. Greenhalgh RM, Taylor GW: Little women with blocked aortas. Br J Surg 61:923, 1975
10. Haimovici H: Atherogenesis. Am J Surg 134:174, 1977
11. Hall R, Bunch GA: Aortoiliac occlusion in women using oral contraceptives. Br J Surg 58:508, 1971
12. Lallemand RC, Brown KGE, Boulter PS: Vessel dimensions in premature atheromatous disease of the aortic bifurcation. Br Med J 2:255, 1972
13. Lallemand RC, Gosling RG, Newman DL: Role of the bifurcation in atheromatosis of the abdominal aorta. Surg Gynecol Obstet 137:987, 1973
14. Malone JM, Moore WS, Goldstone J: Life expectancy following aortofemoral arterial grafting. Surgery 81:551, 1977
15. Maycock W d'A: Congenital stenosis of the abdominal aorta. Am Heart J 13:633, 1937
16. Naide M, Etzel MM: Aorto-iliac occlusion resulting from past trauma. Arch Med 104:298, 1959
17. Quain R: Partial contraction of the abdominal aorta. Trans Path Soc (London) 1:244, 1846–1848
18. Raaf JH, Shannon J: Atherosclerotic coarctation of the abdominal aorta in women. Surg Gynecol Obstet 150:715, 1980
19. Sen PK, Kinare SG, Kulkarni TP, Parulkar GB: Stenosing aortitis of unknown etiology. Surgery 51:317, 1962
20. Siassi B, Klyman G: Hypoplasia of the abdominal aorta associated with the rubella syndrome. Am J Dis Child 120:476, 1970
21. Staple TW: The solitary aortoiliac lesion. Surgery 64:569, 1968
22. Tejada C, Strong JP, Montenegro MR, et al: Distribution of coronary and aortic atherosclerosis by geographic location, race and sex. J Lab Invest 18:509, 1968

TWENTY-NINE

Etiology and Management of Sexual Problems Related to Aortoiliac Disease and Surgery

Ralph G. DePalma

Because of greater general concern with the quality of life, increased interest now exists in disorders of sexual function. A variety of sexual dysfunctions may be associated with aortoiliac disease and surgery to correct occlusive or aneurysmal lesions. This area has been a difficult one for vascular surgeons since current information appears in other specialty literature such as in psychiatric, neurologic, and internal medical journals,[5,10,15,24] and publications concerned with urology.[12,13] It is further complicated in many middle-aged men by interactions among vascular, neurologic, and psychogenic factors. Nonetheless, a tradition of concern with sexual function exists in vascular surgery.

As early as 1923, Leriche[14] recognized the relationship between occlusion of the abdominal aorta and failure of erection. He felt this relationship to be so important that he listed impotence as the first symptom of the syndrome bearing his name. Later, in 1951, Whitelaw and Smithwick[25] described secondary effects of sympathectomy upon erection and ejaculation. In examining results of high or bilateral sympathectomies, they noted significant changes in sexual function in 72 percent of their patients with disturbance of erection in 44 of 118 cases. In 1969, May, DeWeese, and Rob[16] reported changes in sexual function following abdominal aortic operations. They noted impotence in 21 percent of patients after abdominal aortic aneurysmectomy and an incidence of 34 percent of impotence after operations for occlusive disease.

The etiology of erectile dysfunction and other sexual disorders follow-

Supported, in part, by Veterans Administration Grant Number 001.

ing aortoiliac operations is not clear-cut. Some have ascribed it primarily to surgical interruption of genital autonomics[9,21,23]; others emphasized the importance of pelvic perfusion as the primary determinant of postoperative erectile dysfunction.[16,17] It is probably a combination of both factors.[1,3,4,20]

An important source of confusion in the literature in defining postoperative sexual dysfunction has been a lack of clear definition on nomenclature of disorders of sexual function. In addition to failure of penile erection, these disorders also include retrograde ejaculation, diminished intensity or painful orgasm, and, rarely, failure to achieve orgasm in the presence of an adequate penile erection. The latter complaint, considered psychogenic by some, might also be neurogenic in origin. It can prove to be vexing in the presence of a stable relationship.

Generally, postoperative sexual complaints in our society are not mentioned to the surgeon unless specific inquiries are made.[1,21,25] Thus in history taking, they may be vaguely characterized in clinical records making retrospective analyses of data about sexual malfunction difficult. This area is also interesting and controversial because in men with aortoiliac disease, impotence can also be due to psychogenic causes, diabetes, excess alcohol, and drugs used to treat hypertension. Complex interactions of these variables cloud the picture preoperatively and continue to interact postoperatively. In spite of these complexities, a careful history combined with some simple vascular laboratory measurements can be of great assistance.[1-3,11,15,20]

Recently the subject of sexual function has gained visibility because of vascular operations designed to preserve and, in some instances, to restore sexual function.[2-4] Operations such as endarterectomy of the internal iliac orifice or direct corporal revascularization have been undertaken.[3,18] This chapter describes facets of the anatomy and physiology of sexual dysfunction in men, emphasizing neural and vascular problems related to aortoiliac reconstruction. Operative methods to minimize sexual disorders will be considered.

NEURAL PATHWAYS

Normal penile erection depends upon the presence of intact neural pathways and adequate arterial inflow. The neural pathways involved basically achieve integration of afferent signals in the thoracolumbar and sacral erection centers with efferent outflow via autonomic nerves supplying the penis, bladder, and urethra. Weiss[24] has divided the stimuli that elicit erection into two useful categories: psychogenic or reflexogenic. Psychogenic stimuli, such as visual, auditory, or olfactory signals, arouse the erotic centers of the brain to produce erection. Reflexogenic erections are produced by direct genital stimulation or arise from enteroceptive stimuli initiated in the bladder or rectum. These dual interactions can produce interesting and apparently contradictory modes of achieving erection. For example, in certain cases of cord injury in which reflex stimuli are not perceived, erection can be produced by purely psychogenic stimulation. A schematic of the known pathways involved in the integration of these neural impulses is shown in Figure 1.

Although erection is largely a function of the parasympathetic nervous system, the sympathetics appear to be involved as well since extensive sympathectomy alone can provoke impotence.[25] Figure 2 depicts the complexity of interrelationships between the two vegetative systems in their ultimate pathways to the bladder, rectum, and penile corpora. A cause of controversy is that these neural interconnections and their exact locations are still poorly understood.

Some believe that the periaortic neural outflow is involved only with ejaculation. As noted by Whitelaw and Smithwick,[25] it is, however, probable that input to the lumbar erection center is in some way mediated by the high sympathetic lumbar ganglia. The variability of location of the lumbar sympathetics probably accounts for changes in penile erectile function occurring after bilateral high lumbar sympathectomy. When sympathectomy is combined with extensive aortoiliac mobilization, there may also be interference with the parasympathetic outflow via the hypogastric plexi.[4,9,21,23] Figure 3 shows the anatomy of the interrelationships between the sympathetic and parasympathetic neural fibers about the infrarenal abdominal aorta.[19] The reader should note the dominant anterior and left-sided anatomic connections of the neural fibers. The fibers passing with the inferior mesenteric artery are considered to be important in maintenance of normal sexual function as some of these probably course with the blood supply toward perirectal and prostatic plexi. Further anatomic studies of these fibers and their function are required.

These autonomic neural mechanisms are also intimately involved in orgasm and ejaculation. The parasympathetic motor outflow of S2-S4 results in contractions of the muscles about the urethra during ejaculation while the sympathetic motor fibers innervate prostatic smooth muscles and seminal vesicles. Contraction of the internal urethral sphincter muscle occurs mainly by means of sympathetic fibers upon initiation of ejaculation. In retrograde ejaculation into the bladder following sympathectomy or extensive aortic mobilization, the neural lesion is thought to be due mainly to sympathetic denervation. In cases of simple retrograde ejaculation, parasympathetic function and perception of orgasm are unaltered.

In describing sexual dysfunctions following aortoiliac operations,

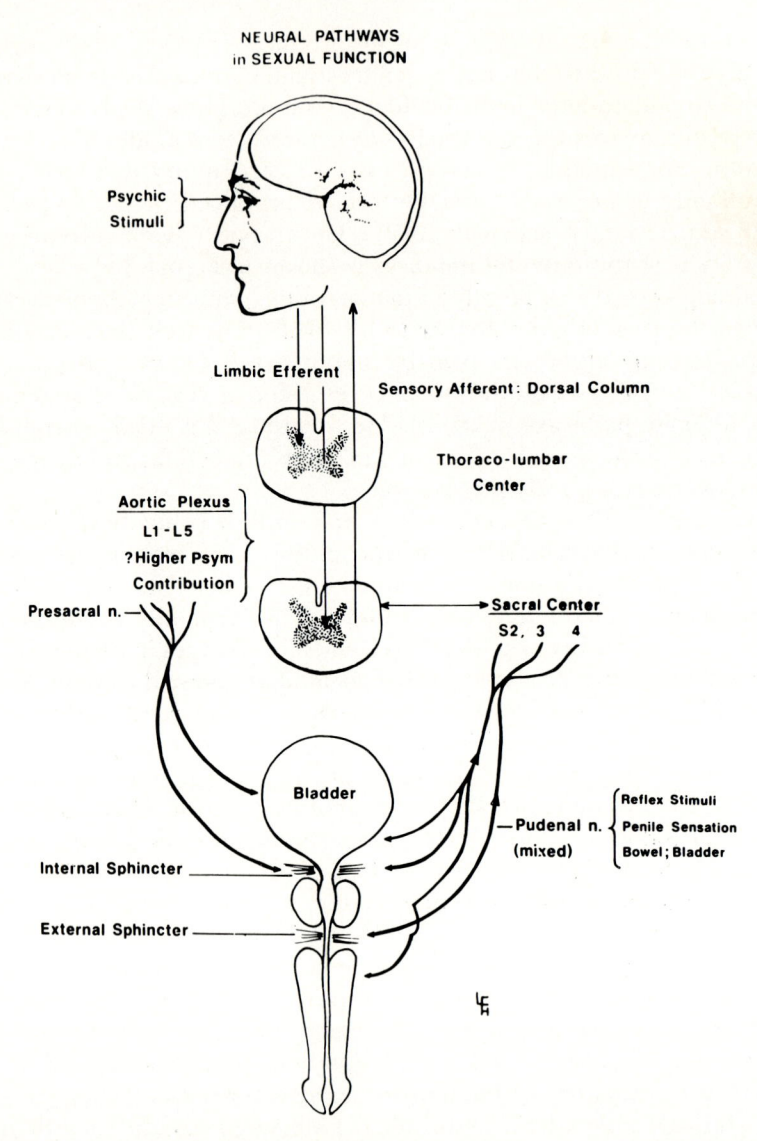

FIGURE 1. Schematic of neural pathways involved in male sexual function. (Adapted from Weiss[24] and Ellenberg.[5])

Hallböök and Holmquist[8] reported interesting data on orgasm in 10 of 31 patients who retained erectile function following operation. They described decreased sensation in six patients, painful orgasm in one, and complete disappearance of orgasm in the presence of normal

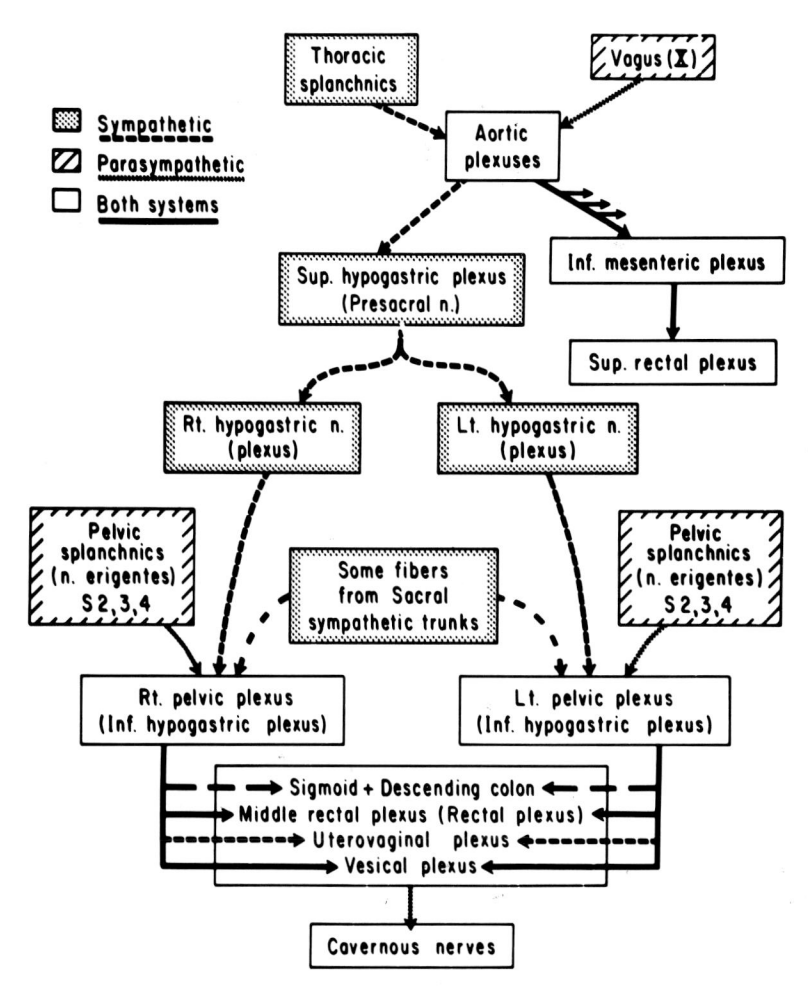

Etiology and Management of Sexual Problems 433

FIGURE 2. Schematic of autonomic outflow showing interconnections between sympathetic and parasympathetic efferent fibers.

erection in three. These dysfunctions as well as impotence can be miminized by reconstructive surgical techniques that spare the periaortic neural fibers. There are patients in whom corporal perfusion is adequate by physiologic measurement and significant sexual dysfunction exists because of neural interruption. We have previously described dissection methods that minimize disturbance of autonomic neural fibers.[3,4] It is worth re-emphasizing that avoiding sympathectomy and limiting aortic dissection to the right side of the aorta are both important steps in preventing postoperative sexual dysfunction including impotence.

434 Critical Problems in Vascular Surgery

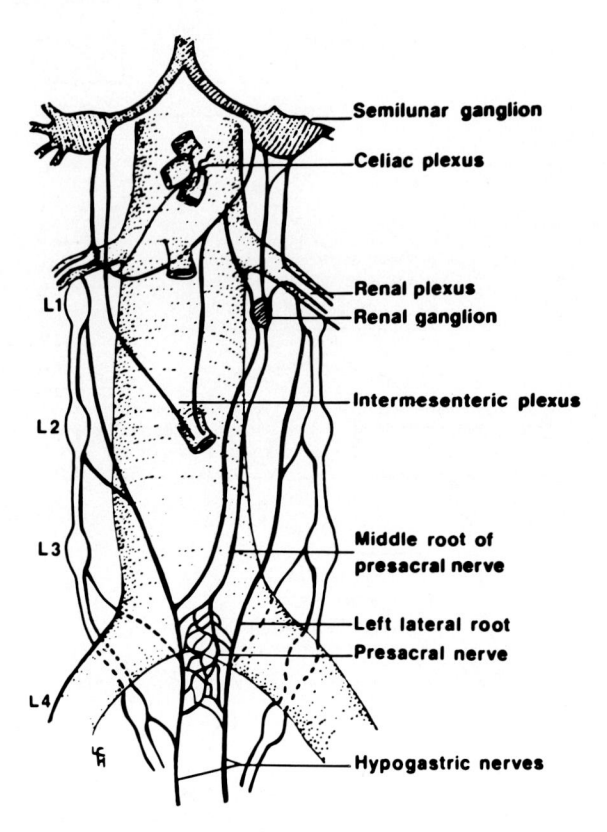

FIGURE 3. Anatomy of neural fibers about the abdominal aorta: Modified from operative observations and after Pick[19] and Whitelaw and Smithwick.[25] Note plexus about inferior mesenteric artery.

VASCULAR FACTORS: PELVIC AND CORPORAL PERFUSION

Methods of maintaining pelvic blood flow to insure adequate penile perfusion are important. To evaluate flow through the three paired arteries that supply the penis, we have found pulse volume recordings (PVR) using a digital Buffington plethysmographic cuff quite useful.[2,3] Typical normal recordings are depicted in Figure 4. May and his colleagues[16] in their original publication attributed loss of erectile function mainly to compromised internal iliac flow. Queral and co-workers,[20] while recognizing neural components, emphasized the importance of internal iliac flow.

Apparently, one normal internal iliac artery is sufficient to sustain

PVR RECORDINGS

Normal Function: Male 48 yrs.

Normal Function: Male 58 yrs.

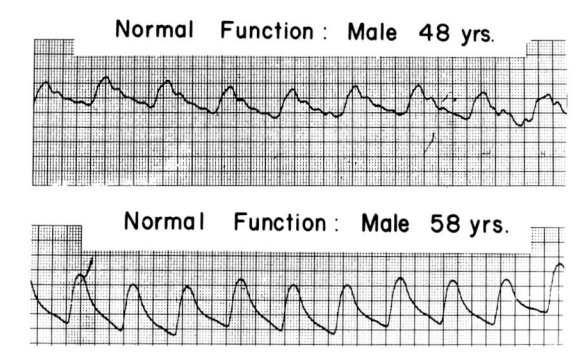

FIGURE 4. Penile pulse volume recordings obtained with digital Buffington plethysmographic cuff inflated to mean arterial pressure; two middle-aged men with normal function. Chart speed 25 mm/second.

erectile function in a young normal male without vascular disease (Fig. 5). In addition, younger men report erectile function after a single renal transplant, but not after a second transplant if both internal iliac arteries are divided and utilized to supply the transplanted kidneys. A single patent internal iliac artery may not be sufficient in older men with diffuse vascular disease. In these patients it is desirable to achieve bilateral flow when possible. To achieve this, vascular anastomoses proximal to the bifurcation of the common iliac artery have been recommended.[16] Unfortunately, atherosclerotic occlusive disease patterns commonly involve the external iliac arteries. This in turn makes the goal of revascularization of both internal and external iliac arterial beds a challenging one that cannot always be achieved. Nevertheless, the surgeon can use a variety of ingenious techniques to overcome this problem. An illustration of a type of modified reconstruction for aneurysmal disease is shown in Figure 6.

In addition to occlusive disease, embolic phenomena to peroneal, gluteal, and genital areas can occur postoperatively, which is a variant of "trash-foot." In the past it was taught that mainstream external iliac circulation took precedence over the pelvic vessels. In fact, an initial flush into the internal iliac system was recommended to rid the graft of minor clot or atheromatous debris. This maneuver should be avoided. It may be more difficult to correct the effects of pelvic vessel emboli than those into the lower limbs. Finally, the utility and simplicity of femorofemoral bypass for unilateral common iliac lesions has much to recommend it in terms of preserving normal sexual function. Table 1

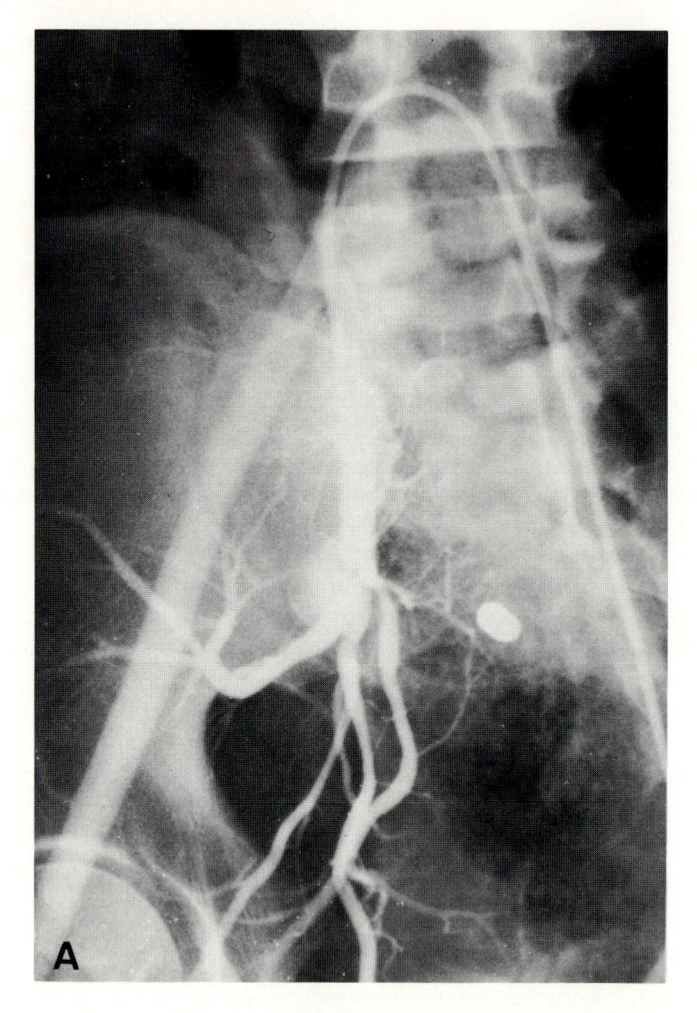

FIGURE 5. A. An angiogram showing injury produced by gunshot wound involving the distal branching of the right internal iliac artery in a 29-year-old male. The patient underwent ligation of this vessel. *(Continued.)*

characterizes a group of 13 patients undergoing a femorofemoral bypass for chief complaints related to unilateral ischemia of the lower extremity. Nine of these patients reported enhanced postoperative erectile function along with relief of their intermittent claudication. These results have been confirmed objectively by improved postoperative penile pulse volume recordings.

A final interventional alternative to be considered is the use of intraluminal dilation or angioplasty as described by Gruntsig and Kumpe[7] for

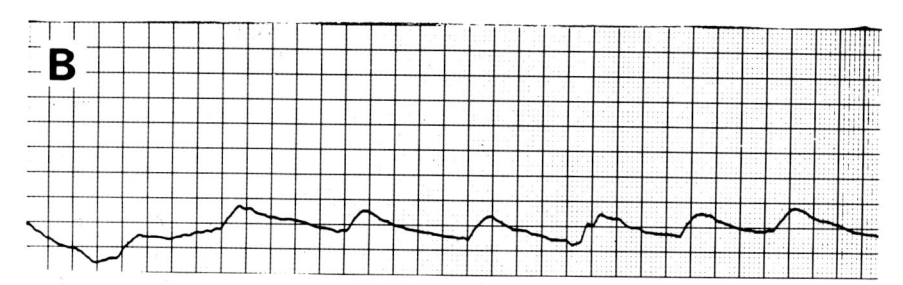

FIGURE 5. **B.** Penile PVR 2 weeks postoperatively. [Male. 29 years. After ligation of right internal iliac (gunshot wound). Reports A.M. erection and function.] Note systolic crest time less than 5 mm; amplitude 6 mm. Chart speed 25 mm/second.

selected isolated lesions involving the common iliac or possibly the internal iliac artery.

FACTORS IN PATIENTS WITH THE PRIMARY COMPLAINT OF IMPOTENCE

Vascular screening of these patients is an important recent development. Men who complain primarily of impotence comprise a distinct population from those who present with ischemia of the lower extremities or aneu-

Table 1. Sexual Function after Femorofemoral Bypass

I.D.	Age	Comment/Anatomy	Sexual Function Preoperative	Postoperative
1	71	Diabetic; diffuse bilat int iliac disease	−	−
2	62	Bilat patent int iliac	−	+
3	69	Single patent int iliac	−	+
4	70	Diabetic, diffuse int iliac disease	−	−
5	52	Postoperative for ruptured aneurysm occlusion int iliacs (embolic in origin?)	−	−
6	72	Bilat patent int iliac	−	+
7	57	Bilat patent int iliac	−	+
8	67	Ca of prostate, orchectomy	−	−
9	48	Bilat patent int iliac	−	+
10	50	Bilat patent int iliac	−	+
11	42	Bilat patent int iliac	−	+
12	69	Bilat patent int iliac	−	+
13	64	Single patent int iliac	−	+

rysmal disease. The former can suffer from isolated pudendal artery lesions; some exhibit impotence due to large and small vessel disease combined. In reviewing screening data related to patients presenting with a chief complaint of impotence to a combined service, we found that among 73 patients examined for this chief complaint, 38 exhibited vasculogenic impotence detected by PVR.[2] Nineteen exhibited glucose intolerance with normal penile PVRs and 14 were due to psychogenic, hormonal, or unknown causes. Trauma or previous surgery including 29 urologic and 3 vascular operations comprised the etiology in the remainder. These proved to be mainly neurogenic in origin.

The surgeon dealing with the chief complaint of impotence will find a multidisciplinary approach useful. Available members of the team should include a psychiatrist, urologist, and internal medical consultants. For the vascular surgeon, a simple first step is utilization of the penile pulse volume recording shown in the screening sequence indicated in Figure 7. The vascular laboratory is not a substitute for an adequate history. As in any diagnostic process, history is paramount. The questions about specific erectile disorders devised by Levine[15] are of value in tentatively characterizing the etiology of the erectile dysfunction.* The surgeon using this technique of history taking can, with experience, recognize organic, psychogenic, or ambiguous patterns of impotence. Patients with a history of risk factors for atherosclerosis and an organic pattern, characterized by the gradual onset of the inability to achieve a firm erection at any time in the setting of an otherwise satisfactory relationship uncomplicated by traumatic life events will frequently have vasculogenic impotence. Along with the history and the PVR vascular screening, a systematic work-up should be done to investigate the other common causes of impotence (Table 2).

Each of these factors should be evaluated before and after aortoiliac surgery. In patients with sexual dysfunction, a normal penile PVR or penile systolic blood pressure greater than 75 percent of arm systolic pressure postoperatively indicates a neurologic deficit related to surgery. If this is the case, the disorder will begin as soon as the patient has had an opportunity for sexual contact after discharge. For these patients,

* Levine's four basic questions are:
1. *What is the physiologic impairment?* Is it the inability to obtain an erection, the inability to maintain an erection during intercourse, or some combination?
2. *How firm does the penis become?* Not firm at all, slightly firm but erection not self-supporting, decreased firmness with coitus still possible, or fully turgid?
3. *Is the impairment constant or episodic?* Under what circumstances is the pattern not present: with other partners, with masturbation, with sleep, upon awakening, during the day, when engaging in other erotic activity?
4. *What life events were occurring when the dysfunction appeared?*

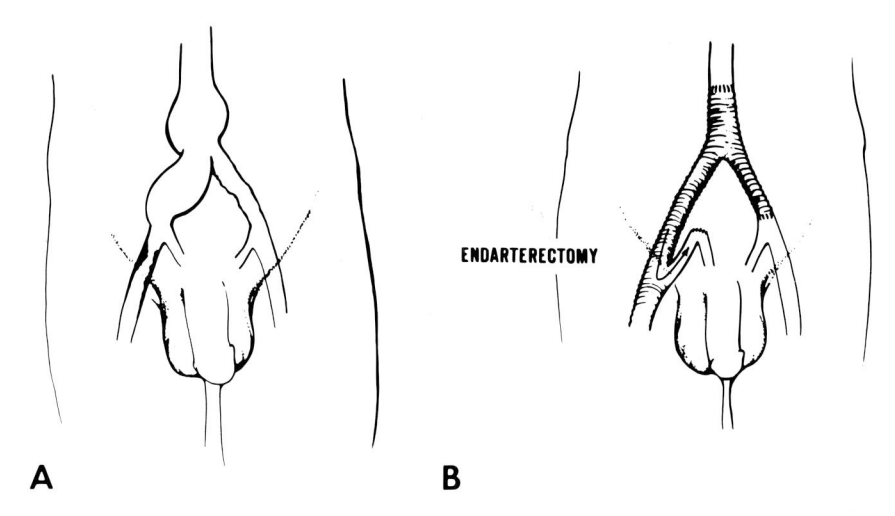

Etiology and Management of Sexual Problems 439

FIGURE 6. **A.** Aneurysmal involvement of the aorta and the right common iliac artery with ulcerated stenotic lesions of the left external iliac artery. **B.** Method of revascularization to perfuse internal iliacs bilaterally. Left external iliac artery was endarterectomized with anastomosis to the common femoral artery.

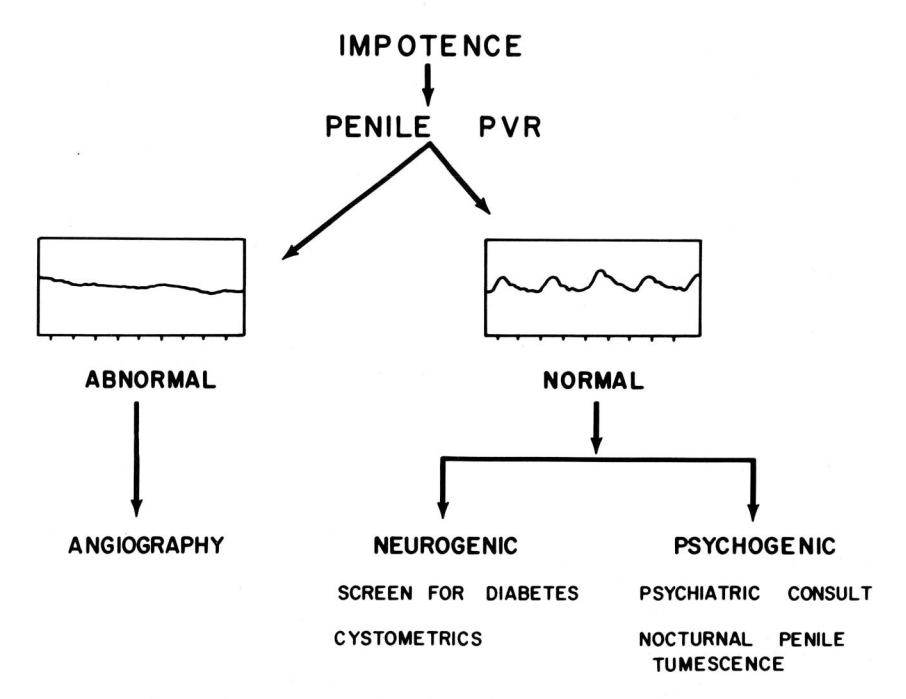

FIGURE 7. Screening algorithm for complaint of impotence.

Table 2. Outline of Common Causes of Impotence

Vasculogenic	Aortoiliac disease
	Pudendal/penile AA disease
	Embolism
	Diabetes
Neurogenic	Trauma/previous surgery
	Diabetes
	Antihypertensive and other drugs
Psychogenic	Traumatic life events
	Alcohol excess
	Depression
Hormonal	Testosterone lack
	Hypothalamic-pituitary
	Gonadal dysfunction

nocturnal penile tumescence monitoring will document the organic erectile malfunction, and then treatment can proceed.[10]

In some diabetics, the neurologic factor is critical. If the PVR is normal, neuropathy can be demonstrated by cystometrics. This assumes that the autonomic pathways involved in micturition and erection are, for practical purposes, identical. Ellenberg[5] has described methods for documenting abnormal cystometrics in diabetics with impotence. It is also possible to diagnose diabetic autonomic neuropathy because the majority of patients with autonomic neuropathy as a cause of impotence exhibit peripheral extremity manifestations as well. For example, among 45 impotent diabetics, 38 had evidence of peripheral neuropathy shown by decreased pain perception, paresthesias, and absent ankle jerks. It is also possible, however, to have neurogenic genital involvement without accompanying peripheral neuropathy. In these cases, cystometrics are indicated. Diabetes can also cause retrograde ejaculation, diminished perception of orgasm, and ejaculation without normal penile erection.

TREATMENT OF VASCULOGENIC IMPOTENCE

A recent observation is that vasculogenic impotence can be due to isolated small vessel disease as well. This process can involve the pudendal artery or even vessels within the corpora themselves. Selective pelvic angiography should be considered to define disease of the small pelvic and pudendal vessels.[6] Operations for direct penile revascularization have been advocated for this problem. Complete discussion of these operations is beyond the scope of this chapter. Currently, experience has been gained in this area and is accumulating, but these operations remain controversial. In any event, for the patient with aortoiliac disease direct corporal revascularization does not appear to be a wise choice. Atherosclerosis has been seen to involve the inferior epigastric arteries used for direct revascularization.[3] Pudendal artery occlusion can also be due to embolic phenomena from ulcerated proximal plaques or aneurysms. In these cases, correction of the proximal disease takes precedence.

In patients with initially satisfactory sexual function after aortic surgery, there may be later impotence. Presumably this occurs after one or more years because of progressive distal disease. For impotence due to diffuse vascular disease, as with neurogenic or other nonvasculogenic impotence, the use of an inflatable prosthetic implant has been found to be a satisfactory method of treatment.[2,3,22]

It is not possible to treat either retrograde ejaculation or orgasmic disturbances because these are due mainly to interruption of neural fibers. Rarely postoperative retrograde ejaculation and orgasmic disorders clear with time, suggesting partial denervation at the time of surgery. Anecdotal reports of regained sexual function have also been brought to the author's attention. Basically, however, the best approach for preventing and treating sexual dysfunction in patients with aortoiliac disease will continue to evolve by using modified operative techniques to minimize neural interruption and to simultaneously maintain or restore internal iliac blood flow.

To achieve these goals it is important that the surgeon make discrete inquiries about sexual function before and after operations for aortoiliac disease. Inquiries can be made without fear of inducing psychic problems. The establishment of a proper relationship will allow assessment of postoperative sexual function and be helpful in guiding treatment. A methodical inquiry in the area of sexual function offers the additional dimension of improving the quality of life for patients suffering from aortoiliac disease. If the sexual dysfunction proves to be untreatable, at the least recognition that the problem is organic and the offer of an explanation does much to allay anxiety.

REFERENCES

1. DePalma RG: Impotence as a complication of aortic reconstruction. In Bernhard VM, Towne JB (eds): Complications in Vascular Surgery. New York, Grune & Stratton, 1980, pp 427–442
2. DePalma RG, Kedia K, Persky L: Surgical options in the correction of vasculogenic impotence. Vasc Surg 14:92, 1980

3. DePalma RG, Kedia K, Persky L: Vascular operations for preservation of sexual function. In Bergan JJ, Yao JST (eds): Surgery of the Aorta and Its Branches. New York, Grune & Stratton, 1979, pp 277–295
4. DePalma RG, Levine SB, Feldman S: Preservation of erectile function after aorto-iliac reconstruction. Arch Surg 113:958, 1978
5. Ellenberg M: Impotence in diabetes: The neurologic factor. Ann Intern Med 75:213, 1971
6. Ginestie JF, Romieu A: Radiologic Exploration of Impotence. The Hague, Martinus Nijhoff, 1978
7. Gruntzig A, Kumpe DA: Technique of percutaneous transluminal angioplasty with the Gruntzig balloon catheter. Am J Roentgenol 132:547, 1979
8. Hallböök T, Holmquist B: Sexual disturbances following dissection of the aorta and the common iliac arteries. J Cardiovasc Surg 11:255, 1970
9. Harris JD, Jepson RP: Aorto-iliac stenosis: A comparison of two procedures. Aust NZ J Surg 34:211, 1965
10. Karacan P: Clinical value of nocturnal erections in the prognosis and diagnosis of impotence. Med Aspects Hum Sex 4:27, 1970
11. Kempczinski RF: Role of the vascular laboratory in the evaluation of male impotence. Am J Surg 138:278, 1979
12. Krane RJ, Siroky MD: The physiology of male sexual function. In Krane RJ, Siroky MD (eds): Clinical Neuro-urology. Boston, Little, Brown, 1979, pp 45–62
13. Lemaire G, Soots G, Espriet G, Patoir G: Les troubles de l'ejaculation. Apres chirurgie due carrefour aorto-iliaque. J d'Urol et de Neph 81:242, 1975
14. Leriche R: Des obliterations arterielles hautes. Obliteration de la terminaison de l'aorte comme cause des insuffisances. Circulatoires des neurbres inferieurs. Bull Mem de la Soc de Chir 49:1404, 1923
15. Levine SB: Marital sexual dysfunction: Erectile dysfunction. Ann Intern Med 85:342, 1976
16. May AG, DeWeese JA, Rob CG: Changes in sexual function following operation on the abdominal aorta. Surgery 65:41, 1969
17. Metz P, Mathiesen FR: External iliac steal syndrome leading to a defect in penile erection and impotence: A case report. Vasc Surg 13:70, 1979
18. Michal V, Kramar R, Pospichal J: Femoro-pudendal bypass, internal iliac thrombo endarterectomy and direct arterial anastomoses to the cavernous body in the treatment of erectile impotence. Bull Soc Intern Chir 33:343, 1974
19. Pick J: Anatomy of the Autonomic Nervous System. Philadelphia, Lippincott, 1970, pp 439–441
20. Queral LA, Whitehouse WM, Flinn WR, et al: Pelvic hemodynamics after aorto-iliac reconstruction. Surgery 86:799, 1979
21. Sabri S, Cotton L: Sexual function following aorto-iliac reconstruction. Lancet 2:1218, 1971
22. Scott FB, Bradley WE, Timm GW: Management of erectile impotence: Use of implantable inflatable prosthesis. Urology 2:80, 1973

23. Weinstein MH, Machleder HI: Sexual function after aorto-iliac surgery. Ann Surg 181:787, 1974
24. Weiss HD: The physiology of human penile erection. Ann Intern Med 76:793, 1972
25. Whitelaw GP, Smithwick RH: Some secondary effects of sympathectomy. N Engl J Med 245:121, 1951

THIRTY

Thrombosis of Aortofemoral, Axillofemoral, or Femorofemoral Grafts

Wesley S. Moore

Aortofemoral, axillofemoral, and femorofemoral grafts represent alternative surgical methods for bypassing occlusive lesions in the aortoiliac system.[2-4,16] Each of these techniques is subject to the complications of early and late thrombosis. This chapter explores the incidence of occlusion complicating each of the three techniques. In addition, the etiology, diagnosis, and management are outlined.

INCIDENCE

In general, of the three alternative methods for bypassing occlusive lesions in the aortoiliac system, aortofemoral grafts have the highest patency rates. Femorofemoral bypass grafts, a technique uniquely reserved for problems involving unilateral iliac artery occlusive disease, have the next highest patency rates. Axillofemoral bypass grafts, with or without a concomitant femorofemoral bypass graft limb, have the poorest patency rates, with the highest rate of thrombosis among the three grafting techniques.[9,12,21] A review of the literature demonstrates a relatively wide spectrum of results depending upon the patient population, the indication for operation (claudication, rest pain, or management of graft sepsis), the presence of significant outflow occlusive disease, and the methods employed for reporting patency or thrombosis rates. With respect to the latter variable, interpretation of the patency rates of axillofemoral bypass grafts presents a problem. The technique of life table analysis, adopted for graft patency, has become the standard statistical method for reporting early and late results. When analyzing graft function in a particular patient, most authors consider a graft to be functioning until a thrombosis occurs; at this point, the graft is deemed a failure and appropriately entered into the statistical calculation. Several authors have recently chosen to alter that pattern of reporting in cases of axillofemoral bypass grafts.[11,12] They reason that, since the graft is a subcutaneous conduit, easily accessible to simple thrombectomy, an axillofemoral bypass that is thrombectomized without an associated revision or angioplasty can be considered "continuously patent." Thus, if an axillofemoral graft occludes, and the patient is returned to the operating room where thrombectomy is carried out successfully, this patient is statistically entered as one having continuous patency. To prevent confusion from this issue, I gathered my own patency data with both types of analyses, but patency results in which thrombectomized grafts are not considered failures are separated from those in which patency is deemed continuous until the first thrombosis.

Patency of Aortofemoral Bypass Grafts

In 1975 we reviewed a 15-year experience with 180 patients undergoing aortobifemoral bypass grafting. This analysis yielded patency and thrombosis data for 360 graft limbs. The immediate patency rate at the time of hospital discharge was 99.2 percent.[14] Table 1 summarizes the early and late patency rates as a function of concomitant peripheral occlusive disease affecting runoff. The compromised runoff is assessed in two ways, one using angiographic criteria and the other using symptomatic

Table 1. Early and Late Patency Rates of Aortofemoral Bypass Grafts (%)

	1 Yr	3 Yr	5 Yr	10 Yr
Overall patency rate	94	90	83	66
Angiographic criteria				
No distal disease	98	95	95	85
Profunda disease with concomitant profundaplasty	97	92	92	—
Profunda disease without concomitant profundaplasty	90	75	62	—
Occlusive disease of the popliteal bifurcation	85	76	64	0
Lesions of both the profunda and popliteal bifurcation	75	70	0	—
Symptomatic criteria				
Asymptomatic postoperative	98	97	97	97
Symptomatic but improved following operation	92	85	72	38

criteria after successful revascularization. It is evident from this table that when peripheral resistance is low, i.e., the quality of outflow is good, late patency from aortofemoral bypass grafting is excellent. When there is significant compromise in runoff, however, the late thrombosis rate is high. For example, the overall five-year patency rate for the entire series was 83 percent. When there was no distal disease seen on angiography, the 5-year patency rate was 95 percent. When there was no distal disease either because of lack of obstruction or good collateral communication as evidenced by the lack of symptoms immediately after operation, the 5-year patency rate was 97 percent. In contrast, when disease was so extensive that both the profunda femoris artery and the popliteal trifurcation vessels were compromised by occlusive disease, no patient went 5 years with a patent graft.

Table 2 presents the patency data on aortofemoral grafts from four major series, subdivided into four intervals: 1, 3, 5, and 10 years. An average calculated from these four series indicates that the patency for aortofemoral bypass grafts at the end of 1 year was 93 percent; 3 years, 88 percent; 5 years, 82 percent; and 10 years, 70 percent. Thus, it is evident that the overall results with aortofemoral bypass graft operations are favorable and that the operation is quite durable.[11,14,20,23]

Table 3 lists the patency data for femorofemoral bypass grafting in three recent series the average of which indicates that 1-year patency was 83 percent; 3 years, 74 percent; and 5 years, 59 percent.[5,9,12] It should be noted that one series did not classify graft thrombosis opened by simple thrombectomy as a failure and another series (the one with the best results) did not state whether patency ended with the first thrombosis or only with failure despite thrombectomy. Nonetheless, patency rates with femorofemoral bypass, while lower than after aortofemoral bypass, appear reasonable when one considers the poor-risk group often selected for the former operation.

Table 4 summarizes patency data reported from five series evaluating the use of axillofemoral bypass grafts for a number of indications.[9-13,21] These data are again difficult to interpret because definitions

Table 2. Summary of Aortofemoral Graft Patency Rates

Series	1 Yr (%)	3 Yr (%)	5 Yr (%)	10 Yr (%)
Papadopoulos et al.[20]	86	81	78	75
Vanttinen and Inberg[23]	96	92	92	—
Johnson et al.[11]	96	87	75	—
Malone et al.[14]	94	90	83	66
Average	93	88	82	70

Table 3. Patency Rates of Femorofemoral Bypass Grafts

Series	1 Yr (%)	3 Yr (%)	5 Yr (%)
Livesay et al.[12]*	82	75	55
Eugene et al.[9]†	74	65	55
Brief et al.[5]	93	82	81
Average	83	74	59

* If graft occlusion could be treated by simple thrombectomy, not counted as failure.
† Continuous patency counted until thrombosis regardless of whether graft could be reopened by simple thrombectomy.

Table 4. Patency of Axillofemoral Bypass Grafts

Series	1 Yr (%)	3 Yr (%)	5 Yr (%)
Ray et al.[21]	83	78	72
Eugene et al.[9]	62	42	41
Lo Girfo et al.[13]			
Unilateral femoral	57	37	33
Bilateral femoral	90	74	74
Johnson et al.[11]*	82	77	75
Livesay et al.[2]*	78	78	—

* Graft thrombosis not counted as a failure if opened by simple thrombectomy.

of what represents a graft failure have differed. Some authors chose not to list a graft thrombosis as a failure if the graft could be reopened by simple thrombectomy, and consequently their data reflect better late patency results than those from authors who chose to report a graft thrombosis as a failure regardless of whether it could be reopened by simple thrombectomy. Finally, some series did not reveal which of these two reporting methods they employed. Accordingly, the 5-year patency data vary from 33 percent to 75, depending upon the author's method of reporting and perhaps other factors.

Despite these variations, it is evident that axillofemoral bypass grafting probably carries a higher thrombosis rate than the other two types of operations.[15]

ETIOLOGY OF GRAFT THROMBOSIS

Factors affecting graft patency or thrombosis tend to be similar regardless of whether aortofemoral, axillofemoral, or femorofemoral grafts are considered. Factors unique to each anatomic location or type of bypass, however, will be dealt with separately. Finally, the subject of graft thrombosis can be divided into categories of factors leading to perioperative or early thrombosis and factors resulting in late thrombosis.

Perioperative Graft Thrombosis

Inadequate Outflow. A predominant cause of early graft thrombosis, inadequate outflow occurs usually when there is concomitant occlusion of the superficial femoral artery and profunda femoris artery disease uncorrected by profundaplasty (Fig. 1).[14]

Technical Error. Technical error is also a common cause of perioperative graft thrombosis. The technical error frequently involves the femoral anastomosis and is related to some misadventure in the handling of the diseased intima. One example is the inadvertent separation of diseased intima from the adventitia at the site of anastomosis which then leads to a direct valvular obstruction of blood flow from subintimal dissection (Fig. 2).[18]

Another source of technical error involving the arterial intima relates to an unsatisfactory end-point following localized endarterectomy of

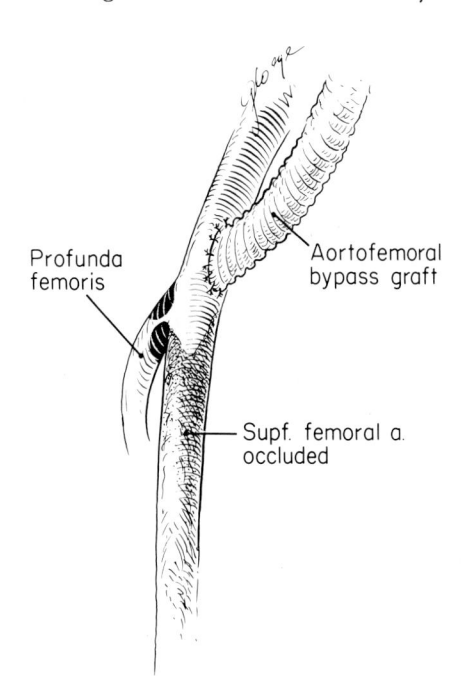

FIGURE 1. An uncorrected lesion of the origin of the profunda femoris artery, combined with occlusion of the superficial femoral artery, will place severe restriction on outflow that will lead to graft thrombosis.

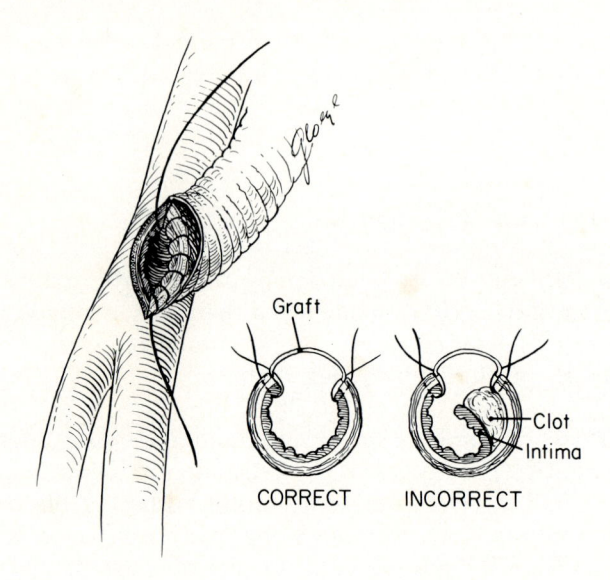

FIGURE 2. The proper construction of an end-to-side anastomosis to the common femoral artery requires that the suture encompass all of the layers of the artery, including the diseased intima. Should a suture inadvertently fail to encompass the diseased intima, it is possible to establish a subintimal dissection leading to valvular obstruction of the outflow tract.

the common femoral bifurcation. The presence of a distal intimal flap can lead to subintimal dissection with obstruction of a major outflow vessel (Fig. 3).

A rare technical error that promptly produces perioperative thrombosis is misalignment of the graft as it is pulled through the subcutaneous or retroperitoneal space. This misalignment or twist compromises blood flow and leads ultimately to thrombosis (Fig. 4).

Patients undergoing axillofemoral bypass grafting are also subject to a particular technical error that may cause an increased incidence of thrombosis, i.e., when positioning a graft with respect to the inferior portion of the rib cage if the graft is brought over the most prominent portion of the costal margin, it can produce obstruction by kinking or angulation at this site (Fig. 5).[7,16]

Incomplete evacuation of blood from the graft before the distal anastomosis has been completed is another technical error. If residual blood is left in the graft, it can clot and become an embolus when flow is re-established into the distal vessels (Fig. 6).

Problems with Arterial Flow. If the lesion being bypassed is insufficient to produce a pressure gradient under conditions of resting blood flow,

Intimal flap with clot formation

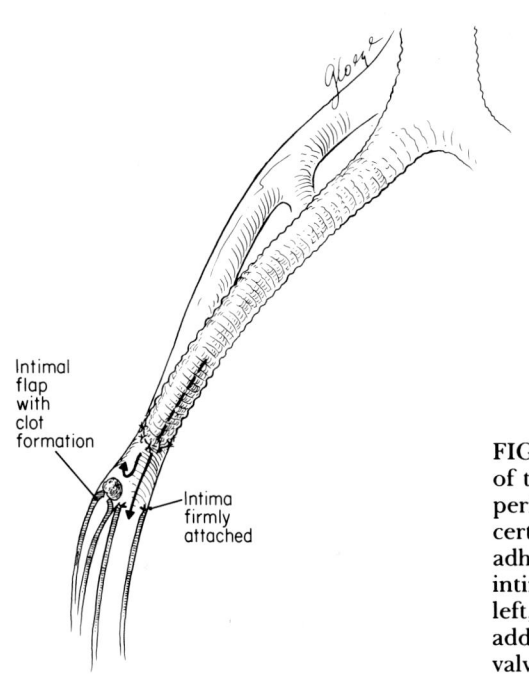

Intima firmly attached

FIGURE 3. If an endarterectomy of the femoral bifurcation is performed, it is necessary to be certain that there is a firmly adherent end point of the distal intima. Should an intimal flap be left, blood flow will cause additional dissection with valvular obstruction.

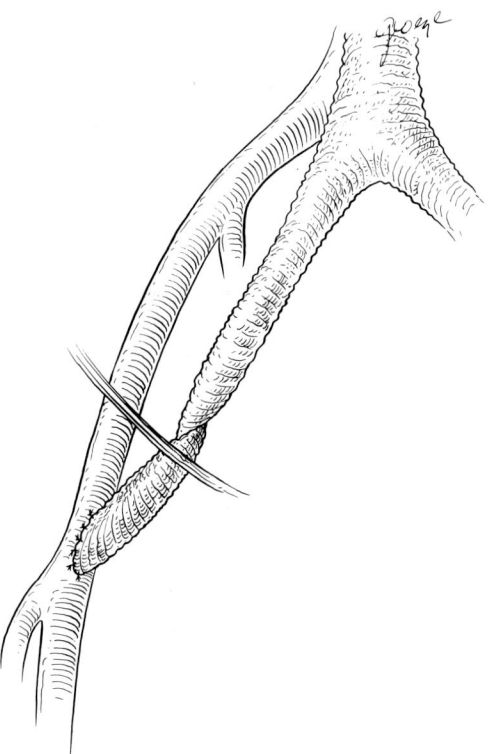

FIGURE 4. Misalignment or a twist in the graft, as it is brought through the retroperitoneal tunnel, will produce a mechanical obstruction to blood flow. Some manufacturers are currently placing a blue line on the graft surface so as to help prevent this complication.

452 Critical Problems in Vascular Surgery

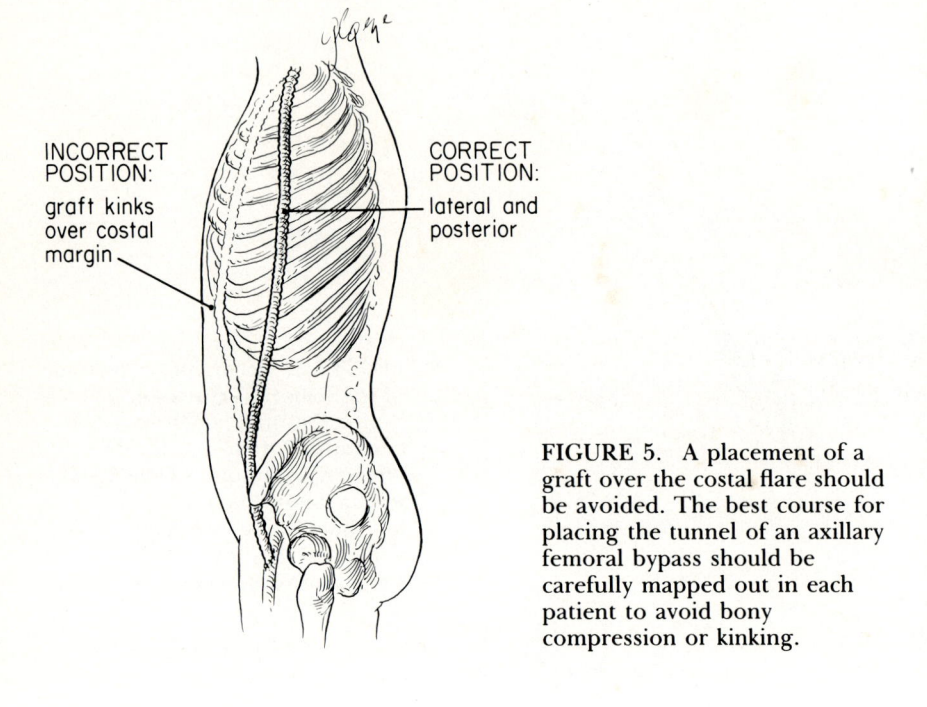

FIGURE 5. A placement of a graft over the costal flare should be avoided. The best course for placing the tunnel of an axillary femoral bypass should be carefully mapped out in each patient to avoid bony compression or kinking.

INCORRECT POSITION: graft kinks over costal margin

CORRECT POSITION: lateral and posterior

FIGURE 6. Residual blood left in the bypass graft will clot during the course of a femoral anastomosis. Thus, when the proximal clamp is released, the clot will embolize and obstruct the outflow tract.

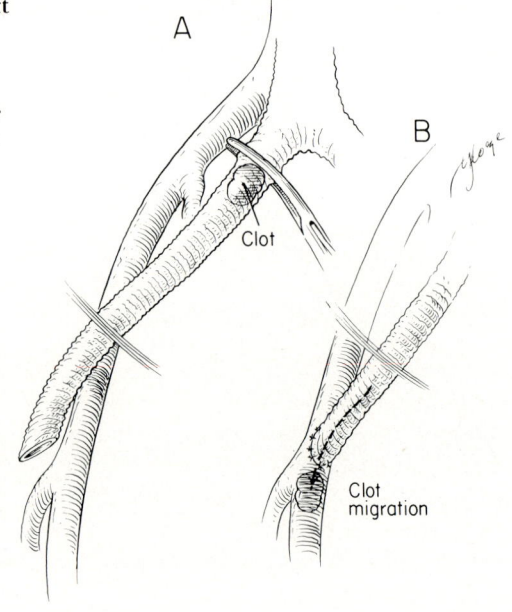

there may be an inadequate flow rate through the graft owing to flow competition with the aortoiliac system, and this can lead to stasis and thrombosis.[17]

In the cases of femorofemoral bypass grafting, misjudging the extent of iliac artery occlusive disease in the iliac artery may reduce flow through the graft and may also lead to thrombosis.

Late Graft Thrombosis

Late graft failure usually stems from compromised runoff through the femoral anastomosis, causing reduced blood flow in the graft, stasis, and ultimately thrombosis.[14,18,19] While this etiology of failure is common to the three anatomic types of bypass, the axillofemoral bypass graft may be more sensitive to small reductions in blood flow because it has the greatest length of prosthetic material.

Neointimal Hyperplasia. Perhaps the dominant cause of obstruction to distal runoff vessels is the tissue buildup at the distal anastomosis, generally termed *neointimal hyperplasia.* While the cause of this abnormal tissue response has not been completely defined, it may in part be a response to mechanical injury occurring secondary to turbulence. It may also be a response to the platelet release reaction occurring when platelets aggregate at the anastomotic site. In any event, once the process starts, it progresses to localized occlusion of runoff vessels at and just distal to the anastomotic site and produces graft thrombosis.

Progression of Atherosclerosis. It has been suggested that the presence of proximal arterial occlusive disease may protect distal vessels from atheromatous degeneration. When the proximal obstruction is bypassed, the forces of increased arterial pressure and flow and perhaps increased turbulence are free to act on the distal (runoff) vessels. These factors may produce arterial injury and may result in an increased progression of atherosclerotic occlusive disease in the more distal vessels. Whether neointimal hyperplasia is a separate entity or an accelerated and modified form of atherosclerosis remains unclear.

Pseudointimal Buildup. The normal response to a discrepancy between large graft caliber and runoff vessel size is a remodeling of the graft lumen by deposition of a compacted fibrin pseudointima so that the graft lumen matches the caliber and flow requirements of the runoff vessels. This caliber remodeling occurs principally at the distal end of the prosthetic graft (Fig. 7). The compacted fibrin layer itself is thrombogenic and may hasten graft thrombosis during the progressive flow reduction phase.

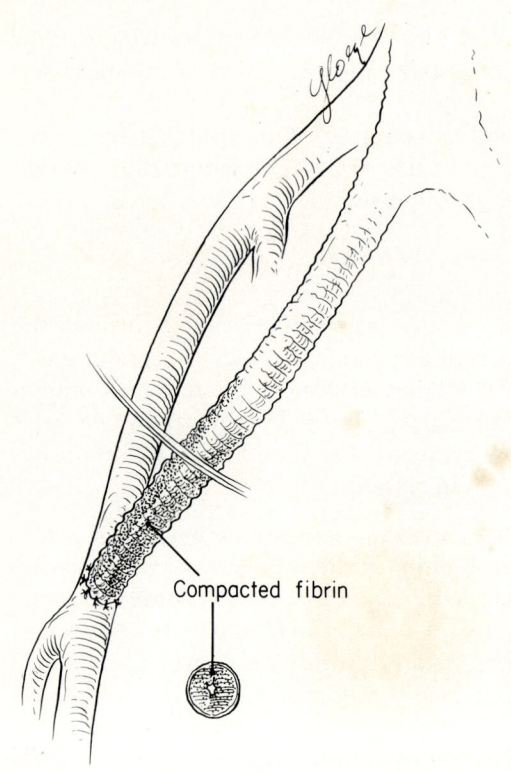

FIGURE 7. A buildup of new pseudointima ultimately occurs in a prosthetic graft. This buildup or remodeling becomes more extensive when there is slow flow due to a compromised outflow.

Compromised Inflow. Reduction of graft blood flow by occlusive disease proximal to the proximal anastomosis is rare in aortofemoral and axillofemoral grafts but more common in femorofemoral bypass operations. Since athero-occlusive disease tends to be a relatively symmetrical process, isolated unilateral iliac artery occlusive disease that is amenable to repair by cross-over femorofemoral bypass grafting is somewhat unusual. Yet, when it does occur and presents an opportunity for treatment by femorofemoral bypass, the atherosclerotic process in the relatively undiseased donor iliac artery may "catch up" once flow demand on that artery is increased by using it as a conduit to both extremities (Fig. 8). This is not always the case, however, as indicated by the late patency rates that have been observed.

Subcutaneous Graft Compression. It is generally thought that grafts placed in a subcutaneous position (axillofemoral and femorofemoral bypasses) are vulnerable to extrinsic compression. Diverse forces, such as a tight belt, sleeping on the graft, and kinking over the costal margin have been implicated in graft compression and subsequent graft thrombosis.

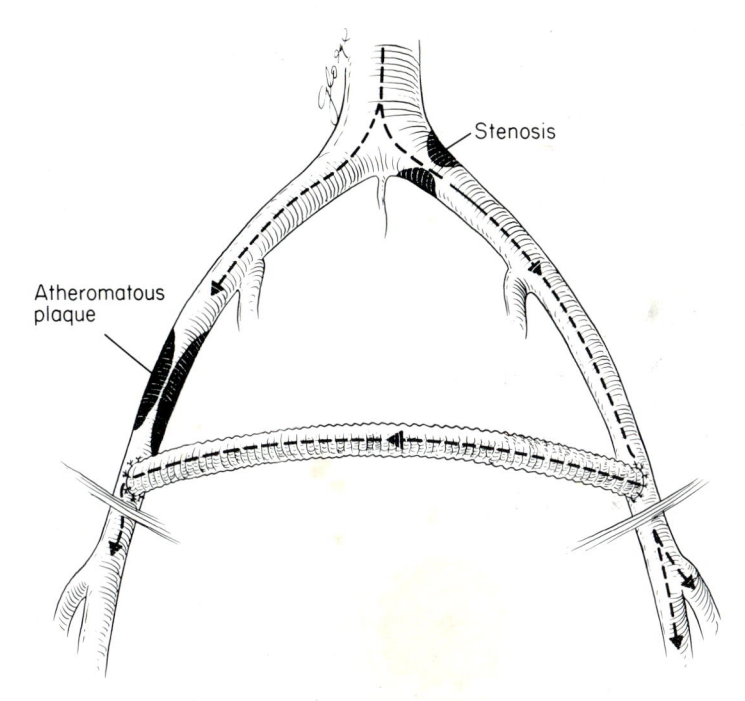

FIGURE 8. Continued function of a crossover femorofemoral bypass graft is dependent upon there being only unilateral iliac artery occlusive disease. Should a stenosis be present or later develop on the contralateral or donor side, the function of the graft will be compromised.

The exact contribution of these extrinsic forces to graft thrombosis in contrast to other causes of graft failure has not been proven conclusively.

MANAGEMENT OF PERIOPERATIVE GRAFT THROMBOSIS

Most instances of graft thrombosis in the early postoperative period are quite obvious from the appearance of deteriorated limb perfusion and loss of peripheral pulses; however, on occasion, an extremity may appear to be poorly perfused on the evening of the operation owing to peripheral vasoconstriction without actual graft thrombosis or peripheral embolization. In this instance, it is valuable to measure ankle/brachial blood pressure indices using a blood pressure cuff and a Doppler flow probe before as well as after operation. If a repeat of these measurements shows deterioration of the index back to preoperative levels, then it is most likely that the graft has thrombosed. If the ankle/brachial index is better than preoperative levels, however, it is probable that the patient is peripherally constricted, and limb perfusion will improve as the patient's general condition and blood volume status improve. While these determinations are in process, a loading dose of heparin (5,000–10,000 units) can be given to the patient intravenously. If the graft is thrombosed, it will help prevent propagation of clot. If it is not thrombosed, heparin may act as a peripheral vasodilator which, combined with a fluid load, may improve limb perfusion. The presence of a pulse along the course of an axillofemoral graft is not a specific guarantee of patency inasmuch as there may be a transmitted pulsation through semiliquid clot.

Once it has been determined that the graft has thrombosed, the patient should be returned promptly to the operating room, and if heparin has not been administered, it should be given at this time.

The entire surgical field is reprepped and draped. When one limb of an aortofemoral graft is thrombosed I recommend reopening the groin incision first, reserving opening of the abdominal incision for a later time and only if necessary. In the case of a thrombosed axillofemoral or femorofemoral graft, it is probably best to reopen all incisions at the onset.

Attention is intially focused on the femoral anastomosis, keeping in mind that the thrombosis is usually due to a technical error at that site. The femoral artery and its branches are mobilized and encircled with vessel tapes. The inside of the anastomosis can be inspected through a transverse graftotomy placed close to the distal anastomosis, or by taking down the distal anastomosis to permit direct inspection. Once the technical problem is identified and corrected, the anastomosis can be redone or the opening in the graft closed. In the case of an intimal flap, the arteriotomy on the superficial femoral artery or the deep femoral artery may require extension to allow sufficient visualization to improve the end point and eliminate the intimal flap. It may be necessary to carry out a patch angioplasty of one or both or these vessels, using a saphenous vein, the arterial tissue harvested from an occluded superficial femoral artery, or the bevel of the prosthetic graft. When the problem is corrected a completion angiogram is recommended to assure a satisfactory technical result and rule out distal thrombosis or embolization of the runoff tract.

MANAGEMENT OF LATE THROMBOSIS

Figure 9 is an algorithm for managing a patient with an established femoral artery bypass graft following acute late thrombosis. When the patient is first diagnosed as having an acute graft occlusion, an intrave-

MANAGEMENT OF ACUTE THROMBOSIS OF AN
ESTABLISHED BYPASS GRAFT TO THE FEMORAL ARTERY

```
                    Aortic graft thrombosis
                             |
                I.V. Heparin, 30-60 min observation
                 _____|_____
                 |                               |
           Nonviable limb                   Viable limb
                 |                   1. Noninvasive diagnosis
         Immediate operation         2. Exercise tolerance
                                _____|_____
                                |                               |
                          Nonlimiting                       Limiting
                          claudication                    claudication
                          observation                          |
                                                          Angiography
                                                               |
                                                        Surgical repair
```

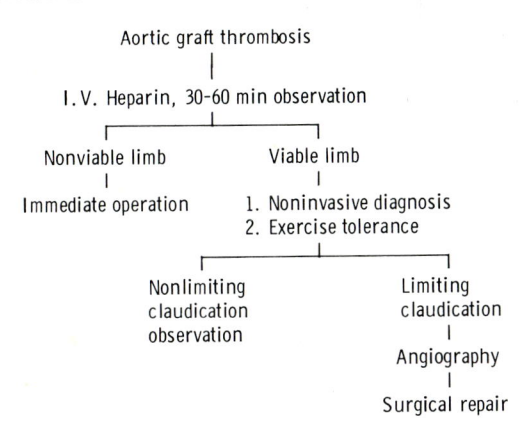

FIGURE 9. Plan for the management of a patient presenting with an acute graft limb thrombosis.

nous bolus injection of 10,000 units of heparin should be administered. The hemodynamic changes that take place in an extremity subsequent to acute arterial occlusion will cause the leg to look worst immediately after the obstruction. This is due primarily to deprivation of blood flow to the extremity but also to a reflex vasospasm that occurs secondary to clot in the femoral artery. Heparin not only prevents propagation of the thrombus, but also serves to reverse this vasospastic process. After administering heparin, the leg should be observed for 30 to 60 minutes, during which time the basic patient work-up can be accomplished and the necessary laboratory data obtained before operation should it become necessary.

After the heparin effect, the leg is reevaluated with respect to its viability. Information concerning sensation, motor power, and capillary refill time will help make that determination. If the leg is clearly nonviable, immediate operation is recommended to repair the outflow tract and reestablish extremity perfusion. I prefer not to obtain preoperative arteriograms in such an event because it would cause delay, but rely instead on arteriography in the operating table as necessary. On the other hand, if the extremity is viable after a period of heparin administration, the evaluation can proceed in an elective and orderly fashion. Patients in this category are evaluated in the same way as during their original presentation with symptoms of arterial occlusive disease. This includes studies in the vascular laboratory where noninvasive segmental pressure data are recorded to document the hemodynamic effect of the arterial lesion. Moreover, exercise tolerance should be evaluated to determine whether or not the patient's symptoms of claudication will cause severe limitation of activity and therefore justify surgical repair, or whether the claudication is nonlimiting in which case operation is not indicated. This determination may require a period of observation. When there is severe disabling claudication, however, elective angiography should be performed to determine the presence and quality of a reconstituted profunda femoris artery as well as of the popliteal artery and its trifurcation vessels. This is done to assess operability and the likelihood of successful secondary arterial reconstruction. If the angiographic findings reveal a satisfactory technical situation, then appropriate surgical repair can be carried out.

Surgical Approach to Late Unilateral Graft Limb Thrombosis of an Aortofemoral Bypass Graft

The patient is prepared and draped for an aortofemoral bypass graft, usually including both extremities, and draping them free if femoropopliteal or femorotibial reconstruction may become necessary.

The incision over the femoral artery is reopened to expose the distal portion of the bypass graft limb. Sharp dissection is used to reidentify the common femoral artery, the superficial femoral artery, and the profunda femoris artery. The graft is then divided just proximal to the femoral anastomosis to facilitate exploration for the cause of outflow obstruction. Thrombus is evacuated from the anastomosis, and the orifices of the superficial femoral and profunda femoris artery are explored. In the event of atheromatous disease progression or obstruction owing to neointimal hyperplasia, the arteriotomy from the common femoral artery can be extended through the localized area of obstruction on to the main trunk of the patent distal vessel, usually the profunda femoris artery. A patch angioplasty, which is best performed with autogenous tissues such as saphenous vein or reconstituted superficial femoral artery, is carried out.

After establishing a satisfactory outflow to the profunda femoris artery, a retrograde thrombectomy of the graft limb is performed. A Fogarty catheter is passed retrograde up the femoral graft limb into the body of the graft, the balloon is inflated, and the thrombus is removed. Success of the procedure becomes apparent with a return of vigorous pulsatile arterial blood flow.[1,6,8,10] If the return is less than expected, then the Fogarty catheter can be reinserted, the baloon inflated to provide inflow control, and a wire loop stripper passed over the Fogarty catheter can be inserted up the graft limb to free any areas of compacted fibrin along the course of the graft limb (Fig. 10b).[18] Once residual thrombotic

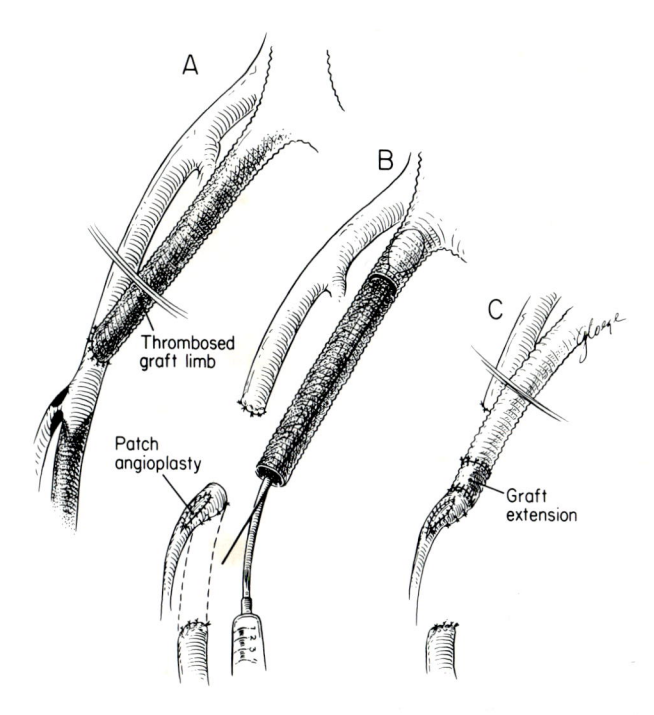

FIGURE 10. The stepwise approach to unilateral aortofemoral graft limb thrombosis includes correction of outflow stenosis, graft thrombectomy, and graft reanastomosis. The occluded superficial femoral artery represents an important source of autogenous material for patch angioplasty of the profunda femoris artery.

debris is removed and satisfactory inflow is achieved, the graft can be anastomosed to the common femoral artery proximal to the autogenous angioplasty (Fig. 10). Satisfactory thrombectomy of the thrombosed graft limb can be assured by performing retrograde arteriography or by using the right angle choledochoscope to directly inspect the course of the graft limb during a period of inflow occlusion provided by inflating the baloon catheter.[22] If it is not possible to disobliterate the graft, inflow can be reestablished by using a crossover femorofemoral bypass graft taken from the opposite patent graft limb.

Late Thrombosis of Both Limbs of an Aortofemoral Bypass Graft

When both graft limbs have thrombosed, the femoral arteries are approached in the manner described above. Once it had been determined that satisfactory outflow can be provided to the profunda femoris artery, the abdomen is reopened in preparation for replacing the aortofemoral bypass graft. Patch angioplasties of the strictured profunda femoris orifices, using autogenous material, are performed bilaterally prior to inserting a new graft.

Management of Late Thrombosis of Axillofemoral or Femorofemoral Bypass Grafts

Surgical preparation of the outflow tract for each of these procedures is the same as that for aortofemoral bypass thrombosis. Although it may be possible to reestablish inflow by simple thrombectomy of the graft, if this proves difficult, there should be no hesitation to replace the graft since this is a subcutaneous operation and replacing the proximal anastomosis does not require entrance to a major body cavity.

REFERENCES

1. Bernhard VM, Lance IR, Towne JB: The reoperation of choice for aortofemoral graft occlusion. Surgery 82:867, 1977
2. Blaisdell FW, Hall AD: Axillary-femoral artery bypass for lower extremity ischemia. Surgery 54:563, 1963
3. Blaisdell FW, Hall AD, Lim RC Jr., Moore WS: Aorto-iliac arterial substitution utilizing subcutaneous grafts. Ann Surg 172:202, 1970
4. Brief DK, Alpert J, Parsonnet V: Crossover femoro-femoral grafts. Arch Surg 105:889, 1972
5. Brief DK, Brennar BJ, Alpert J. Parsonnet V: Crossover femoral-femoral grafts followed up five years or more. Arch Surg 110:1294, 1975
6. Cohn LH, Moore WS, Hall AD: Extra-abdominal management of late aortofemoral graft thrombosis. Surgery 67:775, 1970
7. DeLaurentis DA, Sala LE, Russel E, McCombs PR: A twelve-year experience with axillo-femoral and femoro-femoral bypass operations. Surg Gynecol Obstet 147:881, 1978
8. Ernst CB, Daugherty ME: Removal of a thrombotic plug from an occluded limb of an aorto-femoral graft. Arch Surg 113:301, 1978
9. Eugene J, Goldstone J, Moore WS: Fifteen-year experience with subcutaneous bypass grafts for lower extremity ischemia. Ann Surg 186:177, 1977
10. Harbrecht PJ, Ahmad W, Fry DE: Management of aortic bypass graft thrombosis: Utility of thrombectomy. Am J Surg 136:363, 1978
11. Johnson WC, Logerfo FW, Vollman RW, et al: Is axillo-bilateral femoral graft an effective substitute for aortic-bilateral iliac/femoral graft? Ann Surg 186:123, 1977
12. Livesay JJ, Atkinson JB, Baker D, et al: Late results of extra-anatomic bypass. Arch Surg 114:1260, 1979
13. LoGerfo FW, Johnson WC, Corson JD, et al: A comparison of the late

patency rates of axillo-bilateral femoral and axillo-unilateral femoral grafts. Surgery 81:33, 1977
14. Malone JM, Goldstone J, Moore WS: Autogenous profundaplasty: The key to long-term patency in secondary repair of aorto-femoral graft occlusion. Ann Surg 188:817, 1978
15. Malone JM, Moore WS, Goldstone J: The natural history of bilateral aorto-femoral bypass grafts for ischemia of the lower extremities. Arch Surg 110:1300, 1975
16. Mannick JA, Nabseth DC: Axillo-femoral bypass graft. N Engl J Med 278:461, 1968
17. Moore WS: Reoperation for early and late complications of arterial surgery. In Haimovici H (ed): Vascular Surgery: Principles and Techniques. New York, McGraw-Hill, 1976, p. 584
18. Moore WS, Hall AD, Blaisdell FW: Late results of axillary-femoral bypass grafting. Am J Surg 122:148, 1971
19. Najafi H, Dye WS, Javid H, et al: Late thrombosis affecting one limb of aortic bifurcation graft, Arch Surg 110:409, 1975
20 Papadopoulos CC: Surgical treatment of aorto-iliac occlusive disease. J Cardiovasc Surg (Torino) 17:54, 1976
21. Ray LI, O'Connor JB, Davis CC, et al: Axillo-femoral bypass: A critical reappraisal of its role in the management of aorto-iliac occlusive disease. Am J Surg 138:117, 1979
22. Towne JB, Bernhard VM: Technique of intraoperative endoscopic evaluation of occluded aorto-femoral grafts following thrombectomy. Surg Gynecol Obstet 148:87, 1979
23. Vantinnen E, Inberg MV: Aorto-ilico femoral arterial reconstructive surgery. Acta Chir Scand 141:600, 1975

Index

Abdominal aortic aneurysms, 31–43
  diagnosis of
    by computed tomography, 36–41
    by ultrasound, 31–35
  as a source of infection, 373
Amaurosis fugax, 342, 353
  arteriography for, 347–49
Amputation, 217–26, 229
  below-knee, 219–26, 237–38
    major, 222–26
      vs. femoropopliteal bypass, 224–25
      decision, 226
      rehabilitation, 224
      techniques of, 223
    minor, 219–22
      principles of, 219–22
      rehabilitation, 222
  critical features of, 237
  infection and, 219
  level of, determination, 236–39
    skin blood flow, 236–37
    Ketty-Schmidt equation, 237

Amputation *(cont'd.)*
  level of, determination *(cont'd.)*
    postoperative prosthesis, 238
    with a patent femoropopliteal bypass, 245–46
  pathologic considerations, 217–18
  after profunda femoris angioplasty, 261
  team approach, 238–39
AMTEK/Hunter Tensile Strength Tester, 107
Anastomosis
  earliest reported, 2
  early problems with, 2
Anastomotic neointimal fibrous hyperplasia (ANFH), 151–56
  causes of, 152–55
    delayed endothelialization, 153
    hemodynamic factor, 153–54
    mechanical mismatch, 154–55
    operative trauma, 152
    thrombogenicity of grafts, 152–53
  prevention of, 155–56

Aneurysm
  abdominal aortic
    diagnosis and evaluation of, 31–43
      by computed tomography, 36–41
      growth rates, 35–36
      by ultrasound, 31–35
  dissecting
    first surgical attempt to correct, 19–20
  surgical management, 13–19
  transcatheter therapeutic embolization of, 64
ANFH. *See* Anastomotic neointimal fibrous hyperplasia
Angiography, 59, 74
Annapurna, 7
Antyllus, 14
Aorta, coarctation of, 7
Aortic graft infection, 371–83, 387–97
  autogenous tissues, use in, 387–97
  classification, 374
  diagnosis, 373–78, 389–92
    aids in, 389–91
    groin, 374–76
    intra-abdominal, 376–78
  etiology, 372–73, 387–88
    bacterial contamination, 373
  incidence, 371
  prevention, 371
  surgical management, 391–97
    in abdominal and groin prosthetic grafts, 394–97
    autogenous tissue techniques, 393–94
      advantages of, 396–97
      autogenous graft replacement, 394
      endarterectomy, 393–94
      patch angioplasty, 393
  treatment, 378–83, 391–97
    of infected aortofemoral graft, 380–83
    of infected aortoiliac graft, 380–81
    restricted to groin wound, 378–80

Aortoduodenal fistula, 399–409
  clinical presentation, 402
  diagnosis, 403–404
  pathogenesis, 400–401
  secondary, 400
  surgical management, 404–408
    goals, 404
    results, 408–409
Aortofemoral graft
  patency, 445, 446, 447
  thrombosis of, 445–60. *See also* Graft thrombosis
    incidence of, 445–48
    etiology, 448–55
    late, 453–55
      of both graft limbs, 459–60
      management of, 456–58
      surgical approach, 458–59
    perioperative, 449–53
      management of, 455–56
Aortoiliac disease, sexual problems and, 429–41
Arm vein
  in bypass of inferior vena cava, 208–209
  in femoropopliteal reconstruction, 180–81
Arterial grafts, 25
  early uses of, 2–6
Arterial injuries
  blunt trauma and
    clinical features, 333–36
      carotid injury and, 335
      arteriography, use of, 375–76
      popliteal artery and, 335
    etiology of, 330
    incidence, 329
    location, 329, 330
    methods of repair, 336
      results, 337
    mechanisms, 330–33
    types, 330–33
Artificial heart, 4
Aspirin, 124, 162
  intimal hyperplasia and, 169
  in prevention of neointimal fibrous hyperplasia, 155–56
  reducing incidence of stroke, 365–66

Autofemoral bypass grafts, infection of, 394
Autologous saphenous vein bypass grafts, 242
Autotransplantation, 315
Avitene, 60, 65
Axillofemoral graft
 patency rate, 445, 448
 thrombosis of, 445–60. *See also* Graft thrombosis
  etiology, 448–55
  late, 453–55
   management of, 456–58
  perioperative, 449–53
   management of, 455–56

Baker's cyst, 53
"Bench surgery," 35
Blalock, A., 7
Blalock-Taussig procedure, 125–26
B-mode ultrasound, accuracy of, 33–35
Budd-Chiari syndrome, 201
Buerger's disease, 279
Buffington plethysmographic cuff, 434
Bypass grafts
 failure of, 116–18
 as a replacement for thromboendarterectomy, 12
 use of polytetrafluoroethylene, 116–21
 for venous occlusion, 190–91
Bypass principle, 13

Carotid disease, role of noninvasive testing and imaging in
 accuracy, 341–42
  definition of, 342
 amaurosis fugax, 347–49
 asymptomatic bruit, 352–53
 extracranial carotid surgery, 353–54
 intraoperative monitoring, 355
 methods, 343–47
  combined approaches, 345–47
  physiologic tests, 342–44

Carotid disease, role of noninvasive testing and imaging in *(cont'd)*
 physiologic tests, *(cont'd)*
  accuracy of, 343
 ultrasound, 344–45
  accuracy, 344
 nonlocalizing symptoms, 352
 postoperative follow-up, 355–56
 postoperative monitoring, 355
 proposed roles for, 357
 purpose, 347
 stroke, 349, 352
 transient ischemic attacks, 347–51
Carotid endarterectomy, re-stenosis following
 antiplatelet agents, role of, 365–67
 aspirin, 365–66
 defection, 364
 survey of literature, 362–65
Carotid phonoangiography, 343
Carpal tunnel syndrome, 284
Carrel, A., 2, 20, 152
Causalgia
 clinical manifestations, 322–23
 definition of, 321–22
 etiology, 323–24
 treatment, 324–27
  failure, reasons for, 327
  lumbar block, 325
  results of, 326–27
  stellate ganglion block, 325
  surgical sympathectomy, 326
Chemical sympathectomy, 271
Chronic intestinal ischemia (CMI)
 percutaneous transluminal angioplasty and, 312–17
 symptoms, 312–13
Cid Dis Santos, J., 9, 10
CMI. *See* Chronic intestinal ischemia
Coaxial balloon catheter system, 100
Colchicine, 148
Computed tomography
 abdominal aortic aneurysms, diagnosis of, use in, 31–43
 techniques of, 36–41
 aortic reconstruction and, 39–41
 compared with ultrasound, 41–43

Computed tomogrpahy *(cont'd.)*
  early experience of, 37
  infected aortic grafts, diagnosis of, use in, 389, 391
  time required, 43
Congestive heart failure, 303
Conray, 36, 400
Contrast phlebography
  in diagnosis of deep vein thrombosis, 45–48
    new developments in, 47–48
    postphlebography syndrome, 46
    side effects, 46
Cooper, Sir Astley, 399
Coronary angioplasty, 100–102
Coronary bypass grafts, 124
Coumadin, 148
  after angioplasty, 85

Dacron grafts, 152, 155, 181, 201
  compared to Gore-Tex, 154
  failure of, 151
  femoropopliteal, 170–71
DeBakey, Michael, E., 20
Deep vein thrombosis (DVT), of the lower extremities, 45–56
  diagnosis of, 45–56
    contrast phlebography, 45–48
    Doppler ultrasound, 52–53
    ^{125}I-fibrinogen point scanning, 48–50
    impedance plethysmography, 50–52
    laboratory methods, 55
    radionuclide phlebography, 53–54
    thermography, 53
    thrombus scintigraphy, 54–55
Delbet, P., 9
Diabetes, 258
Digitalis, 303, 309
Dipyridamole, 124, 148, 162
  intimal hyperplasia and, 169, 366
  in prevention of neointimal fibrous hyperplasia, 155–56

Doppler flow signal analysis, 343
Dörfler, J., 2
Dunglison, Robley, 322
DVT. *See* Deep vein thrombosis

Eck, Nikolai, 2
Embolic therapy. *See* Transcatheter therapeutic embolization
Endarterectomy, 133, 145, 315. *See also* Carotid endarterectomy
  in infected aortic grafts, 393–94
"Endoaneurysmorrhaphy," 16
Erection, normal penile, 430–33
  neural pathways of, 430–31
  vascular factors, 434–37

Femorofemoral bypass, sexual function after, 437
Femorofemoral graft
  patency rate, 445, 448
  thrombosis of, 445–60. *See also* Graft thrombosis
    etiology, 448–55
      management of, 455–56
      perioperative, 449–53
      late, 453–55
      management of, 456–58
Femoropopliteal angioplasty, 86
  results of, 88–89
Femoropopliteal bypass
  blind popliteal artery segment and, 241–48
  extension to distal limb arteries, 246–47
  limb loss and, 241–48
  radiographic evaluation, 242
  results, 243–45
  systemic and local risk factors, 245–46
  vs. amputation, 224–26
  Husni's technique, 191
  in occlusion of the superficial femoral artery, 230–32

Femoropopliteal bypass *(cont'd.)*
  and polytetrafluoroethylene, 111–15, 123, 159–71, 241–48
  profunda femoris angioplasty and, 259–60
  saphenous vein, 168
  thrombosis of, 159–71
Femorotibial bypass
  and polytetrafluoroethylene, 123
  profunda femoris angioplasty and, 255–60
5-Fluorouracil, 148
Furosemide, 309

Gangrene, 217, 218
  extent of, 236
  finger, instrinsic small artery occlusive disease, caused by, 286–93
    patient evaluation, 287–89
    patient presentation, 287
    possible causes, 290–91
    treatment and results, 289–91
  management of, 229–39. *See also* Amputation
  profunda femoris angioplasty, success of, and, 257–58
Gelfoam, 60, 65
Gore-Tex grafts, 152, 185. *See also* Polytetrafluoroethylene vascular grafts
  compared with Dacron, 154
  failure of, 151
  strength of, 107–108.
Goyannes, J., 5
Grafts. *See also specific type*
  development of, 105
  failure of, 25, 156. *See also specific problem*
  search for the ideal, 24
  thrombosis. *See* Graft thrombosis
Graft thrombosis, 159–72
  detection of, 159–61
  etiology, 448–55

Graft thrombosis *(cont'd.)*
  etiology *(cont'd.)*
    late, 453–55
      atherosclerosis progression, 453
      compromised inflow, 454
      management of, 456–58
      neointimal hyperplasia, 453
      pseudointimal buildup, 453
      subcutaneous compression, 454–55
    perioperative, 449–53
      arterial flow problems, 450, 453
      inadequate outflow, 449
      management, 455–58
      technical error, 449–50
  polytetrafluoroethylene, 160
    management for, 162–68
    results, 166–68
    reoperation, 168
Gross, Robert, 7
Guanethidine, 286, 291
Guthrie, C.C., 3

Halsted, William Stewart, 16
Heparin, 148, 162
  after angioplasty, 85
  graft thrombosis and, 457
Herzog, Maurice, 7
Holman, Emile, 17
Horner's syndrome, 325–26, 335
Hunter, John, 14, 16
Hydralazine, 305
8-Hydroxyquinoline, 54
Hypersensitivity angiitis, 288
Hypoplastic aortoiliac syndrome, 411–27
  eclampsia and, 423
  intrauterine fetal death and, 423
  materials and methods, 411–15
  measurements, 419–21
  patient clinical history, 412–14
    angiographic studies, 415
    hormonal factors, 413

Hypoplastic aortoiliac syndrome
(cont'd.)
  patient clinical history (cont'd.)
    laboratory data, 414–15
    symptoms, 413
      absence of hypertension and, 414
    treatment, 415–18
      preferred method, 425
      surgical results, 421

^{125}I-fibrinogen point count scanning, 48–50
  advantages of 49
^{125}I-labeled fibrinogen, 45, 49, 54
Impotence, 437–41
  common causes of, 440
  criteria for, 438n
  multidisciplinary approach, 438
  patient factors, 437–39
  screening for, 439
  vasculogenic, treatment of, 440–41
Impra grafts, strength of, 107–108
^{111}Indium, 54
Intimal hyperplasia, 25, 163, 164
  pathogenesis, 133–46
    diabetes and, 135
    experimental data on, 136–46
    hemodynamic factors, 134
    polytetrafluoroethylene and, 115–16, 169–70
  prevention, 146–48
    methods, 148
IPG. See Impedance plethysmography
Ivalon, 60, 65
  disadvantages of, 61

Jeger, Ernest, 13
Jianu, I., 9

Ketty-Schmidt equation, 237
Kunlin, J., 13, 190

Law of LaPlace, 36
Leriche, René, 3, 7, 8, 429
Leriche syndrome, 411. See also Hypoplastic aortoiliac syndrome
Lidocaine, 97
Lindbergh, Charles, 4
Lumbar sympathectomy
  for causalgia, 326
  for lower limb ischemia, 263–73
    arterial reconstruction, use during, 268, 270
    blood flow, effect on, 264–65
    controversy of, 263
    indications, 265–66
      preoperative angiogram, 266
    patient selection, 266
    plethysmography, 268
    predicting results, 266–68
      hemodynamic criteria, 269
      transcutaneous Doppler flow detection, 267–68
    sympathetic innervation of the lower extremity, 264

Mannitol, 309
Matas, R., 16
Mimocausalgia, 322
  cause of, 323
  symptoms of, 323
Myocardial infarction, 302, 305
Myodesis, 224
Myoplasty, 225

New England Society for Vascular Surgery, survey of polytetrafluoroethylene grafts by, 115
Newton, Isaac, 1
Nitroglycerin, 305
Nitroprusside, 305
NMI. See Nonocclusive mesenteric ischemia

Nonocclusive mesenteric ischemia (NMI)
  acute, 302–12
    complications, 310–11
      arterial occlusions, 310
    diagnosis, 302–303
      plain film studies, 305–306
    initial treatment, 303–305
      supportive therapy, 309
      therapeutic papaverine infusion, 307, 309
      vasodilators, 305
    prognosis, 309–310
    selection of patients, 303
    thrombolytic therapy, 311–12
  diagnosis, 301–302
  pathogenesis of, 301
  reversal of, 301

Ocular pressure plethysmography (OPG-Gee), 342, 353, 354, 364
Ophthalmodynamometry, 342
Oudot, Jacques, 7

Palma, Eduardo, 199
Papaverine, 97
  reversal of nonocclusive mesenteric ischemia, use in, 301
  in shock, use of, 305
  therapeutic infusion of, 307, 309
Pedal venous pressure, 55
Percutaneous transluminal angioplasty (PTA), 83–102
  advantages of, 98, 100
  chronic intestinal ischemia and, 312–17
  complications, 95–97
    at the periphery, 95–97
    popliteal artery spasm, 97
    at the puncture site, 95
    thromboembolism, 96
  coronary, 100–102

Percutaneous transluminal angioplasty (PTA) *(cont'd.)*
  historical development and techniques, 83–85
    dilating, 83–84
    instruments for, 84
  peripheral vascular disease and, 85–95
    aortoiliac, 86–87
      success rates, 86
    femoropopliteal, 86, 88–93
      results of, 88–93
    infrapopliteal, 93–95
    renal artery, 97–100
      complications, 98–100
        transplant renal artery stenosis, 98, 100
Peripheral vascular disease, 85–95
Pharmacoangiography, 59
Phenoxybenzamine, 286, 291
Phlebography, 189–90
Phleborheography, 51–52
Photoplethysmography, 187–89, 342
Plethysmography
  impedance (IPG), 50–52
    advantages of, 50–51
    phleborheography, comparison with, 51–52
  strain-gauge, in predicting results of lumbar sympathectomy, 268
Pneumatic cuff technique, 256
Polytetrafluoroethylene grafts (PTFE), 105–20, 123–28
  characteristics, 125
  closure index, 126–28
  criticisms of, 115–16
  differences, 107–108
  evaluation of, 106–107
  description of, 108, 110–11
  failure of, 116–18
    arterial embolization, 117–18
    intimal hyperplasia and, 169–70
      etiology of, 169
  patency rate, 106

Polytetrafluoroethylene grafts
      (PTFE)*(cont'd.)*
   strength of, 107–108
      bursting, 109
      suture retention, 109
   thrombosis of, 160
      management for, 162–68
      saphenous vein femoropopliteal bypasses and, 168–69
      thrombectomy and, 169, 171
   uses of
      arterial replacement, 126
      coronary bypass, 124
      dialysis access, 125
      in extra-anatomic bypass, 118
      in femoropopliteal bypasses, 111–15, 123, 159–71, 241–48
      for vascular access, 118
   venous grafts, 119, 124–25
   vena cava replacement, 201
Posttraumatic pain syndrome. *See* Causalgia
PPCI, 260
Prazosin, 286, 291, 305
Profunda femoris angioplasty, 252–61
   as an alternative to femoropopliteal or femorotibial bypass, 259
   determinants of success, 252
      aortoiliac inflow, 252–53, 259
      diabetes, 258
      extent and pattern of disease, 254–55
      peripheral gangrene, 257–58
      popliteal-tibial run-off system, patency of, 256–57
   mortality, 261
   profunda-popliteal-tibial collateral anastomoses, 255–56
      measurement of, 256
   results of, 258–261
      limb salvage, 259
   severity of stenosis, 253–54
Profunda femoris artery
   angioplasty, 252–61. *See also* Profunda femoris angioplasty
   importance of, 251

Profunda femoris artery *(cont'd.)*
   popliteal-tibial collateral anastomoses, 255–56
   stenosis, 253–54
      extent and pattern of, 254–55
Profundaplasty. *See* Profunda femoris angioplasty
Profunda popliteal collateral index (PPCI), 260
Prostacycline, 155
PTA. *See* Percutaneous transluminal angioplasty
PTFE grafts. *See* Polytetrafluoroethylene grafts
Pulse delay oculoplethysmography (OPG-Kartchner), 342

Radiographic contrast material (RCM), 37–41
Radionuclide phlebography, 53–54
Raynaud's disease. *See* Raynaud's syndrome
Raynaud's phenomenon. *See* Raynaud's syndrome
Raynaud's syndrome, 278–86, 288, 291–92
   associated diseases, 284
   classification, 283
   etiology, 279–82
   evaluation, 282–83
   examination, 284
   history and incidence, 278–79
   laboratory tests, 284–85
   prognosis, 286
   symptoms, 278
   treatment, 285–86
Ray resection, 238
RCM. *See* Radiographic contrast material
Reflex sympathetic dystrophy. *See* Causalgia
Renal artery angioplasty, 97–100
Renal carcinoma, 77
Renografin, 36, 76
Renovascular hypertension, treatment for, 97
Reserpine, 286

Saphenous vein,
  absent or unsuitable, 176–79
    causes of, 177–78
    determination of, 178–79
      preoperative renography, 178
  elective preservation of, 179–80
    cardiac complications of, 180
  femoropopliteal bypass
    thrombosis of, 168–71
      early, 168–69
      late, 170
Sexual problems, aortoiliac disease and, 429–41
  history taking, importance of, 430
  impotence, 437–41
Sjögren's syndrome, 288
SMA. See Superior mesenteric artery
Streptokinase, 311
Stroke, 342, 349, 352, 353
  aspirin and, 365–66
Subclavian venous occlusion, 206, 208
Sulfinpyrazone, 365–66
Superior mesenteric artery (SMA)
  decreased blood flow, 301
  intestinal ischemia and, 300
  percutaneous transluminal angioplasty and, 313
Supraorbital Doppler sonography, 342
Surgery of Pain, 8
Sympathectomy. *See also* Chemical sympathectomy; Lumbar sympathectomy
  as a treatment for causalgia, 324–26
  Leriche and, 8
Syme's amputation, 238
Synthetic grafts, 23
  introduction of, 20–21
  rationale for use, 20–21

99mTc, 53, 54
Tetralogy of Fallot, first operation for, 7
Thermography, 53, 342
Thrombectomy, 9
  and polytetrafluoroethylene femoropopliteal bypasses, 169, 171

Thromboembolism, as a complication of percutaneous transluminal angioplasty, 96
Thromboendarterectomy, 23
  historical background of, 9–13
Thrombus scintigraphy, 54–55
TIA. *See* Transient ischemic attack
Transcatheter therapeutic embolization, 59–80
  applications, 61–64, 79
    gastrointestinal tract, 62
    renal hemorrhage, 63–64
    posttraumatic bleeding, 62–63
  complications, 71–78
    causes of, 71–74
    probability of, 78
    reduce potential of, 78
  factors in the success of, 79
  indications, 80
  results of, 64–71
Transfemoral Seldinger technique, 288
Transient ischemic attack (TIA), 342, 353
  arteriography for, 347–51
  aspirin and, 365–66
  endarterectomy, 362, 365
Transmetatarsal five-digit amputation, 221
Transmetatarsal single-digit amputation, 221
Transphalangeal digital amputation, 220
"Triangulation method," 3
True unreconstructibility, 229–36
  definition, 229
  types of, 230–36
    common femoral bifurcation occlusive disease, 230
    femoropopliteal bypass and, 230–31
    occlusion of the superficial femoral artery, 230–32
    popliteal-tibial occlusive disease, 232–36

Ultrasound
  abdominal aortic aneurysm, diagnosis of, 31–35

Ultrasound *(cont'd.)*
  abdominal aortic aneurysm, diagnosis of *(cont'd.)*
    B-mode, accuracy of, 33–35
    advantages of, 42–43
    A-mode, 32–33
    B-mode real-time, 32–33
    in carotid disease, 344–45
    Doppler, 51–52, 193, 256, 267–68
    computed tomography, comparison with, 41–43
    errors, cause of, 41–42
    in infected aortic grafts, 389–90, 392
    M-mode, 32–33
    obstacles to, 42
Urokinase, 311

Valsalva maneuver, 189–90
Varicose veins, 187
Vascular grafts
  alternatives to, 175–81
  ideal, characteristics of, 175–76
  polytetrafluoroethylene, 105–20, 123–28
Vascular surgery
  historical development of, 1–25
  major breakthroughs in, 21–25
  recent contributions to, 7–9
Venography. *See* Contrast phlebography
Venous grafts
  development of, 5–6
  polytetrafluoroethylene, use in, 124–25.
Venous surgery, reconstructive, 185–96, 199–212
  complications, 211
  diagnostic tests, 186–90
    phlebography, 189–90
    photoplethysmography, 187–89
    techniques of, 188
    venous pressure determinations, 186–87

Venous surgery, reconstructive *(cont'd.)*
  in the iliac and femoral veins, 201–203
  indications, 185–86
  postoperative care, 211
  repair of large veins, 200–201
  techniques, 203–212
    brachial to jugular bypass, 206
    bypass of the inferior vena cava, 208–209
    cross-over saphenofemoral graft, 204–206, 209
      results, 206
    iliac venotomy, 209–211
    saphenopopliteal anastomoses, 206
      results, 207
  types of, 19
    femoropopliteal bypass, 190–91
    valve transposition, 193–94
      results, 194–96
    valvuloplasty, 192
Venous valve transposition, 193–94
  results, 194–96
Venous valvuloplasty, 192
Vinblastine, 148
Vinyon "N" cloth tubes, 21, 24
Visceral ischemia. *See also* Nonocclusive mesenteric ischemia, acute
  cause of, 299
  role of vasoconstriction in, 299–302
  vasodilators, 300

Weibel-Plad bodies, 110

Xylocaine, as a treatment for popliteal spasm, 97